"A 3-pound, 447-page gem, *Getting Stronger* offers well-organized beginning and advanced weight workouts and general fitness programs that will prepare you for 21 different sports. A must for anyone serious about fitness..."

—*Newsday*

"Americans really need this book."

—*Larry Pacifico,* Powerlifter
World Record Holder

"The most informative book I've ever seen or read on bodybuilding."

—*Joe Gold,* Owner,
World Gym, Venice, Calif.

"A crisp, well organized manual for men and women that incorporates reliable guidance for bodybuilders at all levels, programs for general fitness, gym and home training, and routines by top athletes and coaches to fit the requirements of 21 sports. There are illustrated workout charts, cross-referenced to free weight, Nautilus and Universal machine exercises. This large format strength encyclopedia—like Pearl—has no peer."

—*Publishers Weekly*

"A superb piece of publishing, well-written, beautifully designed... Women are going to react very favorably to the equal time given them in the book."

—*Rochelle Larkin,* Editor-in-Chief
Female Bodybuilding Magazine

"Weight training is becoming a big part of baseball. After my third knee operation last season the doctor said without weight training I would not be playing today. I advocate Barry Weinberg's methods in *Getting Stronger;* they will prepare you to be the best player you can be."

—*Larry Parrish*
Texas Rangers
National League All-Star 1979

"GETTING STRONGER is a must for anyone involved in weight training in any sport. Bill Pearl has created the new bible for athletes and bodybuilders of today and tomorrow."

—*Lou Ferrigno*
Two-time Mr. Universe

"The most comprehensive book I've ever read on weight training. It can be used by the instructor as an excellent teaching tool, and by the student as a guide to learning the sport. GETTING STRONGER leaves no questions unanswered. Muscle physiology is explained in detail, allowing the reader to understand the entire process necessary in order to actually get stronger."

—*Diana Buchta,* Strength Trainer
U.S. Triathlon Team

"The most extensive and complete work on weight lifting that I've seen. The piece on volleyball was a carbon copy of our program, with which we've enjoyed great success. Even more interesting was reading the general sections, which presented great 'pearls' to modify or enhance our present program from the 'Pearl' himself."

—*Karch Kiraly*
Captain, 1984 U.S. Olympic
Men's Volleyball Team
(Gold Medalists)

WEIGHT TRAINING FOR MEN AND WOMEN

GETTING STRONGER

SPORTS TRAINING

GENERAL CONDITIONING

BODYBUILDING

BY BILL PEARL

AND GARY T. MORAN, Ph.D.

ILLUSTRATED BY RICHARD GOLUEKE

SHELTER
PUBLICATIONS INC.
PO BOX 279 BOLINAS CALIFORNIA 94924

Distributed in the United States by Random House, Inc.,
New York, and in Canada by Random House, Ltd., Toronto.

Library of Congress Cataloging-in-Publication Data

Pearl, Bill, 1930–
   Getting stronger.
   Bibliography: p.
   Includes index.
   1. Weight lifting. 2. Physical education and training.
3. Physical fitness. I. Moran, Gary T., 1944–
II. Title.
GV546.P32 1986   796.4'1   86-19914
ISBN 0-936070-04-8 (Pbk.)
ISBN 0-679-73948-3 (Random House)

We are grateful to the following publishers for permission to
reprint portions of previously published material:

Contemporary Books, Inc., Chicago, Illinois, for charts appearing
on pp. 61 and 73 from *Aerobic Weight Training* © 1983 by
Frederick C. Hatfield, Ph.D. Reprinted by permission.

Human Kinetics Publishers, Inc., Chicago, Illinois, for material
appearing on pp. 78-79 from *The Athlete's Guide to Sports
Physiology: Mental Skills for Physical People* by Dorothy V.
Harris, Ph.D. and Bette L. Harris, Ed.D. © 1984 by Leisure
Press. Reprinted by permission.

Little Brown and Company, Boston, Mass., for table appearing
on p. 69 from *Lift Your Way to Youthful Fitness* © 1985 by
Terence Todd and Janice S. Todd. Reprinted by permission.

Physical Therapy, Alexandria, Virginia, for table appearing on
p. 16 from *Physical Therapy Review* (36:371), 1956. Reprinted
by permission of the American Physical Therapy Association.

McGraw-Hill, Inc., for material appearing on pp. 338-39 from
The Physician and Sportsmedicine, a McGraw-Hill publication.
Reprinted by permission.

Sports Illustrated, for material appearing on p. 343 from the
July 18, 1983 issue; © 1983 Time Inc., "Pearl Is a Rare Old
Gem" by Terry Todd. Reprinted by permission.

10 9 8 7 6 5 4

First edition - Printed in the United States of America

Additional copies of this book may be purchased for $12.95
plus $2.00 shipping and handling 1st book, $1.00 each additional
book from:

Shelter Publications, Inc.
P.O. Box 279
Bolinas, CA 94924

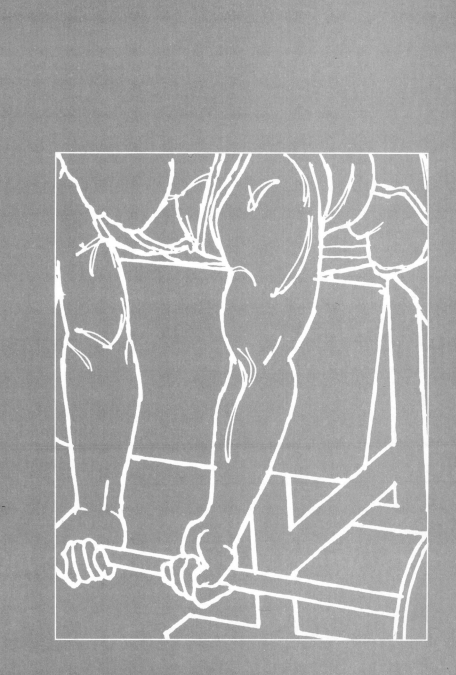

TABLE OF CONTENTS

Introduction, 8

General Conditioning. *12*

Getting Started, 14
- Before You Start, 14
- When You Start, 15
- How Many Sets, Reps? 16
- How Much Weight? 16
- The Seven Most
  Important Muscle Groups, 17

How to Lift, 18
- Stretching, 18
- Proper Position, 18
- Breathing, 19
- Safety, 19

General Conditioning Programs, 20

Weight Training For Women, 26
- Misconceptions of the Past, 26
- Special Training
  Considerations for Women, 27
- The Body Beautiful, 28
- Women's Bodybuilding, 28

Bodybuilding *31*
- Beginning Bodybuilding, 33
- Intermediate Bodybuilding, 38
- Advanced Bodybuilding, 41
- Competitive Bodybuilding, 44
- Posing, 48
- Cautions, 52
- My Routine, 54

Strength Training for Sports. *55*

The Elements of Fitness, 57

Sports Training Principles, 59
- Strength/Power/Speed, 61
- Fast-Twitch/Slow-Twitch, 62
- Isometric/Isotonic/Isokinetic, 63

*Training Concepts
for Advanced Athletes*, 65
- Supersets/Trisets/
  Pyramid Training, 65
- High Intensity Training, 65
- Split Routines, 66
- Super Stretching, 67
- Plyometric Exercises, 68
- Periodization, 68

Cardiovascular Training, 71

Risk Factor Questionnaire, 72

Power of Positive Lifting, 77

Sports Training Programs. *81*
- All-Around Athlete, 84
- Aerobic Dance, 86
- Baseball, 88
- Basketball, 92
- Boxing, 97
- Cycling, 100
- Football, 104
- Golf, 112
- Gymnastics, 116
- Ice Hockey, 120
- Powerlifting, 124
- Rowing, 130
- Running (Distance), 134
- Skiing (Cross-Country), 138
- Skiing (Downhill), 142
- Soccer, 146
- Swimming, 149
- Tennis, 153
- Track & Field, 156
- Triathlon, 165
- Volleyball, 169
- Wrestling, 172

Fine Tuning. *176*
- Muscular Arms, 177
- Strong Back, 178
- Tight Bottom, 179
- Larger Chest, 180
- Shapely Legs, 181
- Broad Shoulders, 182
- Flat Stomach, 183

Exercises for Free Weights........*184*

Body Parts, 186
- Abdominals, 190
- Back, 202
- Biceps, 218
- Calves, 236
- Chest, 244
- Forearms, 258
- Neck, 266
- Shoulders, 272
- Thighs, 284
- Triceps, 300

Exercises for Nautilus Machines.....*311*

Exercises for Universal Machines....*320*

- Universal Aerobic Super Circuit, 323

Stretches for Weight Training,
by Bob and Jean Anderson.......*325*

Fit for Work...................*331*

- Lower Back Pain, 332
- How to Lift, 333
- White-Collar Workers Program, 334
- Blue-Collar Workers Program, 335

Fit for Life...................*337*

Should Kids Lift? 338

Getting Older, 342
- Over-50 Program, 344

Hardware....................*345*

Free Weights vs. Machines, 346

Picking a Gym, 351
- The Home Gym, 352
- Home Gym Dumbbell
  Training Program, 354
- Home Gym Barbell
  Training Program, 355

Muscles.....................*357*

- Inside the Muscle Cells, 359
- The Architecture of Muscle, 359
- Tendons and Ligaments, 360
- Why Muscles get
  Bigger and Stronger, 361
- The Overload Principle, 362

Injuries......................*365*

- Strains and Sprains, 366
- Treatment of Injuries, 368
- Rehabilitation of Injuries, 370
- Preventing Injuries, 371

Nutrition....................*373*

- Protein, Carbohydrates, Fats, 374
- Vitamins, Minerals, Water, 377
- Nutritional Supplementation, 380
- "Natural Foods", 381
- A Vegetarian Bodybuilder? 382

Drugs.......................*387*

A Brief History of
Resistance Exercise
by Terry Todd, Ph.D.......... *397*

Appendix *416*

Training Card, 417

Language of Lifting, 418

Bibliography, 424

Exercise Index — Drawings, 426

Exercise Index — Titles, 433

Index, 438

Credits, 443

About the Authors, 444

INTRODUCTION

I'll never forget the day the circus came to town. The town was Yakima, Washington, the year was 1938 and I was an impressionable 8 years old. Fliers were posted throughout the town, showing the usual elephants, lions, clowns and best of all . . . the strongman! He was an impressive sight: handlebar mustache, leather wrist straps, powerful muscles and a seemingly immense barbell held overhead at arm's length with one hand. From that time on, I wanted to be a bodybuilder. My friends dreamed of being policemen, firemen or baseball players, but not me.

My father owned a restaurant and our entire family worked long hours there. I celebrated my 11th birthday by standing against the wall of the restaurant kitchen, marking my height and noting that I weighed 111 pounds. I started training at that early age by taking gallon cans of corn or green beans and pressing them overhead like dumb-bells. I would also lie on the floor, haul a gunny sack full of potatoes onto my chest and press it up as many times as I could. I kept a record of how many times I could do this and tried to lift more weight each day.

A few years later my dad sold the restaurant and bought a tavern and pool hall. This freed my brother, sister and me from the hard work of helping run a restaurant, since minors were not allowed on the premises. My training devices were now left behind so I graduated to heavy manual labor where I could lift heavy objects and build the muscles I was hoping for. I found summer work digging ditches, working in lumber yards or doing concrete work. I don't know how much actual muscle I got for my efforts, but I do know that I never had any trouble eating whatever was put in front of me. I also learned, when I was quite young, that if anything is worth having, it usually takes a lot of work to get it!

One day in 1944 my best friend Al Simmons, who knew of my Superman dreams, rode over to my house on his bike with an issue of *Strength and Health* magazine—eager to tell me that he had *found the secret.* What a revelation—here were black and white photos of strongmen John Grimek, Clancy Ross and Steve Sanka lifting beautiful barbells and dumbbells—a far sight from my cans of beans and sacks of potatoes!

Al and I—then 14 years old—resolved to get a set of weights and with another friend, Pete Trusley, agreed to buy a York Big-10 Special (a 110-lb. set), splitting the cost three ways. I worked hard that summer saving up my one-third of the $38.95 and we sent off for the weights. However, York's ad had failed to mention the iron shortage in those war years and we had to wait nearly a year for our set to arrive.

The three of us agreed to meet in my basement Monday, Wednesday and Friday to work out for an hour. We also agreed that, if one of us quit, the weight set would remain intact so the other two could continue to train. The third stipulation was that if I quit training, either Al or Pete would get to take the set home. But I knew in my heart that *no way in hell* was I going to let that set out of my sight.

I studied the instructions that came with the set and followed them to a "T." Even though my muscles didn't grow as fast as I'd hoped, I stuck with it. I never missed a workout. Eventually Al and Pete lost interest, but I kept on training. Even when the football, track, swimming and wrestling seasons came along, my weight training was first and foremost. By this time I had added a couple of apple boxes and a four-foot-long plank for a bench, extra plates, expansion springs and grippers—giving me what was probably the only home gym in town.

One day, cold weather forced me to train in the living room. I felt I had been making progress so I thumbed through some back issues of *Strength and Health* as I looked at my physique in the mirror. After close observation I called Al to come over and have a look. I was sure I looked as good as some of the guys in the magazine.

Al came over on his bike in sub-zero weather and agreed that, although I may have lost a little of my "pump" waiting for him, I did look about as good as some of them. That was close enough for me!

• • • • •

By the time I was 16 I felt I was also getting stronger. In the summer months I'd take the weights out on the front lawn and practice the "clean and snatch" (where the weight is raised from ground to overhead at arm's length in one rapid motion). I got to where I could do this with 110 pounds. The whole practice infuriated my father, since for every one time I'd get the weight overhead, I'd drop it about ten times on the lawn. The front lawn looked like it had bomb craters.

From the time we were quite small, my brother and I always wrestled with my dad and we continued to do so as we grew up. One night I came home later than my curfew and my dad started wrestling with me, trying to get me on the floor. I knew that I was getting stronger from my weightlifting and when I got my dad down with a figure-four wrestling hold I kept telling him I'd back off if things got too rough. He didn't say a word and I kept applying pressure until it dawned on me he was no longer struggling. I had squeezed him so hard he had passed out! I felt terrible and apologized and gave him a hug as soon as he got his breath back.

My weight training eventually graduated from the house to a local YMCA gym in Yakima. The "Y's" weight room wasn't much better than what I had at home, but there were people to talk to and working out with others provided inspiration and encouragement. Another person who used this gym was Eric Beardsley. Eric was a few years older than me, the best athlete in the valley and the "best-built" man in town. Eric was my first idol. When I'd hear he was working as a lifeguard at a public pool, I'd ride my bike down to admire his physique. It seemed he rippled with every step.

One summer day I was standing near the fence at the pool and I overheard one of Eric's friends remark that if Eric didn't spend more time training "that Pearl kid over there" was going to pass him by. Man! I was out of the pool, on my bike and heading for the weight room.

●　●　●　●　●

The day after I graduated from high school I started hitchhiking south to Fullerton, California to visit my brother. It took two days just to get to Sacramento and rather than spend another night roaming the streets I checked into the YMCA. After cleaning up and resting a few hours I asked if there was a weight room and was told to go down to the basement. I put on my shorts and T-shirt, went downstairs and opened the door to the first real weight room I'd ever seen. It was Monday night and the place was packed with bodybuilders and lifters and ten times as much equipment as I'd ever seen. I couldn't believe my eyes! Everyone looked like a monster!

One person I remember well was Tommy Kono, a former world record holder and Olympic weightlifting champion. Tommy weighed 148 pounds then and during that particular workout was doing military presses with two 110-pound dumbbells, squats with over 400 pounds and bench presses with 320 pounds. After his workout he took off his shirt and struck a few poses. He was the most muscular person I'd ever seen.

I was so overwhelmed by the whole scene—the muscles, the equipment, the energy and camaraderie—that I just stood around staring for an hour or so, an 18-year-old country boy star-struck at the sights of the "big city." I didn't even consider working out there. Finally I went back to my room and pulled on my set of expander springs until I was ready to drop. What I'd seen had given me a vision of the future and the incentive to work even harder.

That summer back home, I dug sewer ditches for $1 an hour and gave swimming lessons on the weekends. I had made up my mind to go to college (I had been offered 14 scholarships for football and wrestling), but my friend Al intervened, insisting that we go down to the local Navy recruiting office and talk to the recruiter. At this time the United States was approaching the Korean war and we were both of draft age.

As we came out of the recruiting office we ran into some friends. "Guess what," said Al. "We just joined the Navy." By the time we got back to the swimming pool all our friends had heard about it. The next day, to save face, we went down and enlisted.

I spent two years at the Whidbey Island Naval Air Station in Washington and was then transferred to a station in San Diego, California. The best thing about being in San Diego was meeting Leo Stern and working out in his gym. Leo had trained one of my heroes,

Clancy Ross (Mr. America, 1942) and rapidly became the most important influence on my career. Not only did he teach me how to train, he also taught me how to run a gym. He instilled in me the importance of setting realistic goals, and helped open the doors to my lifelong dream of a career in physical fitness.

In 1952, under Leo's guidance I entered my first bodybuilding competition and placed third in the Mr. San Diego contest. It was one of the proudest moments of my life and I was so inspired that I practically lived in Leo's gym when I wasn't aboard ship. Leo gave me a key to the club so I could come and go as I pleased. Each weekend I would sleep on the couch and have the gym all to myself on Sunday. I was on my way.

In 1953, I won the Mr. Southern California, Mr. California, Mr. America and the amateur Mr. Universe titles. I started getting requests for magazine articles, photos and posing exhibitions. I got calls to appear at grand openings, stock car races and I even got a few movie roles. One producer wanted me to become the new Superman; he suggested that I appear at different events, wearing a cape and tights for the publicity. I had to pass on that one . . . I didn't think the Navy would approve.

o o o o o

My enlistment ended in 1954. I had saved $2800 by buying war bonds with my Navy salary, I had some gym equipment I had made and a burning desire to run a gym. Since I didn't want to compete with Leo's gym in San Diego, I moved to Sacramento and opened a gym there. Before long I expanded to nine gyms, but soon cut it back to one when I learned I didn't have the ability to manage such a large operation. Eventually I sold the Sacramento facility and opened a gym in Los Angeles. During these years I continued to compete. My last competition was when I won the professional Mr. Universe contest in 1971 at age 41.

By then I had been a professional bodybuilder for over 30 years and had trained literally thousands of people. But the pressures of living in Los Angeles and the long hours I spent each day running my business were getting me down. I started thinking about moving out of the city.

At this time the great American fitness revolution was picking up steam, and there was an unprecedented interest in all types of exercise. I knew I couldn't train enough people personally and also that there was a need for a reference manual—something that anyone could use, with or without a teacher, to illuminate the somewhat garbled concepts of a mysterious and generally misunderstood activity. I hit upon the idea of producing a book on weight training—one that would allow me to serve many more people than could ever come into my gym for one-on-one instruction and selling the book, along with a personalized training program, by mail.

There had been mail-order training programs before but never a reference book listing several hundred exercises. This would allow me to communicate with anyone who could speak English, and anyone in the world could become a member of my mail-order course.

My wife Judy (also a bodybuilder) and I set to work on the book. (If we'd known what we were getting into we probably would never have started!) We took photographs of me doing the various exercises and an illustrator did pen and ink drawings from the photos. But for each exercise we documented we realized there were a dozen more to show. As long as we had gone that far we decided to show every exercise on every piece of equipment that anyone could use under any circumstances for bodybuilding.

o o o o o

A project we thought would take six months took us four years and cost over $200,000. We ended up with *Keys to the Inner Universe, An Encyclopedia on Weight Training,* a 638-page, five-pound book with 1500 exercises and over 3000 drawings. We invested every penny we could scrape up and printed 10,000 copies. We began selling the book at $32.95.

The book sold surprisingly well. Most people also bought our personalized training course in which I designed a program tailored to their needs. They would start on the program, send me feedback and I sent revisions when necessary. This soon started getting out of hand, as in a few years I was getting 100-150 letters a week asking for advice. I simply couldn't type long enough and fast enough each day to answer all those questions.

One day I showed the book to a good friend, Jim Morris, an ex-Mr. America who also ran a gym. "My God, Bill," he said, "I'd love to have the book for my gym. You could sell thousands." I didn't think anyone would buy a book this specialized in a store, but Jim disagreed and eventually talked me into distributing the book through fitness and weight training stores.

Jim was right. We started selling the book wholesale (although not in bookstores) and the orders started coming in. There are now over 60,000 softcover books and 10,000 hardcover books in print.

We did finally move—in 1980—to a small town near Medford, Oregon. We bought a ranch with 2½ acres, fruit trees and a barn where I set up my own gym. I opened up a general conditioning store nearby that sold weightlifting equipment, vitamins and nutritional supplements. One day, as the sales of the book were increasing, it dawned on me that if there was this much demand for a $32 book on just one aspect of weight training—bodybuilding—there was an even greater need for a book that also covered weight training for sports and general conditioning. I had seen the fitness revolution start and blossom in America to the point where the town of Medford (60,000 population) had 20 health food stores, three fitness stores, seven health clubs and two YMCAs. I'd also seen the phenomenal increase in the use of weight training by athletes; top competitors in almost every sport were using weights to increase strength, muscular endurance and flexibility and to speed up recovery from injuries.

From my 40-odd years of bodybuilding and training others, I knew I could create good programs for general conditioning and bodybuilding. I had also worked with a variety of athletes in achieving their individual aims. But I knew that by consulting specialists in each sport, we could devise weight training programs that would pinpoint the muscular needs of each sport. Twenty-four of the country's top coaches, trainers and athletes—including two world record holders and 11 Olympic coaches—have helped us develop the strength training programs on pages 82-175.

Since many aspects of athletics, including weight training, have been studied and analyzed by scientists in recent years and more sophisticated training methods are evolving every day, Gary Moran, a runner, triathlete and weight lifter with a doctorate in human anatomy and kinesiology and a master's degree in exercise physiology has helped provide the book with a scientific overview. Knowing what goes on inside the muscles when you work out, how food and drugs affect performance and how to diagnose and treat injuries are all part of the modern athlete's commitment to understanding, achievement and excellence.

Weight training is one of the most versatile of all athletic activities. It can be used for a variety of purposes: getting stronger, improving looks, losing fat, strengthening weaknesses or preventing injuries. It is an excellent foundation for improved performance in almost every sport and can be a cornerstone in the development of good health. I sincerely hope this book will help you to begin, continue or supplement a lifelong program of physical fitness.

To Your Very Best Health,

Bill Pearl

GENERAL CONDITIONING

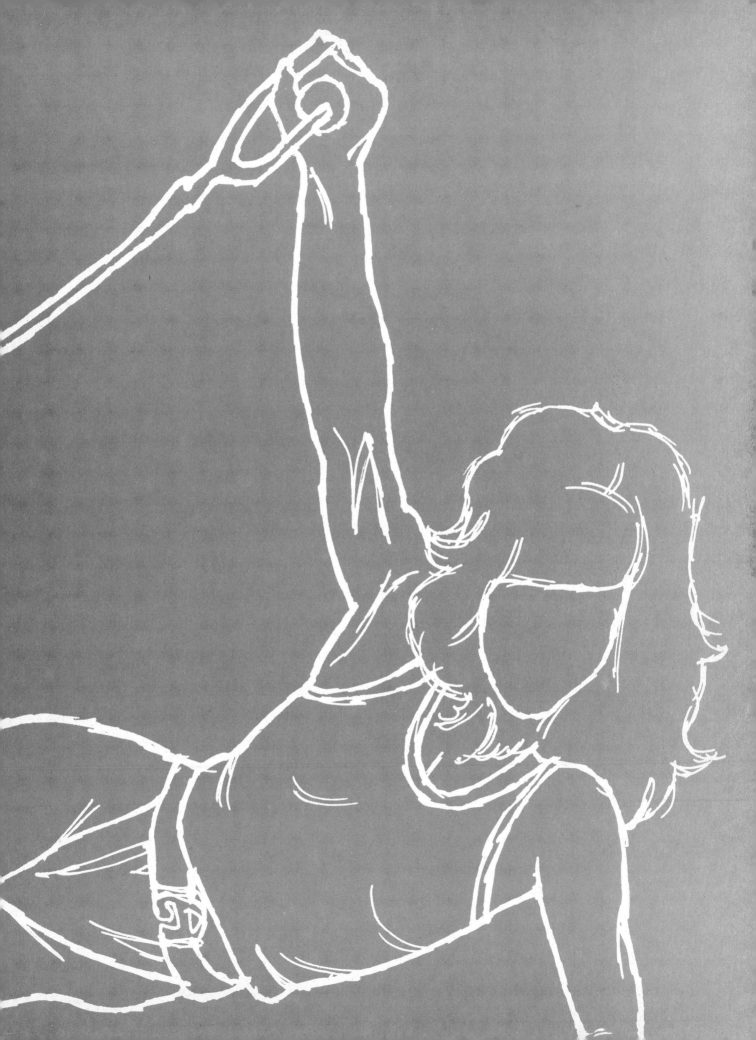

GETTING STARTED

This section of the book—"General Conditioning"—can be used for:

- Getting started with a weight training program
- Getting back into shape after a long layoff
- A first step to getting in shape for either a bodybuilding program (see pp. 32-34) or a sports training program (see p. 82)
- An on-going general fitness program where you work out three times a week, 45 minutes a day, and don't want to put any more time than that into weight training.

The General Conditioning Program will enable you to:

- Develop muscle tone
- Improve circulation
- Start building strength and endurance
- Start replacing fat with muscle
- Develop the capacity to work out harder
- Feel good

Before You Start

1. *Get a physical* from your doctor, especially if you are overweight or have not exercised for a while. In addition, if you are over 35, you should have an exercise stress test. Weight training is vigorous and demanding and you must be in good health to get good results.
2. *Stick to one program*—this one—at least in the beginning. Don't be influenced by what you read or by your friends in the gym, it can be confusing.

    In all the books and articles on bodybuilding and weightlifting, everyone has a different philosophy, training method and surefire guarantee of success. I've found that often the most rigid opinions are held by those with the least knowledge.

    In spite of all the claims, there is no one method that works best for everyone. I've seen people make progress with all *kinds* of training programs. (Just about *anything* you do is better than nothing.) But in recent years, along with the surge of interest in fitness, there have been certain principles and guidelines that have come to light that seem to work for everyone in maximizing progress. Our approach is simple and it works.
3. *Keep a record.* Plan your workouts at the beginning of each week and write them down for each day. After each workout write down sets, reps and poundages of each exercise. This eliminates "guesswork," shows your progress and can help eliminate weak spots. (On p. 417 is a card you can photocopy for this purpose.)

Setting Goals

Set goals that you can reach. If your goals are too high, you're likely to become discouraged, or worse, injured. On the other hand, if you set goals that are too low, you will not make enough progress. Set a long-term goal—perhaps a year in advance—and then several short-term goals to keep things moving along. Also, put a time limit on your goals. Don't just say, "Some day . . . ." But promise yourself that on July 1st, or whatever day, the goal will be achieved.

When You Start

1. *Be sure to warm up and stretch* (see pp. 325-330).
2. *Take it easy.* Don't watch others in the gym and try to handle the same weights they do. This can be discouraging and cause injuries. Also, you don't have to copy the top competitive athletes. They push their bodies to the absolute limits and are often on the edge of injury. The average person does not have to train like this to be in good shape and feel good.
3. *Pay attention to previous injuries.* If it's hurting, don't "work through the pain." Switch to an exercise that works the same area but isn't painful. A light, non-painful workout of an injured area gets the blood moving, helps clean out wastes and speeds healing.
4. *Don't worry about your body weight* when starting. You may *gain* weight at first, since muscle weighs more than fat.
5. *Don't worry about diet* when you're just starting. It's not a good idea to change everything at once. I never tell people to change their eating or drinking or smoking habits when they're starting. Because I know from experience that if you try too big a change in lifestyle all at once, you're more likely to drop the program. Once you get encouraged by some results the other things will fall into place.
6. *Watch for the development of muscle tone*—a slight yet constant tension in the muscles. This will be one of the first positive and exciting effects of your new training program.

How Often Should You Lift?

Rule of Thumb: Three workouts a week, 45-75 minutes a session, with a rest day following each workout. It's the same as running or cycling; you get best results when you apply stress in a hard day/easy day routine. This allows for cellular changes to occur on the rest days, for the muscles to recover from stress and automatically rebuild stronger. Thus, workouts are Monday/Wednesday/Friday or Tuesday/Thursday/Saturday.

Don't skip the rest day. It's important. Gary Moran, an all-around athlete and veteran weight lifter, fractured his leg skiing and had to quit his usual running, swimming and racquetball games. "I put all my energy into lifting, as it was the only exercise I could do." He lifted five or six times a week and doubled the usual number of sets. In about six weeks he found he could only bench press 210 lbs., compared to his usual 250 and he lost ground (about 15%) in the other lifts as well. He also had soreness in the tendons and ligaments of his shoulders.

    His mistake was in increasing his workload too drastically and not giving his body time enough to recover from the added weight training stress. He quit the new program, took a week off, returned to his normal program and within three weeks was back to pressing 250.

How Many Sets?

A set is a fixed number of repetitions (reps), or repeated movements of an exercise.
     The best strength gains come from three to five sets per exercise, as shown in the following chart:

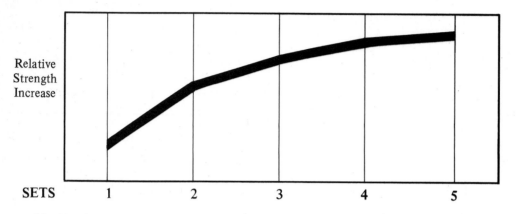

Relative
Strength
Increase

SETS   1   2   3   4   5

     Notice that you get more rapid strength increases with one, two and three sets and then the curve starts leveling off. Four to five sets give you gains, but you have to work harder for less results—the law of diminishing returns. After five sets the curve flattens out and you get less for your efforts.
     In our beginning program you will do one to three sets per exercise.

How Many Reps?

In the beginning program stick to 10 reps (except for abdominals).

How Much Weight?

Rule of Thumb: Use as much weight as is comfortable for 10 reps. The last rep should be fairly hard to perform. Use the first few weightlifting sessions primarily as testing sessions so you can see how much weight you can handle.

When To Increase Weights?

Once you're able to do more than 10 reps, increase the weight.

Two Types of Lifting

There are two basic types of lifting; they produce different results.

Low reps/high weights = strength

High reps/low weights = endurance

     These principles become much more important when you are training for a sport, but they are mentioned here so you can start thinking about them. When you want to develop *strength,* or the ability of the muscles to produce force, you train with relatively high weights and few repetitions.

When you want to develop muscular *endurance*, or the ability of your muscles to produce force repeatedly over a period of time, you train with lighter weights and high repetitions. The latter also produces "the pump," an increase in blood flow to the muscle. This is described in more detail in "Sports Training Principles," pp. 59-64.

The Seven Most Important Muscle Groups

In each session you'll work the seven most important muscle groups, the larger groups before the smaller. Why? If you fatigue the smaller muscle groups first, you can't work the larger ones adequately. For example, if you first do barbell curls, you fatigue your arms (small group). Then when you do a bench press to work the chest and back muscles (large groups), the limiting factor is not the chest muscles, but the fatigued arms.

A typical order of exercises:

1. *Abdominals.* Start here for a partial warm-up.
2. *Thighs.* Since the legs automatically bring the muscles of the lower back into play, be sure you are thoroughly warmed up before working thighs. This is the largest muscle group in the body.
3. *Chest.*
4. *Back.* Again, be thoroughly warmed up before working this large muscle group.
5. *Shoulders.*
6. *Triceps.*
7. *Biceps.* Work triceps and biceps last, as they are small muscle groups.

Cardiovascular Training

Cardiovascular training is an important component of general conditioning. It refers to exercises that strengthen the heart, lungs and circulatory system. You *can* get your cardiovascular training in the gym, by moving rapidly from one exercise to another, but it is more efficient to run, swim, cycle (or exercycle), hike, or walk briskly. You should also do some type of cardiovascular activity for at least 30 minutes, three times a week. A good time is a day when you are not weight training. For details, see "Cardiovascular Training," pp. 71-76.

Warning!! Remember to rest. The benefits from your training program will be so clear and there will be such noticeable changes that you will be tempted to overtrain. If you do not rest enough, you will soon be plagued by injury. If you are injured, you can't work out. If you can't work out, you can't improve. Sounds obvious but many people make the mistake of pushing too hard too fast. Do not overtrain. Listen to your body. When you are tired—rest!

The General Conditioning Program

Skip forward to pp. 20-25 and look at the general conditioning programs. They are meant to be photocopied and taken into the gym. Before doing this, look up the instructions for each exercise on the pages indicated so you will know the proper form and procedure for each one.

What To Do if You Want to Graduate to Harder Training?

Turn either to the intermediate or advanced bodybuilding programs on pp. 38-43 or the "All-Around Athlete" program on pp. 84-85. □

HOW TO LIFT
Techniques of Lifting

Proper technique will improve performance, minimize workout time, speed up improvement and help prevent injuries.

Stretching

Stretch *before* lifting:

• To prepare the joints for motion
• To extend the range of motion of the muscles
• To help avoid injuries

Stretch *after* lifting:

• To taper off the stress on muscles, to "wind down"
• To relax
• To reduce soreness

How to Stretch:

• Stretch until you feel a *slight* tension. Hold a position for 10-20 seconds. Relax a moment, then extend the stretch slightly farther for another 10-20 seconds.
• Relax.
• Don't bounce or jerk.
• No pain. Back off if it hurts. If the stretch is painful you'll actually tighten up the very muscles you're trying to loosen.

Stretches for Weight Training. The best book on the subject is *Stretching* by Bob Anderson, 1980. See pp. 326-30 for Anderson's special stretches for weight training.

Warming Up. Warming up prepares your joints and muscles for activity. Often lifters do a light first set to warm up—this brings the blood to the specific muscles to be worked. Others warm up more thoroughly by doing push-ups or light calisthenics, running, exercycling, etc. If the weather is cold, or you're sore from previous workouts, be especially sure to warm up well. The head and feet are the body's air conditioning units. Keep them covered in cold weather to keep the body warm.

Proper Position

Stance. When lifting in a standing position (curls, overhead press, etc.) your feet should be:

• A little wider than shoulder width apart
• Balanced fore and aft

   Many lifters wear shoes or boots with a heel to help offset the shifting of their center of gravity when lifting heavy weights. Sometimes a board is placed under heels when doing squats to help maintain balance.

Head. Keep head and neck straight during your lifts. Many injuries are caused by twisting the head, neck or trunk. Leverage is reduced and muscle injuries can occur when the spine is twisted.

Breathing

- Do not hold your breath throughout the entire exercise. It can stop the flow of oxygen to your brain and cause you to pass out. This is extremely dangerous if you have heavy weight overhead.
- Breathe *both in and out* through your nose and mouth. By breathing in only through your nose, you may not get enough oxygen.

How to breathe: Inhale during the beginning of the lift, *momentarily* hold your breath during the most difficult part, then exhale as you finish the lift. When doing a bench press, for example, inhale as you lower the weight to your chest, momentarily hold your breath as you begin to press the weight up and then exhale during the latter part of the movement.

Flexibility and Range of Motion

If you exercise through the whole range of motion of the joints, you will maintain and probably increase your flexibility. Testing has shown that top bodybuilders and weight lifters are among the most flexible athletes.

Safety

1. Try not to train alone. Even at home, try to have someone there to help if it is needed. Most serious weight training injuries occur when the lifter is training alone.
2. Always have a spotter for bench presses and squats when you are getting close to your strength limit. Serious accidents have occurred when lifters have been pinned by the weight doing bench presses.
3. Use collars on barbells. If you don't, the weights can slip off one end, causing the other end to dive for the floor, throwing you off balance and possibly injuring your back or other joints or muscles. Take the few seconds to put on the collars.
4. Use proper positions for all exercises. Study the positions shown in this book.
5. Do not jerk or twist when lifting. These movements increase stress and can lead to injury.
6. Be especially careful doing the following exercises:

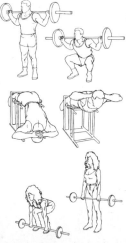

- Full squats, especially with heavy weights. This puts great stress on the lower back and the ligaments and tendons in the knee.

- Back hyperextensions, especially with heavy weights. Although these are good for strengthening the lower back, using too much weight too soon can cause muscles to tighten and spasm. Start light and add weight gradually.

- Dead lift. Keep your back straight and lift with the legs. Keep your head up, eyes on ceiling, squeeze buttocks and tighten abdominals. □

General Conditioning Program #1

8 Weeks

Do in this order:		See p. no.	Rest between sets	Week 1	Week 2	Weeks 3-8
1. Abdominals		193 mid.	30 sec.- 2 min	1 set 15 to 20 reps	1 set 15 to 20 reps	1 set 15 to 20 reps
2. Abdominals		190 top	30 sec.- 2 min.	1 set 15 to 30 reps	1 set 15 to 40 reps	1 set 15 to 50 reps
3. Abdominals		192 bot.	30 sec.- 2 min.	1 set 15 to 30 reps ea. side	1 set 15 to 40 reps ea. side	1 set 15 to 50 reps ea. side
4. Thighs		289 bot.	30 sec.- 2 min.	1 set 10 reps ea. leg	2 sets 10 reps per set ea. leg	3 sets 10 reps per set ea. leg
5. Chest		244 top	30 sec.- 2 min.	1 set 10 reps	2 sets 10 reps per set	3 sets 10 reps per set
6. Shoulders		274 top	30 sec.- 2 min.	1 set 10 reps	2 sets 10 reps per set	3 sets 10 reps per set

How often?
Once a week: You can maintain a reasonable amount of fitness. *Twice a week:* You will make a definite improvement. *Three times a week:* You will see noticeable improvement.

For best results: Train M-W-F or T-Th-Sat.

How long? 45-60 minutes per workout

How much weight? As much as is comfortable for reps shown. Last rep should feel difficult.

When to increase weight? Once doing sets and reps fairly easily, increase poundages so last rep is again difficult.

How to breathe? Inhale at beginning of exercise, exhale at end.

Do NOT lift to failure.

Feel any pain? *Stop!* Find another exercise that works same area, but causes no pain.

Do in this order:		See p. no.	Rest between sets	Week 1	Week 2	Weeks 3-8
7. Back		202 mid.	30 sec.- 2 min	1 set 10 reps	2 sets 10 reps per set	3 sets 10 reps per set
8. Triceps		300 top	30 sec.- 2 min.	1 set 10 reps	2 sets 10 reps per set	3 sets 10 reps per set
9. Biceps		225 mid.	30 sec.- 2 min.	1 set 10 reps	2 sets 10 reps per set	3 sets 10 reps per set
10. Chest		252 top	30 sec.- 2 min.	1 set 10 reps	2 sets 10 reps per set	3 sets 10 reps per set

Staying on this program:
If you do not want to increase intensity of workouts, you can stay on this program indefinitely. However, change exercises, sets, reps, poundages or any of these combinations every 6-8 weeks.

What to do if you want to advance to a harder training program:
Turn to "General Conditioning Program No. 2," which is slightly more difficult.

General Conditioning Program #2

8 Weeks

Do in this order:	See p. no.	Rest between sets	Week 1	Week 2	Weeks 3-8
1. Abdominals	*193 mid.*	30 sec.- 1 min	1 set 15 to 20 reps	1 set 15 to 20 reps	1 set 15 to 20 reps
2. Abdominals	*190 top*	30 sec.- 1 min.	1 set 15 to 30 reps	1 set 15 to 40 reps	1 set 15 to 50 reps
3. Abdominals	*193 bot.*	30 sec.- 1 min.	1 set 20 to 30 reps ea. side	1 set 20 to 40 reps ea. side	1 set 20 to 50 reps ea. side
4. Abdominals	*201 bot.*	30 sec.- 1 min.	1 set 15 to 20 reps ea. leg	1 set 15 to 25 reps ea. side	1 set 15-30 reps ea. leg
5. Chest	*248 bot.*	30 sec.- 1 min.	2 sets 8 to 10 reps per set	2-3 sets 8 to 10 reps per set	3 sets 8 to 10 reps per set
6. Chest	*251 top*	30 sec.- 1 min.	2 sets 8 to 10 reps per set	2-3 sets 8 to 10 reps per set	3 sets 8 to 10 reps per set

How often?
Once a week: You can maintain a reasonable amount of fitness. *Twice a week:* You will make a definite improvement. *Three times a week:* You will see noticeable improvement.

For best results: Train M-W-F or T-Th-Sat.

How long? 45-60 minutes per workout

How much weight? As much as is comfortable for reps shown. Last rep should feel difficult.

When to increase weight? Once doing sets and reps fairly easily, increase poundages so last rep is again difficult.

How to breathe? Inhale at beginning of exercise, exhale at end.

Do NOT lift to failure.

Feel any pain? *Stop!* Find another exercise that works same area, but causes no pain.

Do in this order:	See p. no.	Rest between sets	Week 1	Week 2	Weeks 3-8
7. Back	205 top	30 sec.-2 min	2 sets 8 to 10 reps per set	2-3 sets 8 to 10 reps per set	3 sets 8 to 10 reps per set
8. Shoulders	278 bot.	30 sec.-2 min.	2 sets 8 to 10 reps per set	2-3 sets 8 to 10 reps per set	3 sets 8 to 10 reps per set
9. Triceps	304 bot.	30 sec.-2 min.	2 sets 8 to 10 reps per set	2-3 sets 8 to 10 reps per set	3 sets 8 to 10 reps per set
10. Biceps	218 mid.	30 sec.-2 min.	2 sets 8 to 10 reps per set	2-3 sets 8 to 10 reps per set	3 sets 8 to 10 reps per set
11. Thighs	288 top	30 sec.-2 min.	2 sets 10 to 12 reps per set	2-3 sets 10 to 12 reps per set	3 sets 10 to 12 reps per set
12. Thighs	291 bot.	30 sec.-2 min.	2 sets 15 to 30 reps per set	2 sets 15 to 30 reps per set	3 sets 15 to 30 reps per set

Staying on this program: If you do not want to increase intensity of workouts, you can stay on this program indefinitely. However, change exercises, sets, reps, poundages or any of these combinations every 6-8 weeks.

What to do if you want to advance to a harder training program: Turn to "General Conditioning Program No. 3," which is slightly more difficult.

GETTING STRONGER ©1986 Bill Pearl & Shelter Publications, Inc.

General Conditioning Program #3

8 Weeks

Do in this order:		See p. no.	Rest between sets	Week 1	Week 2	Weeks 3-8
1. Chest		*244 top*	30 sec.- 2 min	1-2 sets 8 to 10 reps per set	2-3 sets 8 to 10 reps per set	3 sets 8 to 10 reps per set
2. Shoulders		*275 bot.*	30 sec.- 2 min.	1-2 sets 8 to 10 reps pers set	2-3 sets 8 to 10 reps per set	3 sets 8 to 10 reps per set
3. Abdominals		*190 mid.*	30 sec.- 2 min.	1 set 25 to 35 reps	1 set 25 to 40 reps	1 set 25 to 50 reps
4. Back		*205 mid.*	30 sec.- 2 min.	1-2 sets 8 to 10 reps per set	2-3 sets 8 to 10 reps per set	3 sets 8 to 10 reps per set
5. Back		*206 mid.*	30 sec.- 2 min.	1-2 sets 8 to 10 reps per set	2-3 sets 8 to 10 reps per set	3 sets 8 to 10 reps per set
6. Abdominals		*191 bot.*	30 sec.- 2 min.	1 set 25 to 35 reps ea. side	1 set 25 to 40 reps ea. side	1 set 25 to 50 reps ea. side
7. Triceps		*303 bot.*	30 sec.- 2 min.	1-2 sets 8 to 10 reps per set	2-3 sets 8 to 10 reps per set	3 sets 8 to 10 reps per set

How often?
Once a week:
You can maintain a reasonable amount of fitness.
Twice a week:
You will make a definite improvement.
Three times a week:
You will see noticeable improvement.

For best results:
Train M-W-F or T-Th-Sat.

How long?
45-60 minutes per workout

How much weight?
As much as is comfortable for reps shown. Last rep should feel difficult.

When to increase weight?
Once doing sets and reps fairly easily, increase poundages so last rep is again difficult.

How to breathe?
Inhale at beginning of exercise, exhale at end.

Do NOT lift to failure.

Feel any pain?
Stop! Find another exercise that works same area, but causes no pain.

Do in this order:		See p. no.	Rest between sets	Week 1	Week 2	Weeks 3-8
8. Biceps		*219 top*	30 sec.- 2 min	1-2 sets 8 to 10 reps per set	2-3 sets 8 to 10 reps per set	3 sets 8 to 10 reps per set
9. Abdominals		*196 mid.*	30 sec.- 2 min.	1 set 15 to 20 reps	1 set 15 to 25 reps	1 set 15 to 30 reps
10. Triceps		*302 top*	30 sec.- 2 min.	1-2 sets 8 to 10 reps per set ea. arm	2-3 sets 8 to 10 reps per set ea. arm	3 sets 8 to 10 reps per set ea. arm
11. Biceps		*225 top*	30 sec.- 2 min.	1-2 sets 8 to 10 reps per set	2-3 sets 8 to 10 reps per set	3 sets 8 to 10 reps per set
12. Abdominals		*195 top*	30 sec.- 2 min.	1 set 15 to 20 reps	1 set 15 to 25 reps	1 set 15 to 30 reps
13. Thighs		*284 top*	30 sec.- 2 min.	1-2 sets 8 to 10 reps per set	2-3 sets 8 to 10 reps per set	3 sets 8 to 10 reps per set
14. Thighs		*289 top*	30 sec..- 2 min.	1-2 sets 15 to 25 reps per set ea. leg	2-3 sets 15 to 25 reps per set ea. leg	3 sets 15 to 25 reps per set ea. leg

Staying on this program:
If you do not want to increase intensity of workouts, you can stay on this program indefinitely. However, change exercises, sets, reps, poundages or any of these combinations every 6-8 weeks.

What to do if you want to advance to a harder training program:
Turn to either "Intermediate Bodybuilding" (p. 40) or one of the sports programs.

GETTING STRONGER ©1986 Bill Pearl & Shelter Publications, Inc.

WEIGHT TRAINING FOR WOMEN

In 1972, Mary Peters, the great Irish track and field champion came to the United States to train for the women's pentathlon in the Munich Olympics. Mary stayed with my wife and me in Pasadena and trained in my gym each day. I started helping her in her field workouts and it was then that I had a startling realization of how strong and powerful a woman could become. When Mary practiced the shotput, or high jump, or hurdles I was her "gopher." I placed the high jump bar up at six feet, realizing I could never come close to jumping that height. I watched her run a sprint and saw that I would hardly be out of the starting blocks before she was halfway to the finish line. When she put the shot, I had to pick it up and walk back 20 feet and then roll it back to her. Mary was 36 at the time and weighed about 160; I was in my early 40s and weighed 235.

One day, one of the "heavies" in my gym got a shock from the "weaker sex." Mary always came into the gym dressed neatly, her hair down, and looking very feminine. She went into the back room where the heavy weights were and asked Buck, a big strong bodybuilder, if she could work with him on bench presses. He said, "Well, I've got 135 pounds on here and I don't want to break it down."

Mary said that would be fine and they started lifting, alternately, and adding weights. Buck was flabbergasted that a woman could keep up with him and became increasingly uncomfortable as the weight got up to over 225. When they got to 250, Mary handed Buck the bar and he couldn't push it up. Then she got on the bench, he handed her the bar and she pressed it twice and put it back in the rack. Buck was very unhappy, got his clothes on and left the gym.

Mary was capable of cleaning and pressing 110-pound dumbbells and could do a quarter-squat with over 800 pounds. A lot of the serious male lifters wouldn't train when she was there. Thankfully for all of us, those days and those attitudes are changing. Many women athletes—no longer afraid to train with heavy weights—are making rapid progress in a variety of sports.

Misconceptions of the Past

For years, weight training and bodybuilding were considered primarily male activities. Why was this?

• Men, with their bodybuilding contests and attendant publicity, got the lion's share of attention. Of course, there were often women's beauty contests along with the men's events, but there was little regard for muscular development.
• A persistent myth inhibited women from training hard: that heavy lifting would produce bulging muscles, that it would make women less feminine. So those women who *did* train generally planned programs with light weights and high repetitions.

In the last few years though, a revolution has taken place in women's weight training. Many of the old myths have been dispelled and women everywhere are now coming to recognize that:

• Anything traditionally considered a good health practice for men applies equally to women.
• Weight training is the fastest, easiest and best way to improve the shape, tone and strength of the body, female or male.
• It is physiologically very difficult, if not impossible, for women bodybuilders to develop the huge, bulging muscles of their male counterparts (without anabolic steroids).
• Lean muscle gives a woman curves and shape. When women lose fat and gain muscle tissue, the feminine physique truly emerges.

Special Training Considerations for Women

Any woman can use this book to improve her health, figure, athletic ability, strength and physical fitness. In most respects women and men follow the same training rules. However, there *are* differences that must be noted:

Physiology. Cardiovascular training has the same benefits for women as for men. In skeletal muscular training, however, there is a big difference–primarily due to hormonal influence. Both men and women secrete the male sex hormone testosterone and the female sex hormone estrogen, but men have a much higher level of testosterone (as do women estrogen) circulating within their bodies.

Testosterone, along with weight training, increases muscle mass (hypertrophy). Thus women seldom experience dramatic muscular development from weight training–unless they have an unusually high level of testosterone or use anabolic steroids (see "Drugs," pp. 387-95.) This is why most women can increase strength, add muscle tone and improve endurance from weightlifting without becoming "masculine" looking.

Bone Structure. The bone structure of the female pelvic girdle is proportionally wider than a male's, to facilitate childbirth. Women's knees, however, are the same distance apart as men's. Thus there is a greater convergence angle and stress, and women are more likely to have knee problems doing exercises such as deep or full squats. You can minimize this problem by doing half-squats and *gradually* increasing resistance.

Menstruation. Women who train very hard for long periods sometimes cease menstruation. The medical term for this is *amenorrhea*. The evidence is not clear, but recent studies indicate that low body fat (8-10%) and a combination of heavy training and/or mental stress can cause this condition. The significance of amenorrhea is not known. There appear to be no immediate physiological problems, but there have been no long-term studies. If a woman wants to reverse this condition, she should cut back on training, try to reduce mental stress and raise body fat to above 10%.

Pregnancy. Women who are physically fit are said to have fewer problems and more comfortable pregnancies, with shorter and easier labors. Exercise during pregnancy will produce better cardiovascular response, better muscle tone, reduction of tension and a higher level of stamina.

It's best to be fit prior to pregnancy and not suddenly start a strenuous activity program after conception. During pregnancy women should avoid extreme exertion and overheating and, of course, stop if they feel faint. The level of training should decrease as the pregnancy advances and should increase again gradually after birth. (An excellent book is *Essential Exercises for the Child Bearing Year* by Elizabeth Noble, 1982, Houghton Mifflin, Co.) *If you are pregnant or contemplating having a child you should consult your doctor before beginning any new exercise routine.*

Body Fat. Women have a higher percentage of body fat than men. This is true in the general population (men 14-18%, women 18-24%) as well as in comparing male and female athletes (men 4-10%, women 10-14%). Exercise can reduce body fat for both sexes.

Diet. Quick weight loss results in loss of muscle tissue and is not the way to achieve ideal proportions. Since women have less muscle mass, extreme diets are even more damaging to the female physique than to the male. When you cut back on food intake enough to reduce thighs and hips, the upper body usually becomes emaciated, muscles flat and stringy. A loss of over two pounds a week means you are losing some muscle. With weight training, and the muscle it develops, you can achieve harmonious body proportions.

The Body Beautiful

*It is highly dishonorable for a Reasonable Soul to live in so
Divinely built a Mansion as the Body she resides in, altogether
unacquainted with the exquisite structure of it.*
Robert Boyle, 1627-1691

Weight training is the fastest, easiest and best way to improve the shape, tone and strength of a woman's body. Running, swimming, cycling and aerobics classes are excellent cardiovascular conditioners and burn calories, but they can't compare with weight training for developing a shapely body.

When you begin a weight training program—and stick with it—you notice changes in a few weeks. Even if you don't lose weight, you'll find that clothes you may have grown out of will begin to fit once again. This is because *muscle weighs more than fat* and as you gain muscle and burn off the fat, your mirror and your clothes will tell you more than the bathroom scale.

As your abdominal muscles become stronger, your stomach will become flatter. Flabby areas will decrease: the triceps, or back of upper arms will tighten up and *cellulite*, the fatty dimpled deposits on the thighs and buttocks will diminish and gradually be replaced by firm, toned muscles. Small-breasted women often increase their bust size and women with larger breasts often find their breasts have become firmer and sag less.

Women's Bodybuilding

Women's bodybuilding is a very recent phenomenon. The first real women's bodybuilding contest was held in Canton, Ohio, in 1977, and contestants were judged "just like the men," based upon muscular development and overall physique development. The winner of the contest was Gina LaSpina.

Then in 1978 Doris Barrilleaux, then 47 and sensationally fit from 20 years of bodybuilding, founded the Superior Physique Association. The SPA was the first women's bodybuilding association and put out a newsletter devoted to promoting the sport for women. The SPA's aim was to give credibility to women's bodybuilding and to initiate women's contests that emphasized women's muscles and were not merely beauty contests.

The efforts of Doris and the SPA coincided with the needs and determination of a shy, nervous young woman who decided to take up bodybuilding in the late 70s. Inspired by Arnold Schwarzenegger, Lisa Lyon joined the mecca of male bodybuilders, Gold's Gym in Santa Monica, California, and began working out with drive and dedication. Within months, Lisa transformed herself into a powerful, strong athlete and became the first World Women's Bodybuilding Champion in 1979. She showed women everywhere that a strong, hard body and well-defined muscles did not have to detract from a woman's femininity or attractiveness. An intelligent and articulate spokesperson, Lisa won over many of the skeptics and helped secure a place for women's bodybuilding in the American consciousness. In 1981, she published *Lisa Lyon's Body Magic*, an attractive and inspiring book for women bodybuilders.

An even more recent boost for women's bodybuilding came in 1984 with the book *Pumping Iron II: The Unprecedented Woman* and the movie. Both the book and the movie chronicled the background, preparation and competition at the first International Federation of Bodybuilder's Miss Olympia contest in 1980. The public got a look at what goes on in training, preparing and competing in a women's bodybuilding contest. One of the most stunning contestants in the event was Rachel McLish, an exotic looking bodybuilder from Texas who seemed to communicate to other women the possibility of combining beauty, grace and muscles. The show also introduced the public to such outstanding bodybuilders as Carla Dunlap, Lori Bowen, Laura Combes and the incredibly muscular Australian power lifter, Bev Francis.

Hard Training

In the past, women often gave up weight training shortly after starting. And no wonder. When two sets of 20-30 repetitions on the "butterfly" chest machine didn't improve their bust size as fast as the spa manager promised, they would feel the training was useless. Or if they lost 10-15 pounds jogging or dieting, the low-weight/high-rep routine didn't get rid of the flabbiness. This is because you simply cannot build muscle or tone your body—to any degree—doing too many reps with too little weight.

Remember, building and toning take place when the muscles are challenged by heavy resistance. See the "overload principle," pp. 362-63.

Behind every worthwhile curve, there is a muscle.
Dr. Lynn Pirie
Getting Built □

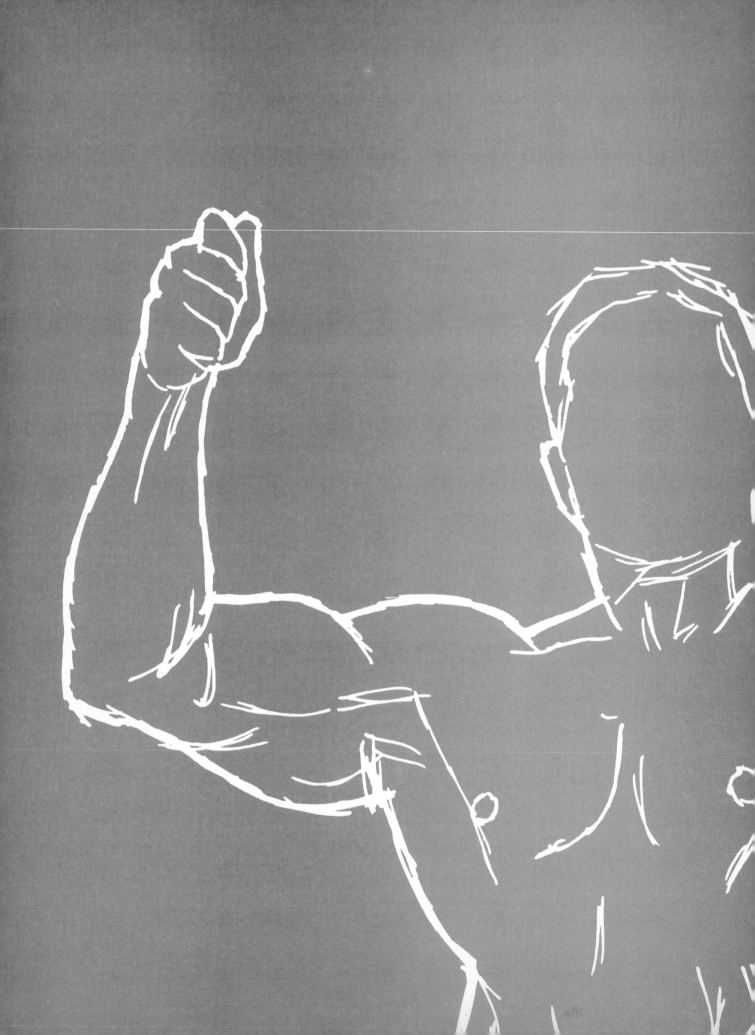

BODYBUILDING

BODYBUILDING

*A sound mind in a sound body is a short but full description
of a happy state in this world.*

John Locke, 1693

Bodybuilding is the primary reason that most people today go into gyms. Not bodybuilding of the competitive or Mr. Universe variety, but the use of weights to change
looks, to improve physical appearance. Bodybuilding is practiced on many levels: people
who simply want to tone up and look better; models, actors and actresses whose appearance helps ensure a job; and competitive or professional bodybuilders such as myself.

I'm going to share some secrets I've learned in over 40 years of bodybuilding. I've
tried just about every path known to man—the extremes, the fads, the trends—as well as
the tried and true. I've worked with literally thousands of people as a trainer and seen
every variety of human being, male and female, young and old try just about every
variety of exercise. I've seen some amazing transformations—lives turned around—and
also some abject failures. Out of all this experience—all the stories I've heard, the
successes and failures I've seen—I've developed some very simple techniques that are
going to help you achieve your goals, whatever they may be.

How Do These Programs Differ From the General Conditioning Programs?

Although many features of the general conditioning and bodybuilding programs are
similar (exercises, poundages, sets, reps), the difference here is your approach. The
bodybuilding section of this book is designed for the person who wants to begin a
steady but continuing improvement in health and fitness, as opposed to maintaining
a given level.

Each training session should be made a little more difficult than the previous one.
This is why keeping a record book is so important. You can do this by adding a few
more repetitions in the abdominal exercises, increasing the weights in other exercises,
resting less between sets, etc.

If however, you are not able to continue increasing the difficulty of each workout,
or not able to do what you have previously done, you are probably training too hard and
should cut back on the intensity until the muscles recover enough for you to pick up the
pace again. If you *do* feel low in energy, it is better to do a light workout than to skip a
training day completely.

The Bodybuilding Programs

There are programs on the following pages for four levels of bodybuilding:

1. Beginning
2. Intermediate
3. Advanced
4. Competitive

Before you get started on the bodybuilding programs you should read the following
chapters, as they apply to bodybuilding as well as general conditioning:

- "Getting Started," pp. 14-17.
- "Techniques of Lifting," pp. 18-19.

I'd also suggest you look at the chapter "Muscles", pp. 357-64, to get an idea of what
makes your muscles respond, and study the "Body Parts" drawings on pp. 186-89 that
will tell you what exercises to do for specific body parts.

Next, I suggest that you stick with these programs. I guarantee they will work. It's all too easy to get diverted by a magazine article or friends in the gym promising instant success with the latest technique. If you follow these programs and the general principles in this book I promise you better looks, greater strength and the improved confidence and self-esteem that accompany any such improvement in overall health.

BEGINNING BODYBUILDING

This program is very simple. You're not going to revolutionize all your habits. You're not going to worry about:

- Diet
- Drinking or smoking
- Weight

The object is to develop MUSCLE TONE. That's your only goal right now. This will:

- Improve circulation
- Start reducing fat and building muscle
- Give you the ability to work harder
- Start making you feel better

Here are 12 tips for a beginning bodybuilder:

1. *Get a physical:* Check with your family doctor before embarking on any new exercise program, especially if you are overweight, have high blood pressure or a history of heart disease, or have been sedentary for some time.
2. *Be realistic:* Set up a training program that you'll be able to stick with on a regular basis. Exercising a few days, then laying off, may be worse than no exercise at all. It can cause joint and ligament soreness, muscle strain and even high blood pressure. It's better to start out at three 45-60 minute sessions a week than to start by training two hours a day.
3. *Get your cardiovascular training:* Run, swim, exercycle, go to aerobics classes, etc., at least three times a week and work up to at least 30 minutes or more per session to condition your heart and lungs (see pp. 71-76).
4. *Add variety:* For your mind and body, change your routines every four to six weeks. This will keep you interested, and is good for your muscles. If an exercise becomes stale, change it.
5. *Start light:* At the beginning, use weights of about half your maximum effort. After training awhile, increase to about two-thirds of your maximum effort. The last week in each program you should be up to about 90% of maximum.
6. *Rest when you need to:* If you feel tired, cut back each exercise by one set, or drop back on weights or reps. You should feel fired up after a workout and rarin' to go for the next session.
7. *Work on your weaknesses:* Too many people work only on their strengths and don't make overall improvement. The best trainers concentrate on weak areas to achieve overall balance and symmetry.
8. *Zero in:* Mentally focus on the body parts you're exercising. If you're doing a biceps exercise, mentally concentrate on the biceps, trying to make it do as much work as possible.
9. *Dress right:* Wear shoes while training and wear warm enough clothes so your body doesn't divert energy from the exercising to keeping you warm.

10. *Take some photos:* It's a great way to chart your progress, especially in the beginning. Photos do not lie! Take some "before" shots: natural poses, front, side and back views.

11. *Take your measurements,* using a tailor's tape:
    - Height and weight
    - Chest, inflated and deflated. Pass tape around nipples.
    - Waist. Pass tape 1" above navel.
    - Hips at widest part
    - Thigh, flexed, directly below buttocks
    - Triceps/Biceps. Pass the tape perpendicular, around widest part.

12. *"A sound mind in a sound body . . .".* Work on improving yourself mentally, socially and spiritually just as you work on your body. They are all equally important.

In bodybuilding, you wear your sport.

Beginning Bodybuilding Program #1

8 Weeks

Do in this order:	See p. no.	Rest between sets	Week 1	Week 2	Weeks 3-8
1. Abdominals	190 mid.	30 sec.-2 min.	1 set 10 to 20 reps	1 set 10 to 30 reps	1 set 10 to 50 reps
2. Thighs	291 bot.	30 sec.-2 min.	1 set 10 to 20 reps	2 sets 10 to 20 reps per set	3 sets 10 to 20 reps per set
3. Back	212 bot.	30 sec.-2 min.	1 set 10 to 20 reps	2 sets 10 to 20 reps per set	3 sets 10 to 20 reps per set
4. Chest	244 top	30 sec.-2 min.	1 set 12 reps	2 sets 12 reps per set	3 sets 12 reps per set
5. Shoulders	272 top	30 sec.-2 min.	1 set 12 reps ea. arm	2 sets 12 reps per set ea. arm	3 sets 12 reps per set ea. arm
6. Chest	251 top	30 sec.-2 min.	1 set 12 reps	2 sets 12 reps per set	3 sets 12 reps per set
7. Triceps	300 top	30 sec.-2 min.	1 set 12 reps	2 sets 12 reps per set	3 sets 12 reps per set
8. Biceps	225 top	30 sec.-2 min.	1 set 12 reps	2 sets 12 reps per set	3 sets 12 reps per set

How often?
Once a week:
For reasonable level of fitness.
Twice a week:
Definite improvement.
Three times a week:
Noticeable improvement.

For best results:
Train M-W-F or T-Th-Sat.

How long?
45-60 minutes per workout.

How much weight?
As much as is comfortable for reps shown. Last rep should feel difficult.

When to increase weight?
Once doing sets and reps fairly easily, increase poundages so last rep is again difficult.

How to breathe?
Inhale at beginning of exercise, exhale at end.

Do NOT lift to failure.

Feel any pain?
Stop! Find another exercise that works same area, but causes no pain.

For a harder program:
Turn to "Bodybuilding Program No. 2," which is slightly more difficult.

GETTING STRONGER ©1986 Bill Pearl & Shelter Publications, Inc.

Beginning Bodybuilding Program #2

8 Weeks

Do in this order:	See p. no.	Rest between sets	Week 1	Week 2	Weeks 3-8
1. Abdominals	190 top	30 sec.-2 min.	1 set 15 to 20 reps	2 sets 15 to 20 reps per set	2 sets 15 to 30 reps per set
2. Chest	248 top	30 sec.-2 min.	2 sets 10 to 12 reps per set	3 sets 10 to 12 reps per set	4 sets 10 to 12 reps per set
3. Back	203 bot.	30 sec.-2 min.	2 sets 10 to 12 reps per set ea. arm	3 sets 10 to 12 reps per set ea. arm	4 sets 10 to 12 reps per set ea. arm
4. Shoulders	279 bot.	30 sec.-2 min.	2 sets 10 to 12 reps per set	3 sets 10 to 12 reps per set	4 sets 10 to 12 reps per set
5. Triceps	304 mid.	30 sec.-2 min.	2 sets 10 to 12 reps per set	3 sets 10 to 12 reps per set	4 sets 10 to 12 reps per set
6. Biceps	218 mid.	30 sec.-2 min.	2 sets 10 to 12 reps per set	3 sets 10 to 12 reps per set	4 sets 10 to 12 reps per set
7. Thighs	288 top	30 sec.-2 min.	2 sets 10 to 12 reps per set	3 sets 10 to 12 reps per set	4 sets 10 to 12 reps per set
8. Thighs	289 top	30 sec.-2 min.	2 sets 10 to 12 reps per set ea. leg	3 sets 10 to 12 reps per set ea. leg	4 sets 10 to 12 reps per set ea. leg

How often?
Once a week: For reasonable level of fitness. *Twice a week:* Definite improvement. *Three times a week:* Noticeable improvement.

For best results: Train M-W-F or T-Th-Sat.

How long? 45-60 minutes per workout.

How much weight? As much as is comfortable for reps shown. Last rep should feel difficult.

When to increase weight? Once doing sets and reps fairly easily, increase poundages so last rep is again difficult.

How to breathe? Inhale at beginning of exercise, exhale at end.

Do NOT lift to failure.

Feel any pain? *Stop!* Find another exercise that works same area, but causes no pain.

For a harder program: Turn to "Bodybuilding Program No. 3," which is slightly more difficult.

Beginning Bodybuilding Program #3

8 Weeks

Do in this order:	See p. no.	Rest between sets	Week 1	Week 2	Weeks 3-8
1. Abdominals	*195 top*	30 sec.-2 min	1 set 10 to 20 reps	2 sets 10 to 20 reps per set	3 sets 10 to 25 reps per set
2. Thighs	*284 mid*	30 sec.-2 min.	3 sets 8 to 10 reps per set	4 sets 8 to 10 reps per set	5 sets 8 to 10 reps per set
3. Chest	*245 bot.*	30 sec.-2 min.	3 sets 8 to 10 reps per set	4 sets 8 to 10 reps per set	5 sets 8 to 10 reps per set
4. Shoulders	*272 bot.*	30 sec.-2 min.	3 sets 8 to 10 reps per set	4 sets 8 to 10 reps per set	5 sets 8 to 10 reps per set
5. Back	*205 top*	30 sec.-2 min.	3 sets 8 to 10 reps per set	4 sets 8 to 10 reps per set	5 sets 8 to 10 reps per set
6. Chest	*251 top*	30 sec.-2 min.	3 sets 8 to 10 reps per set	4 sets 8 to 10 reps per set	5 sets 8 to 10 reps per set
7. Triceps	*300 top*	30 sec.-2 min.	3 sets 8 to 10 reps per set	4 sets 8 to 10 reps per set	5 sets 8 to 10 reps per set
8. Biceps	*222 top*	30 sec.-2 min.	3 sets 8 to 10 reps per set ea. arm	4 sets 8 to 10 reps per set ea. arm	5 sets 8 to 10 reps per set ea. arm

How often?
Once a week: For reasonable level of fitness. *Twice a week:* Definite improvement. *Three times a week:* Noticeable improvement.

For best results: Train M-W-F or T-th-Sat.

How long? 45-60 minutes per workout.

How much weight? As much as is comfortable for reps shown. Last rep should feel difficult.

When to increase weight? Once doing sets and reps fairly easily, increase poundages so last rep is again difficult.

How to breathe? Inhale at beginning of exercise, exhale at end.

Do NOT lift to failure.

Feel any pain? *Stop!* Find another exercise that works same area, but causes no pain.

For a harder program: Turn to either "Intermediate Bodybuilding" or one of the sports programs.

INTERMEDIATE BODYBUILDING

By following the beginning program, you've felt some of the benefits of your new activity: improved muscle tone, better circulation and greater strength. You can actually stay with the beginning program if you want to, just changing the exercises every six weeks. If you don't want to put any more time in on it, this (along with some cardio-vascular conditioning) will provide a good minimal level of fitness and improved looks. However, if you want to work harder and improve your appearance further, you can move along to this, the intermediate stage.

In the beginning stage, I told you not to worry about diet, weight, smoking, drinking, etc. *Now*, however, those things become important. To increase your energy output and effort and achieve a healthy lifestyle, you now start bringing these things into line.

1. *Diet.* What you eat is important now. Your body will need enough calories, protein, vitamins and minerals to build new muscle and help you recover from training stress. (See the chapter on nutrition, pp. 373-85 for specifics.)
2. *Rest and sleep.* You need seven to nine hours sleep a night depending on your metabolism and how you train. Progress = stress + rest. Don't neglect the *rest* part of that equation.
3. *Drinking and smoking.* I'm not going to preach. The better your condition, the more in tune you'll be with your body. Harmful habits will drop by the wayside naturally.
4. *Variety.* With an increased level of activity, variety is even more important. Boredom is the most common cause of quitting. Do anything you can to keep it interesting. Change exercises. Set new goals. Put time limits on your goals.
5. *Higher intensity.* If you want to make progress beyond the beginning program, get stronger and build more muscle, do one or more of the following:

   - Add sets.
   - Add reps.
   - Add more weights.
   - Cut back on rest between sets.
   - Add more exercises.

Various techniques for increasing intensity have been employed by bodybuilders over the years. Lately they have been used by athletes in other sports as well. These techniques seem to phase in and out of popularity:

- Supersets
- Trisets
- Pyramid training
- Forced reps
- Partial reps
- Negative reps
- Multi-poundage system
- Cheating

They are described in detail in "Advanced Training Concepts," pp. 65-70.

In addition, you may want to read the chapter "Muscles," pp. 356-64, for a description of what takes place *inside* the muscles that causes them to grow bigger and stronger from the stresses of weight training.

Training to Failure

A fad in recent years has been the idea of "training to failure," doing each exercise to the point where you are in great pain with your last rep and you cannot possibly lift the weight one more time. There are two things wrong with this idea:

1. It's hard on your body—it's too exhausting, it takes away from your next workout and you run the risk of injury.
2. It's hard on your mind—you're working toward a goal of failure and it subtly produces a negative rather than a positive attitude.

Every gym manager faces the problem of keeping members motivated. When training to failure was popular, many people who practiced it quit training. Going to failure on every set meant maximum effort and pain from 30 to 60 times per training session—someone pulling the bar off their chest, etc. Few people could take that kind of physical and mental strain for long.

(See Intermediate Bodybuilding Program, next page.)

Intermediate Bodybuilding Program

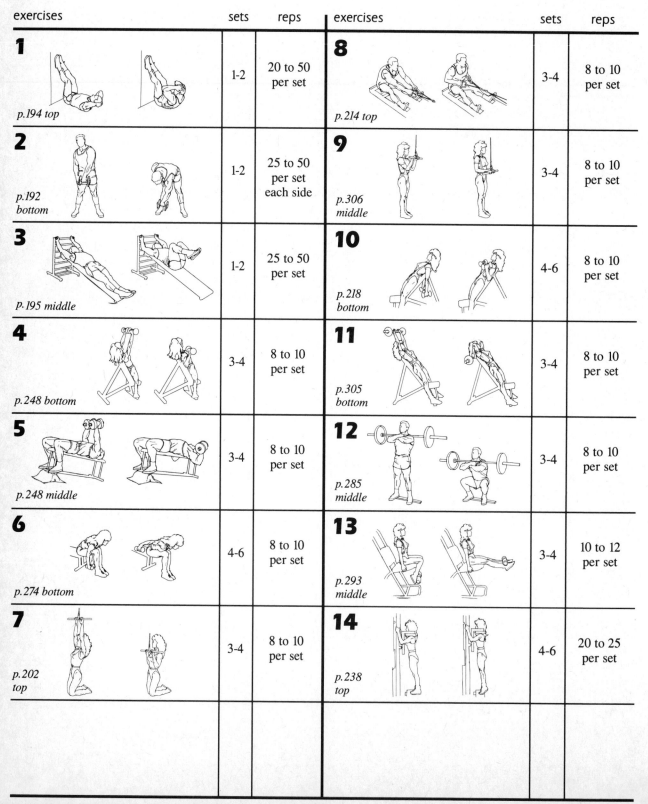

exercises	sets	reps	exercises	sets	reps
1 p.194 top	1-2	20 to 50 per set	**8** p.214 top	3-4	8 to 10 per set
2 p.192 bottom	1-2	25 to 50 per set each side	**9** p.306 middle	3-4	8 to 10 per set
3 p.195 middle	1-2	25 to 50 per set	**10** p.218 bottom	4-6	8 to 10 per set
4 p.248 bottom	3-4	8 to 10 per set	**11** p.305 bottom	3-4	8 to 10 per set
5 p.248 middle	3-4	8 to 10 per set	**12** p.285 middle	3-4	8 to 10 per set
6 p.274 bottom	4-6	8 to 10 per set	**13** p.293 middle	3-4	10 to 12 per set
7 p.202 top	3-4	8 to 10 per set	**14** p.238 top	4-6	20 to 25 per set

ADVANCED BODYBUILDING

These programs are for serious, hardcore bodybuilders. Only 5% of all bodybuilders fit into this category. Here are some characteristics of being an advanced bodybuilder:

- *Priority:* Weight training may be your number one priority.
- *Time required:* You will be training five or six times a week, two to three hours per session.
- *Lifestyle change:* Bodybuilding is no longer a hobby, or just a way to keep in shape, but a lifestyle.
- *Diet and sleep* are even more important. You need adequate nourishment and rest to maintain the intense level of exertion.
- *Maintenance:* Once you have developed an outstanding physique, a high level of intensity and frequent training will be required to maintain it.
- *Family, friends, social life* may suffer because of the time required and the high priority given to bodybuilding.
- *Narcissism* is the real danger with serious bodybuilders. If you don't watch it, you'll find you're starting every conversation with an "I" and ending with a "me."

Hardcore bodybuilding is a serious undertaking. While it has its rewards for those who are so inclined, there are a few pitfalls along the way. It is a heavy commitment, one which I made a long time ago and that has been wonderful for me. But it is certainly not for everyone.

On the next two pages is a six-days-per-week program for advanced bodybuilders.

Advanced Bodybuilding Program

M-W-F

exercises	sets	reps	exercises	sets	reps
1 p.194 middle	1	50 to 100	**8** p.274 middle	4-5	8 to 10 per set
2 p.191 middle	1	50 to 100	**9** p.255 top	4-5	8 to 10 per set
3 p.197 top	1-2	15 to 25 per set	**10** p.251 top	4-5	6 to 8 per set
4 p.192 top	1	25 to 50	**11** p.209 bottom	4-5	8 to 12 per set
5 p.245 top	4-5	6 to 8 per set	**12** p.251 top	4-5	8 to 10 per set
6 p.275 bottom	4-5	8 to 10 per set	**13** p.213 top	4-5	15 to 25 each side
7 p.246 bottom	4-5	6 to 8 per set	**14** p.238 top	6-9	20 to 25 per set

Advanced Bodybuilding Program

T-Th-Sat

exercises		sets	reps	exercises		sets	reps
1 p.194 top		1-2	25 to 50 per set	**8** p.218 bottom		4-5	6 to 8 per set
2 p.192 bottom		1	25 to 50 each side	**9** p.307 bottom		4-5	8 to 10 per set
3 p.194 bottom		1-2	15 to 25 per set	**10** p.224 bottom		4-5	6 to 8 per set
4 p.198 bottom		1	25 to 50 each side	**11** p.293 middle		4-5	10 to 15 per set
5 p.306 middle		4-5	8 to 10 per set	**12** p.291 top		4-5	15 per set
6 p.220 bottom		4-5	6 to 8 per set	**13** p.292 bottom		4-5	10 to 15 per set
7 p.305 bottom		4-5	8 to 10 per set	**14** p.242 middle		6-9	20 to 25 per set

GETTING STRONGER ©1986 Bill Pearl & Shelter Publications, Inc.

COMPETITIVE BODYBUILDING

Weight training for competitive bodybuilding is extremely demanding and not many people can hold up to the strain for an extended period of time. The long hours of training, the mental concentration and the restricted diet can easily lead to burn-out. Even champion bodybuilders are not in contest form 12 months of the year. They periodically back off and adjust their training, diet and attitude.

Often, ironically, very little physical progress (increase in muscle mass) is made when the bodybuilder is training for competition. Sometimes the competitor becomes overly concerned with the ratio of body fat to muscle mass and cuts back too far on caloric intake. Also, much time that would ordinarily go into training is spent on practicing posing and getting a tan. Your energy is more scattered, so the poundages and intensity of training will drop. All this is not conducive to increasing muscle size.

If you are aware of these pitfalls, however, you can sidestep them and go into training with the best possible weapon: positive mental attitude. If you convince yourself that each workout will bring physical improvement, that you are becoming stronger and adding muscle size with each workout, you should be able to maintain approximately the same body weight while increasing muscle mass and losing body fat.

Your diet should consist of 70% complex carbohydrates, 15% fat and 15% protein, with little or none of the simple sugars found in desserts, canned foods and other sweets. This will keep your energy level at a high pitch, help reduce body fat and still supply you with enough protein and fat for muscle growth and repair.

I like to train a little faster and not handle maximum poundages when preparing for competition. I try to do about 30 sets of exercises per hour. I concentrate intensely on the muscle groups I am working and focus on getting a complete contraction and extension of the particular muscles with each rep.

If I find an exercise or two getting stale, I change them for others that work the same area. It's important to keep your interest alive and your spirits high. If you have an injury, select exercises that work but do not irritate the injured area.

Because of the stress of training for competition, I suggest training in a wholesome and supportive atmosphere. Try to keep negative thoughts at bay and forget about training once you are finished for the day. The mind needs a rest too!

Set a mental goal for where you want to place in the contest and work toward achieving that goal. I have found that success comes as much from mental attitude as from physical training. As someone once said, "You are what you think."

A six-days-per-week program for Competitive Bodybuilding is on the next three pages. Naturally you will alter, subtract or expand on this according to your individual goals, strengths and weaknesses.

Competitive Bodybuilding Program

M, Th

exercises		sets	reps	exercises		sets	reps
1 p.194 middle		1	50 to 100	**9** p.202 bottom		5	8 to 10 per set each arm
2 p.193 top		1	25 to 50 each side	**10** p.246 bottom		5	8 to 10 per set
3 p.197 top		1	15 to 30	**11** p.250 bottom		5	8 to 10 per set
4 p.193 bottom		1	25 to 50 each side	**12** p.246 top		5	8 to 10 per set
5 p.195 top		1	20 to 50	**13** p.206 middle		5	8 to 10 per set
6 p.257 top		5	5 per set	**14** p.260 middle		5	20 to 25 per set
7 p.216 top		5	8 to 10 per set	**15** p.270 middle		5	15 to 20 per set
8 p.255 top		5	8 to 10 per set	**16** p.238 top		9	20 to 25 per set

Competitive Bodybuilding Program

T, F

exercises		sets	reps	exercises		sets	reps
1 p.194 top		1	25 to 100	**9** p.276 bottom		5	8 to 10 per set
2 p.191 top		1	25 to 50	**10** p.292 bottom		5	10 to 12 per set
3 p.201 top		1	15 to 30 each leg	**11** p.275 bottom		5	8 to 10 per set
4 p.191 bottom		1	25 to 50 each side	**12** p.294 bottom		5	10 to 12 per set
5 p.195 middle		1	15 to 30	**13** p.277 bottom		5	6 to 8 per set
6 p.293 middle		5	10 to 12 per set	**14** p.260 top		5	15 to 20 per set
7 p.278 top		5	6 to 8 per set	**15** p.266 bottom		1	complete set
8 p.286 bottom		5	8 to 10 per set	**16** p.242 middle		9	20 to 25 per set

GETTING STRONGER ©1986 Bill Pearl & Shelter Publications, Inc.

Competitive Bodybuilding Program

W, Sat

exercises	sets	reps	exercises	sets	reps
1 p.195 bottom	1	50 to 100	**9** p.225 middle	5	6 to 8 per set
2 p.191 middle	1	50 to 100 each side	**10** p.304 top	5	8 to 10 per set
3 p.201 middle	1	15 to 30	**11** p.221 top	5	6 to 8 per set
4 p.198 bottom	1	25 to 50 each side	**12** p.307 bottom	5	8 to 10 per set
5 p.194 bottom	1	15 to 30	**13** p.222 top	5	6 to 8 per set ea. arm
6 p.303 top	5	8 to 10 per set	**14** p.263 top	5	Ground to top each set
7 p.233 bottom	5	6 to 8 per set	**15** p.269 middle	5	20 to 25 per set
8 p.306 middle	5	8 to 10 per set	**16** p.243 bottom	9	20 to 25 per set

POSING

Bodybuilding is a sport, but posing is an art. In the past very few bodybuilders went so far as to enter contests. However, these days there is a surge of interest in both body-building and contests—among both men and women.

Just as all football games are not the Super Bowl, not all contests are for the Mr. America or Miss Universe crown. There are thousands of bodybuilding contests each year, for all ages, sizes and categories. For example, there are contests by territory (local, regional, state, national, international); by height (small, medium, tall); by drug use (natural physique or open contests); pairs contests; combination lifting and posing contests; etc. If you are thinking of competing (or if you just want to pose at home in front of a mirror), here are some tips on the art of posing.

Learning to Pose

There are two main reasons the average bodybuilder does not pose well:

- Not enough practice
- Failure to understand anatomy and one's own body

You don't have to wait until you're ready to enter a contest to start practicing. Regular practice will both teach you voluntary muscle control and actually improve muscle tone: posing is hard work! A 30-minute posing session where you contract and extend nearly every muscle can be as good a workout as a two-hour training session.

Begin by studying physique photographs. Pick out people and poses that seem to fit your body type and try to duplicate them. A word of caution: don't try to copy a completely different body type. I've seen countless beginners try to imitate Lee Haney or Rachel McLish to no avail. Practice only those poses that compliment your bone structure and musculature.

If you train in a club where you can get some advice from an active competitor, by all means do so. Or ask advice of your training partners. Choose 8-10 poses and practice them until you could do them in your sleep. Learn each individual pose before you try blending them into a routine. Your first posing routine should then consist of these 8-10 poses.

Something to remember: In most physique contests, you are judged not only by your own routine, but by certain mandatory poses each contestant must use, such as: standing semi-relaxed to the front, right side, straight-on back, left side, and again to the front position. In addition to these unseemly poses, there may be more mandatory poses to strike so the judges can make comparisons.

Use a Mirror

Don't just stand in front of the mirror admiring yourself. Make each session constructive: look for faults or weak points. Using a camera is another good way to correct your faults.

Try to find a full length distortion-free mirror of good quality glass. If you are going to compete, you'll need to devote 30 minutes three or four days a week to practicing. Practice only poses that are easy to fall into. Flex all your muscles, but only from the neck down: never tense your face. If your face is twisted or painful it destroys the beauty of a pose. Also, avoid excessive smiling; it looks artificial.

The Basics

- *Keep it simple.* The most common error a novice makes is in trying spectacular or fancy poses. Stick to the standard, easy-to-do ones. Very few posers can look good doing swirling, whirling poses.

- *Keep it harmonious.* Many beginners try to show all the muscles without regard to form or symmetry. The body should be shown as a unit with all muscles harmoniously displayed. A mark of poor posing is taking a position that emphasizes only arms and chest and neglects the rest of the body. Accentuate your best features but not at the expense of the overall effect.
- *Take several positions* to display the body well. Don't try to show off all the muscles at their greatest muscularity in a single pose.
- *Proper stance and body symmetry* are crucial. Look at photos of the champions. Each pose is a work of art. They have complete control and can contract their muscles fully without strain. The novice, on the other hand, usually flexes too hard—to the point of shaking.
- *Go for the "flow"* of posing. Only practice will teach you how to bring out maximum muscularity without appearing strained.

How to Flex

- *Watch your face* when practicing. When you look strained, relax, take a few breaths and start again. It takes lots of practice to have your face relaxed while all other muscles are flexed.
- *Start relaxed.* First get your feet and arms in the exact position of the pose while relaxed. When your body is in harmony with the pose, then flex.
- *Flex in stages.* Once you have the feeling of the pose, start tensing the muscle groups one by one: legs, abdomen, chest, arms, etc. Don't start out trying to flex everything at the same time. Once all the groups are under control, tense them more and more. Relax and repeat, each time tensing harder until you can reach maximum contraction with an unstrained facial expression.
- *Don't be discouraged* if your first attempts are clumsy and stiff. It takes lots of practice to be graceful.

Developing a Routine

Once you have developed some poses, you're ready to work them into a routine. A good routine can be worked out with as few as six to eight poses. In fact, I won the Mr. America contest in 1953 with four poses: front, side, back and an optional. No matter how many (or few) poses, they should be blended so you go from one to another smoothly and gracefully. The poses on page 51 are arranged in an order so that going from one to the next is natural and smooth.

Men and women may use the same basic poses, but there are differences. Women often use more of the stage than men and may add twists and twirls for a more artistic approach. Women often take a slightly different stance. For example in a side pose a woman may tilt her hip upward and crouch a little more, for a more feminine look.

Because women are usually more flexible than men, they often emphasize their agility when posing. This can be overdone, but a certain amount of it is certainly impressive. Many women who are not heavily muscled include dance movements in their routines, depending upon grace, symmetry and proportion rather than mass.

Remember that everything you do on stage is important. Go from one pose to another smoothly by pivoting on the balls of your feet with a minimum of motion. Show your best features and cover up weak points.

One other point: It is difficult to change directly from a front to a back view. It is too awkward. In the routines shown I have you moving gradually from a front, to a side, to a 3/4 back pose...etc.

On the Platform

"All the world's a stage..." and now you're on it! Timing is important. You want to hold each pose long enough for the judges to view it, but not too long: you may shake from too much tensing or worse, the judges may start looking for weak points if you're up there too long. Hold each pose four to six seconds, longer if you're in good control.

Move from pose to pose slowly, taking about two seconds to get into the next one. Practice this to music with a 4/4 beat and think of your routine as a dance step.

Don't stay up on the stage too long, with too many poses. "Always leave them wanting more."

Hair and Skin

Shave excess body hair with an electric razor. This allows you to tan better and shows more muscularity. A good sun tan, either from the sun or a tanning bed (which has harmful rays removed) gives your skin a healthy look.

Oil

Application of a light oil brings out highlights and muscularity and gives the skin a glow. Many bodybuilders use baby oil. Don't apply too much oil. It is actually better to use none than too much.

Building a body that is healthy, strong, vigorous and beautifully developed is a goal worth striving for. The art of posing, which enables you to display it in the best possible manner can inspire others to reach for the same goals.

12 BASIC POSES

Here are 12 poses, selected for the flow of movement and for minimal leg movement. To do all these on a stage in a contest takes about one minute.

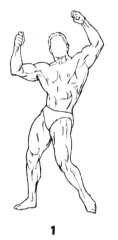

1

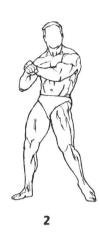

2

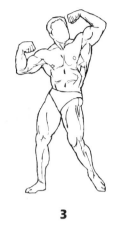

3

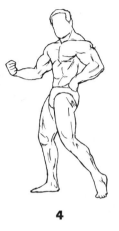

4

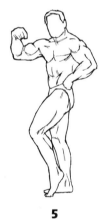

5

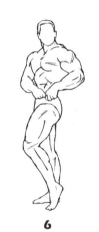

6

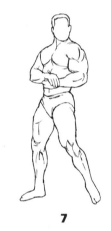

7

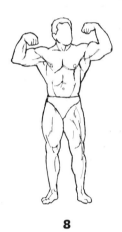

8

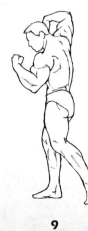

9

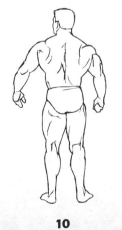

10

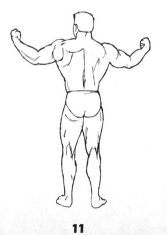

11

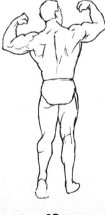

12

CAUTIONS

Weight training, bodybuilding or gains in strength can produce some powerful changes in your life. But, like any new and exciting activity, there are pitfalls along with the benefits.

Obsession

Ron was a bodybuilder who got carried away with training. At age 21 he decided bodybuilding was more important than anything else. He'd get a job, like parking cars for Hertz or Avis and work six months, just long enough to qualify for unemployment. Then he'd do something to get himself fired and collect unemployment payments for the next six or nine months. He'd live frugally during those nine months and center his life on training. He'd work out twice a day, lie in the sun, work on his posing and think only about his body. When the unemployment payments ran out he'd go out and get another job for six months and start the cycle over again.

Ron did this from age 21 until his early 30s. He had a wife and child he couldn't support so he deserted them. He took to living in the gym, sleeping on an exercise mat. That was his home. One day he finally woke up: he was going nowhere. The only job he could find was driving a truck. So he started competing in the job market when he was 31, not 21, and he was 10 years behind everyone else. Now he drives a truck and doesn't train anymore. He went from one extreme to another.

Ron's story is not unique in the world of bodybuilding. (Or other sports for that matter—running, cycling, swimming, triathlons, etc.) The gains are spectacular. The enthusiasm is exhilarating. To make visible progress is inspiring. With newly-found self-confidence and the feeling of well-being it's all too easy to get carried away. I've seen many, many people waste the best years of their life this way. Either they (unrealistically) thought they were going to be Mr. America, or they just fell in love with working out and getting bigger muscles. They'd center their life around training, diet compulsively and sometimes take dangerous drugs in an effort to gain even more muscles and strength.

When I see a weight lifter getting carried away like that, following a pattern like Ron's, here's my usual advice: Look, you're probably not going to be a Mr. or Miss America. Face the facts. Don't waste precious years of your life chasing rainbows. But you can still train and make some wonderful improvements in your life. You don't have to give up your family, friends, or your job. Weight training can be an important *part* of a whole life if you don't get carried away, if you keep your life balanced.

Unrealistic Goals

To be the *best* at any sport is usually expecting too much. To improve yourself is a much more realistic goal—one we can *all* accomplish.

Success is the best motivator. Your goals should be reachable, so don't aim for the moon. Be patient—remember that you can benefit from weight training for the rest of your life. You can't reach your full potential in a week, a month, a year. There is nothing wrong with dreaming, but always chasing rainbows will leave you disappointed. A 150-pounder will not be bench pressing 450 pounds. Tailor your expectations to your own abilities—not to the abilities of some sports superstar or personal idol. You want to feel inspired to continue, not so frustrated that you quit.

Burning Out

Some people never miss a day's training. For a world-class athlete this might make sense. But most people need a break once in a while.

All athletes know the overload principle—overload the muscles with stress and *with enough rest* they'll build up stronger. But many people skip the rest part of the formula; they don't realize that rest is just as important as stress. Like everyone else, you undoubtedly have stress and pressure in your life: money or family problems, increased responsibility, job pressure. Adding obsessive training to these everyday worries creates additional stress and can lead to injuries, to burning out.

There are early warning signs. If you're tired, run down, on edge, if you're not sleeping well, back off from training. Listen to your body. Use common sense. Don't look for an excuse to miss a workout, but be wise enough to rest when you need to. If you can avoid injury and burning out, you will improve. Work with your body, not against it. □

The Original Iron Man

Most people interested in bodybuilding are aware of the popular four-color mainstream bodybuilding magazines, such as Joe Weider's *Flex* and *Muscle and Fitness* in the U.S. and Dave Williams' and Chris Lund's *Bodybuilding Monthly* in England. An outstanding bodybuilders' and weight lifters' magazine—lower in profile, but highly respected and well loved by most serious practitioners of the "iron game" — is *Iron Man*. Published in Alliance, Nebraska by Peary and Mabel Rader, *Iron Man* recently celebrated its 50th anniversary. A one year's subscription (6 issues) is $12.50, from Iron Man Publishing Company, P.O.Box 10, Alliance, Nebraska, 69301.

MY ROUTINE

Tuesday

1-21-86
1 AMF LEG PRESS   6 x 17
2 LEG BI-CEPS   6 x 12

3 DECLINE CAMBERED   6 x 10
4 STANDING FRONT PRESS   6 x 10

5. T-BAR ROWS   6 x 10
6 MOON PULL OVERS   6 x 10

      (FLOOR)
7 EZ CURL BAR TRI-EXTENSIONS 6 x 10
8 GLOBAL BI-CEPS   6 x 10

1. 140 lbs ↑ 5 lbs ea set   5. 135 lbs ↑ 2½ lbs ea set
2. 75 lbs ↑ 2½ lb ea wk   6. 90 lb 0.0 ↑ 5 lb ea wk
3. 125 lbs ↑ 5 lb ea set   7. 80 lbs ↑ 2 lbs ea set
4. 115 lbs ↑ 5 lb ea set   8. 80 lbs ↑ 2 lbs ea set

Wednesday

1-22-86
1 INVERTED LEG PRESS   6 x 17
2 LEG-BICEPS   6 x 12

3 CAMBERED FLAT   6 x 10
4 BENT OVER REAR DELT B.B 6 x 10

        (FRONT)
5 WIDE GRIP PULL DOWNS   6 x 10
6 D.B PULLOVERS ON BENCH   6 x 10

      (HIGH CABLE ON WALL)
7 STANDING TRI-CEPS EXT.   6 x 10
8 STANDING E.B.B CURLS   6 x 10

1. 200 lbs ↑ 5 lbs ea set   5. 175 lbs ↑ 5 lbs ea wk
2. 75 lbs ↑ 2½ lb ea wk   6. 100 lbs ↑ 5 lbs ea wk
3. 165 lbs ↑ 5 lbs ea set   7. #8 ↑ 5 lbs ea wk
4. 60 lbs ↑ ea wk   8. 85 lbs ↑ #3 lbs ea wk

Each of us has only 24 hours a day. It's not a matter of someone having 22, and another 26. Twenty-four is all we've got, so it's important to make those hours count.

Since I have to work at a regular job like everyone else from 9:00 a.m. to 5:00 p.m., I have to get in my training early in the morning. Over the years I've readjusted my "biological clock" so that I go to bed at 8:00 p.m. and get up at 3:00 a.m. to get in my 2½-3 hour workout before work. I have been doing this for over 25 years, and many people seem either intrigued or skeptical about it. Clarence Bass, a champion bodybuilder and lawyer from New Mexico, visited us and when he returned home he started working out early in the morning. He was amazed at how much time he had left in the evenings. Here is my early morning routine, in case you are interested:

I get up at 3:00, have a cup of tea and maybe an orange or nectarine, and read a little. I start getting psychologically prepared for the day ahead. At about 3:45 I go up to my gym in a barn behind my house. I'll hang upside down for two or three minutes using my inversion boots and then do 100 situps from this inverted position. Then on Monday, Wednesday and Friday I'll ride a stationary bike for 30 minutes and on Tuesday, Thursday and Saturday I'll use the rowing machine for half an hour. By that time my training partners will arrive: my wife Judy, loyal friends and various visitors from time to time. There have been as many as 12 of us and as few as one. At 4:30 sharp we start bodybuilding.

We follow a program that I work out and change every four or five weeks. Each person does the same exercise, with the same number of sets and reps, but we adjust the poundages according to each person's strength.

By 7:00 a.m. we finish training. By 8:45 we'll have showered, had breakfast and are feeling great, ready for the day. □

STRENGTH TRAINING FOR SPORTS

STRENGTH TRAINING FOR SPORTS

The race is to the swift;
The battle to the strong.
John Davidson, 1857-1909

One of the most exciting things going on now in athletics is the use of weight training for sports. Weights are used to develop strength and muscular endurance, to correct muscular weakness and imbalance, to prevent or rehabilitate injuries, and to improve technique and performance in virtually every sport, from baseball to wrestling.

It wasn't always this way. Back in the '50s, weight training was strictly for body - builders, power lifters and Olympic lifters (plus a small contingent of health and strength-minded pioneers). The first use of weights for other sports that I can recall was with track and field star Dave Sime in the early '50s. Sime, a top sprinter who made the 1952 and 1956 Olympic teams, proved that weights at least didn't *hurt* performance. Billy Cannon, an All-American running back for LSU in 1959, owed much of his success to weight training. He and his LSU teammates were pioneers in the use of weights in sports.

As the years passed, there was a ripple effect as more and more trainers and players discovered what weight training could do:

- Supplement and complement traditional training
- Produce gains in strength or size that could not be achieved any other way
- Balance strength of different body parts
- Prevent injuries
- Often provide the quickest and safest way to recover from an injury

It's surprising to most people, especially those who remember the '50s and '60s, just how extensive weight training in sports has now become. Coaches now have their own weight training programs or consult with strength coaches for the appropriate exercises for their particular sport. On pages 82-175 some of the top trainers, coaches and athletes in the country have provided training programs for 21 different sports. Each of these people has a different approach but the message is the same: To be competitive in most sports today, weight training is mandatory.

Obviously, different sports require different skills and therefore different training programs. But there are certain elements of fitness and generalized principles that apply to all athletic training.

Note: For a brief explanation of what takes place *inside* the muscles due to the stresses of weight training and a discussion of the "overload principle," see the chapter "Muscles," pp. 356-64.

THE ELEMENTS OF FITNESS

What does it take to be in shape? What are the basic qualities of fitness? Just as a farmer needs the four elements for his crops to grow—water, sun, soil and air—*you* need the following four elements to be in good shape:

- Strength
- Muscular endurance
- Cardiovascular endurance
- Flexibility

Understanding these elements of fitness, especially how you train to achieve each one, is very important if you are to get the most out of your weight training.

Strength

Strength is the ability of a muscle to produce force. It is measured by the amount of weight you can lift in one repetition; for example, the most amount of weight you can bench press or lift in the squat.

Pure strength is the most important ingredient in many sports: shot-putting, discus-throwing, jumping high in basketball, having a powerful tennis serve, driving a golf ball, throwing a baseball, etc. Strength is also the key to sports where you have to meet an opponent with a lot of force, such as wrestling or football.

Power is something different.

$$Power = Strength + Speed$$

A person may have a lot of strength at the bench press, but not be able to put the shot well. He doesn't have the speed of movement that, combined with strength, generates the necessary power for a long toss.

Muscular Endurance

Muscular endurance is the ability of a muscle to produce force repeatedly *over a period of time.* It is measured by the number of repetitions of the movement or skill. If you can do only one or two push-ups, then for you it's a strength movement. If you can do 35 push-ups, then for you it's a muscular endurance exercise. Sports requiring muscular endurance are wrestling, hurdling, rowing, sprinting and sprint swimming. These sports differ from strength sports in that you have to apply force for a longer period of time.

An athlete can continue to produce muscular force for only a limited period of time before the energy stores in the muscle are depleted. In movements that apply maximum force (strength), such as lifting a heavy weight, the energy stores are quickly depleted. If less than maximum force is required, and the athlete must ration strength (as in a wrestling match or sprint), energy stores are depleted more gradually and the movement can continue for a longer period (muscular endurance).

Cardiovascular Endurance

Cardiovascular endurance is the capacity of the respiratory system (lungs and blood vessels) and the circulatory system (heart, arteries, capillaries and veins) to supply oxygen and nutrients to the muscle cells so an activity can continue for a long period of time.

This type of fitness is necessary for sports like distance running, cross-country skiing, cycling, distance swimming, triathlons, rowing and soccer. (These sports are also the best exercises for *improving* cardiovascular endurance.) Here the amount of force required of a particular muscle or muscle group is low and the movement is rhythmic. This means that one muscle group is resting while another takes over. For example, in rowing you pull with your back muscles in the power stroke and push with chest muscles on the return stroke; while one group is resting, the blood stream is bringing in nutrients and whisking away waste products. These alternating rest periods allow the movement to continue for a long time. See "Cardiovascular Training," pp. 71-76.

Flexibility

Flexibility, the fourth element of fitness, refers to the range of motion possible in the joints. This is controlled by muscles, tendons and ligaments.

It is well known that flexibility can be increased by stretching. However, there are two important factors to keep in mind:

1. *Every individual differs in flexibility.* Some are loose-jointed, some tight. A loose-jointed person is obviously well-suited for gymnastics, but is liable to get injured in contact sports. A tight-jointed person can better withstand the impact stresses of contact sports, but tends to have great difficulty at gymnastics. Most people are somewhere in between and can modify their flexibility to coincide with the demands of the sport and their body type.
2. *Each sport has different flexibility requirements.* You don't always want *maximum* flexibility in every direction. Example: football players are susceptible to blows from the side of the knee, and skiers often fall and twist their knees. These athletes should do quadriceps exercises to provide stability for the knee, and make themselves *less* flexible in side-to-side knee motion. On the other hand, gymnasts need full body flexibility, since good performance involves going to the extreme range of motion for the joints.

As a general rule, *you need enough flexibility to go through the range of motion required· in your sport without restrictions in movement.*

Many people think that weight lifters are inflexible or "muscle-bound." On the contrary, weight training improves flexibility. In a study that compared flexibility for champion college gymnasts, champion college wrestlers, and average 16-year-old boys along with national champion weight lifters and bodybuilders, the weight lifters were slightly more flexible (in measurements of 30 different joint movements) than the gymnasts and much more flexible than the wrestlers or 16-year-olds.*

See pp. 325-30 for Bob Anderson's "Stretches for Weight Training."

To repeat, the elements of fitness are:

1. *Strength:* Maximum force in a short burst
2. *Muscular Endurance:* Power that is repeated for a period of time, not just a short burst
3. *Cardiovascular Endurance:* Force applied over the long haul
4. *Flexibility:* Range of movement in joints □

---

*Flexibility Characteristics of Three Specialized Skill Groups of Champion Athletes. Jack Leighton, Ph.D. *Archives of Physical Medicine*, 1957, Vol. 38, No. 9.

SPORTS TRAINING PRINCIPLES

Weightlifting is just about the most versatile of all athletic activities. You can lift to look good and feel good—for general conditioning. You can train to get back into shape or to lose weight after years of inactivity. You can lift to get a more attractive physique or for bodybuilding. You can build pure strength and power, as for competitive lifting or other power sports. And as shown on pages 82-175 you can use weightlifting to improve performance in just about any sport.

In the last chapter we talked about the four basic elements of fitness:

- *Strength*
- *Muscular endurance* } Best improved by weight training

- *Cardiovascular endurance*
- *Flexibility* } Best improved by other methods

The two elements best improved by weightlifting are strength and muscular endurance. Cardiovascular endurance *can* be improved in the weight room but running, swimming, walking, exercycling, etc., are more efficient ways to strengthen the heart and lungs. Flexibility can also be improved by weight training, but again, stretching is the obvious tool for getting looser and increasing range of motion.

The Most Important Principles in Weight Training for Sports

- *Low reps/high weights = Strength*
- *High reps/low weights = Muscular Endurance*

Or in other words:

- *Heavy resistance with low repetitions builds strength.*
- *Light resistance with high repetitions builds endurance.*

The following chart shows you how to train for different goals. At the left is the low rep/high weight training for strength. At the right is the high rep/low weight training for muscular endurance. In the middle is the medium rep/medium weight approach for most athletes.

SPORTS TRAINING CONTINUUM

	Strength Training	All Around Sports Training	Muscular Endurance Training
Goal	Strength & power	General conditioning (Strength + endurance)	Muscular endurance (Stamina)
Who trains this way	Power lifters Olympic lifters Football linemen Shot putters Etc.	Most athletes General population	Swimmers Rowers Cyclists Distance runners Cross-country skiers Etc.
Physiological changes	Increase in size of muscle fiber	Some increase in both size of muscle fiber and vascularization	Increase in vascularization, blood supply to muscle
Type of lifting	Low reps (2-4-6) High weights	Medium reps (8-10-12) Medium weights	High reps (15-25) Low weights

1. To develop *strength* you need to work as many fibers at one time as possible. Thus you lift heavy weights for a few reps. This causes maximum neurological stimulation of the muscle, causing many fibers to contract at the same time.
2. To develop *muscular endurance* you lift lighter weights for many reps. Here fewer fibers contract at one time and alternate their contraction in an on/off fashion. This allows the muscle fiber to recover on the off cycle and the movement to continue through many reps.
3. *Weight training* can be used to *supplement* other training. The athlete can train to develop the elements of fitness not acquired during normal training. Examples: runners would work on developing muscular endurance for their arms, skiers would strengthen quadriceps to prevent knee injuries, cyclists should work on upper body endurance to delay fatigue.
4. Many strength coaches have their athletes *exercise opposite muscle groups* for muscle balance and to prevent injury. They feel that many injuries occur by building up one set of muscles and not the opposing set. For example, they recommend that if you do leg extensions for the quads you should then do leg flexions or other exercises for the hamstrings. Here are some major muscles and their opposite groups:

- Chest/Upper back
- Shoulders/Lats
- Biceps/Triceps

5. *Key for athletes:*

- Analyze the needs of your sport.
- Analyze your own strengths and weaknesses.
- Work on the weaknesses. Many athletes work only on their strengths (it hurts to work on the weaknesses). A chain is only as strong as its weakest link, and you won't make maximum progress until you correct the deficiencies.

Number of Reps the Athlete Should Perform at Various Intensities

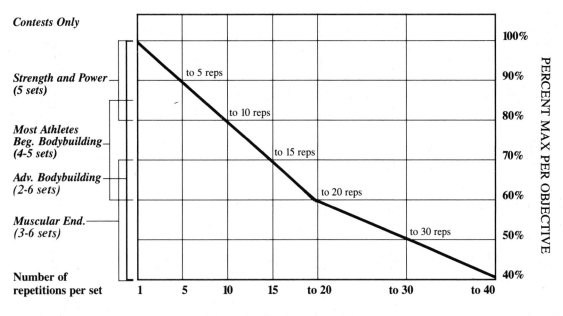

Table adapted from Aerobic Weight Training *by Frederick C. Hatfield, Ph.D. (Contemporary Books, Inc., 1983.)*

Note: The table shows, among other things, that:

- If you are doing one rep only, it should be at 100% effort.
- There is a wide range for advanced bodybuilders, from low reps/high weights to high reps/low weights, depending on their goals.
- Most athletes need both strength and endurance, so they stay in the 7-20 rep zone. Ten reps generally gives you proportional amounts of strength and endurance.

Strength/Power/Speed

In the previous chapter we defined power as strength + speed and mentioned that strength in and of itself does not guarantee high performance. For example, the strongest football lineman may not be the best. If he doesn't have enough speed, agility, balance or co-ordination he may be outmaneuvered and outleveraged despite his greater strength. Or consider the difference between the two types of competitive lifting—powerlifting and Olympic lifting. In powerlifting (bench press, squat, dead lift), speed is not nearly as important as it is in Olympic lifting (clean and jerk, the snatch), where speed is critical. Olympic lifters must have explosive speed to perform.

   The quickness of the first step in basketball, changing direction on a dime in football, and explosiveness out of the starting blocks in sprinting are all examples of power.

Quickness is a function of several factors:

- *Strength*, which is a measure of force. The more force you can produce, the greater your speed (so long as you maintain good form).
- *Resistance.* In some sports the resistance is another person (football, wrestling, boxing). In other sports, the resistance is an object (shotput, javelin, barbell). In many sports, the resistance is your own body, how much you weigh. If you are light and strong you will be faster than if you are heavy and weak.
- *Nerve stimulation.* The speed of nerve impulses affects speed of movement. It is difficult to improve this with training, but plyometric exercises (see p. 68) can help, and weight training can improve nerve transmission by increasing the number of neural endings in the muscles.
- *Fast-twitch/slow-twitch fibers.* All people have both fast- and slow-twitch fibers. Fast-twitch fibers contract faster and can produce more explosive movements. You cannot change the ratio of fast- to slow-twitch fibers in your body, but weight training can maximize development of those fast-twitch fibers you do have (see below).
- *Biomechanics.* Getting yourself in the best position to move can increase speed. This is why baseball and basketball players stay on the balls of their feet and sprinters use crouch starts.
- *Anticipation.* Thinking of a movement beforehand helps the nervous system to respond and make the movement faster.

Fast-Twitch/Slow-Twitch

Within the last 10 years researchers have discovered that human muscle is composed of two major types of fiber: fast-twitch and slow-twitch.* The terms "fast" and "slow" indicate the speed at which they can contract.

Fast-twitch fibers are white, slow-twitch are red. For example, a chicken drumstick is dark meat while the wing and breast are white. That's because the domestic chicken walks and runs but does very little flying. Her leg muscles (red, slow-twitch fibers) have endurance and stamina for all-day locomotion. Her wings and breast muscles (white, fast-twitch fibers) are for flapping rapidly and short flights to escape predators.

Human muscles contain both fast- and slow-twitch fibers. We all have a mixture of both types, but some people have more of one than another.

Fast-twitch: Sprinters, shot-putters, Olympic lifters have a high percentage of fast-twitch fibers.

Slow-twitch: Marathoners, distance swimmers or cyclists and cross-country skiers have a high percentage of slow-twitch fibers.

Fast-twitch fibers contract two to four times faster than slow-twitch and also fatigue faster. They generate energy anaerobically (without oxygen). They are best suited for high-intensity events that don't last long, like running a hundred-yard dash, or broad jumping.

Slow-twitch fibers contract slower and also fatigue slower. They contain more and larger mitochondria (the "power plants" of the muscle cells which convert food into usable energy) and generate energy aerobically (with oxygen). This makes them suitable for prolonged aerobic exercise. One study shows that world-class distance runners had an average of 80% slow-twitch fibers in their thighs.

*There are actually four types of fibers: Type I, Type IIA, Type IIB and Type IIC. However, the three Type II fibers differ from Type I in not having the capacity for long-term endurance and are classified as fast-twitch.

Here are microscopic photos of fast-twitch and slow-twitch muscles:

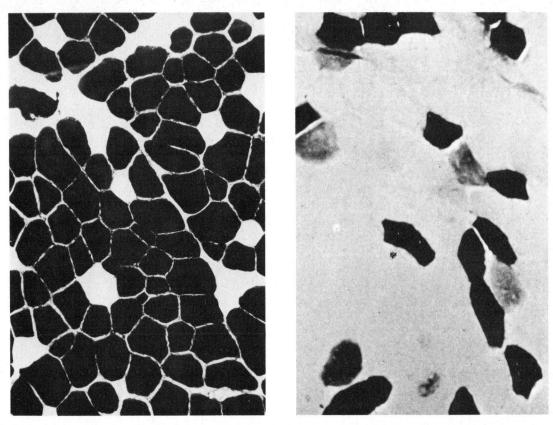

Cross section of skeletal muscle samples from a male sprinter who ran the 100 meter sprint in 10 seconds (left) and an elite distance runner (right). The fibers are stained to show the fast-twitch fibers as dark, the slow-twitch fibers as light. Note the preponderance of fast-twitch fibers in the sprinter's muscle and the reverse for the distance runner. Courtesy Phillip D. Gollnick, Ph.D.

What's the point of this discussion about fast/slow-twitch muscle fibers?

1. *Distribution:* Research indicates you're born with a ratio of fast- to slow-twitch fibers and that it's genetically determined. Until recently it was thought that you could not change this by training, but current research has shown that you can train one type of fast-twitch fibers (fast twitch IIA)—through aerobic training—to respond like slow-twitch. This aids in endurance events.
2. *Changes in size:* You *can*, however, increase the *size* and *capacity* of both fast- and slow-twitch fibers by different types of training: slow-twitch by aerobic training (distance running, swimming, etc.), fast twitch by anaerobic training (sprinting, weightlifting, etc.).

Isometric/Isokinetic/Isotonic

There are three types of progressive resistance weight training that are so named for their different effect on the muscles. The prefix "iso-" is from the Greek *isos* meaning equal.

> Isometric: equal length
> Isotonic: equal weight
> Isokinetic: equal speed

In the past 20 years various forms of these three types of exercises have come in and out of fashion.

Isometric. "Dynamic Tension," as touted by Charles Atlas in the comic books in the '50s was the best-known form of isometric exercise. You could transform yourself from a skinny wimp into a muscular hero with Atlas's mail-order course. And no weights were necessary!

In isometric training you push or pull against an immovable object such as a wall or an anchored bar. Muscle tension is increased but there is little or no change in muscle length. Research in the '50s showed that a maximum isometric contraction produced more force than lifting weights. This was thought to be a breakthrough in training and in the early '60s many pro football teams practiced isometric exercises.

The advantages of isometric training are:

- Maximum muscular contraction (as opposed to isotonic or free weight training).
- The exercises can be done anywhere, at any time, since virtually no equipment is needed.
- They take very little time, three to six seconds per exercise.

Later research, however, turned up some disadvantages:

- Isometrics can hamper or decrease muscular *endurance* because such static exercises do not entail the pumping action of the blood normally associated with muscle movement, and in fact, the muscles' blood supply can be diminished.
- There can be a significant rise in blood pressure which could be dangerous for people with heart and vascular problems.
- Strengthening a limb in a static contraction can also lead to reduction in the *speed* of movement.
- Athletes found the exercises boring. There was no feedback, as in knowing how much they were lifting.

Today, isometrics are rarely used in athletic training. The primary use today is in rehabilitation. The patient can develop force and work the muscles without moving the joints or limbs (for example, if one's leg is in a cast).

Isotonic means equal tension or weight. In this type of training there is a change in the length of the muscle. Lifting free weights (barbells and dumbbells) is the classic form of isotonic exercise. As contrasted to isometric training, where maximal muscular contractions are possible throughout the exercise, in isotonic training resistance during the entire lift is not consistent. There is an easy part and a hard part. The hard part—the "sticking point"—is the weakest spot in the range of motion (where the weakest muscles or joint angles come into play). This feature is important to understand when comparing isotonic training with isokinetic training.

Isokinetic is a newer form of exercise and is a specialized type of isotonic exercise where there is an "accommodating resistance."

In lifting free weights (isotonic) there is an easy part and a hard part to the lift. When you curl a dumbbell, the hardest part of the exercise is at the beginning—you must overcome the inertia of the weight and the poor anatomical leverage. As you continue the lift, the movement becomes easier and is at its easiest at the end of the lift when the weight is moving and leverage is improved.

What does the lifter do when he wants to lift the maximum weight? He chooses a weight he can lift through the part of the exercise where his muscles are weakest—the first half of a biceps curl, for example. During the rest of the lift, his muscles are not working to their fullest.

If, however, you could develop an exercise machine that would increase resistance throughout the lift then you could lift "to the max" throughout the entire range of motion. This is exactly what has been attempted with the Nautilus, Cybex, Biokinetic and other machines. Accommodating resistance means the machine theoretically provides resistance proportional to whatever effort you apply to it.

A full description of free weights vs. machines (and the limited uses of accommodating resistance machines for athletes) is on pp. 346-50. □

TRAINING CONCEPTS FOR ADVANCED ATHLETES

As knowledge about weight training increases, and coaches and trainers become more sophisticated in their use of this knowledge, advanced training techniques and principles are evolving to meet the needs of serious, competitive athletes.

Workout Techniques

These three techniques are used to provide variety, increase resistance or maximize workout time in daily workouts:

1. Supersets
2. Trisets
3. Pyramid Training

Supersets. A superset is when you do one exercise right after the other, with little or no rest until the second set is completed. These are usually done with opposing muscle groups, such as the biceps and triceps, or chest and back. For example, you might do a bench press followed by a rowing exercise, then a rest of one to two minutes, followed by the remaining sets.

Supersets can reduce workout time, or allow you to pack more exercises into a given training session. However, you must be in good shape and work into them slowly to avoid injury.

For an example of a superset program, see "Cycling," pp. 101-02.

Trisets. A triset is a group of three exercises, each done after the other with little rest in between. Trisets can be used to work three different muscle groups, to work different areas of the same muscle from three different angles, and to work the same area of a muscle (from the same angle).

Pyramid Training. Here you start with high reps, low weight (to warm up) and then decrease the reps as you add weight. Following is an example with the bench press:

Sets	Reps	Weight
1	12	135
1	8	185
1	6	225
1	4	245
1	2	275
1	1	300

Then you work your way back down, taking off weight and adding reps. (Scale the weight down or up, according to your ability.)

You can do any number of reps for the desired number of sets as long as you follow the high rep/low weight progression to heavier weights and less reps.

High Intensity Training

The following techniques have been developed to create a maximum muscle overload. They are used by hardcore bodybuilders or athletes.

Warning: These methods are effective, but should be used only if you are already in good shape and preferably with the aid of an experienced partner or trainer. *Proceed with caution!*

Note: Some of these techniques (forced reps, partial reps, multi-poundage system) have not proven as effective as was originally believed. The theories had merits, but in actual practice, many lifters did not hold up to the stress. Of these five, cheating has produced the best results and is the most widely used.

1. Forced reps
2. Partial reps
3. Negative reps
4. Multi-poundage system
5. Cheating

Forced Reps. A partner helps you to do a few more reps when you can't do any more alone. This is done by giving you a *slight* amount of assistance, for example, by helping you raise the barbell in a bench press. Your partner must judge how much strength you have left and give you only enough help to get you through the toughest part of the lift. The object is to have *you* do as much of the work as you can.

Partial Reps. After the last rep of the last set—when you are unable to do another full rep—you concentrate on doing half- or quarter-reps. For example, on a bench press you would lower the weight half-way or quarter-way down and press upward. You continue this until you can do no more.

Negative Reps. This technique works the muscle during the eccentric (lengthening) phase—when the weight is lowered. Physiologists have found that the muscle can produce the most force during this phase. A partner helps you raise the weight; then you lower it as slowly as possible. Again, without a partner you couldn't get the weight back up. This puts great stress on the tendons and ligaments and increases risk of injury, so be very careful.

Multi-Poundage System. After you get to the maximum weight or after you finish your normal number of sets, you immediately (without rest) take some weight off the bar and do an additional set. Then again—without rest—you decrease the weight and do another set. You repeat this for one to five sets with descending weights. This exhausts the muscle and provides more of an overload.

Cheating. Cheating is when you alter a position so you can lift more weight. An example is arching your back on a bench press. This changes the line of pull of the muscles and improves leverage, allowing you to lift more weight. Another example is when you lean back when doing a curl.

Cheating is an advanced technique and should only be used by experienced lifters. When starting to lift, use the form indicated in the instructions. Even advanced lifters don't cheat on all sets, but sometimes on just the last few sets, or last reps of the last set.

Cheating is used by advanced lifters to handle heavier weights than they can normally handle in the strict position. This can eventually lead to them being able to lift that weight with standard form. Thus there is a place for cheating but it should be used sparingly and carefully.

Split Routines

With split routines you work the upper body one day and the lower body another day. As we have explained, muscles need a day of recovery between workouts. This means that if you work all the major muscles one day, you must rest the next day. With a split routine, however, you can work out on successive days, since the upper body is getting a rest while you're working the lower body, and vice versa. Here are some examples of split routines:

4-day*	5-day*	5-day	6-day*	6-day, 2 per day
M: Upper	M: Upper	M: Chest	M: Upper	Mon a.m.: Chest
T: Lower	T: Lower	T: Shoulders	T: Lower	Mon p.m.: Back
W: Rest	W: Upper	W: Back	W: Upper	Tue a.m.: Shoulders
Th: Upper	Th: Lower	Th: Rest	Th: Lower	Tue p.m.: Upper legs
F: Lower	F: Upper	F: Tri/Bic	F: Upper	Wed a.m.: Triceps
	Reverse cycle following week	S: Legs	S: Lower	Wed p.m.: Biceps
		Work abs and calves each day or minimum three days, but fewer sets		Th a.m.: Chest
				Th p.m.: Back
				Work abs and calves each day or minimum three days, but do fewer sets

Note: Work abdominals each day.

Here are some other techniques and concepts aimed at maximizing athletic performance.

Super Stretching

PNF—*proprioceptive neuromuscular facilitation*—is a stretching technique that has been used successfully for a number of years by gymnasts, dancers, track and field athletes and physical therapists. It involves fatiguing a muscle or muscle group through an isometric contraction and then (usually with the help of a partner) stretching the muscle. The athlete can generally achieve a greater range of motion or stretch once the muscle has first been fatigued.

For example:

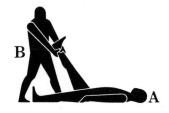

Athlete (A) lies on his back and tries to bring his leg to the ground. His partner (B) holds the leg and resists the movement. (A) holds the contraction for 8-10 seconds, then relaxes. Then (B) pushes (gently) upward on A's leg, stretching the hamstrings—increasing the range of motion of the hip.

The procedure is repeated up to five times and you should be able to go farther with each progressive stretch.

Most muscle groups can be stretched in a similar way. PNF exercises are also being used by physical therapists and athletic trainers for treatment and rehabilitation of both athletic and non-athletic injuries and conditions.

Note: Your muscles are protected from overstretching by an automatic mechanism called the *stretch reflex:* when you stretch too far or too quickly the muscles will automatically contract to prevent tearing. PNF overrides the stretch reflex and thus you must be very careful. Go slowly, concentrate on how it *feels*—there should never be pain. Your partner should be sensitive and not jerk or push too hard, too far or too fast.

Plyometric Exercises

Plyometric exercises are being used increasingly these days by athletes in sports that require speed, quickness and jumping ability. Plyometrics can improve both strength and speed—explosiveness—when combined with a good weight training program. A typical *lower body* plyometric exercise is jumping from a box onto the ground then rebounding onto the box as quickly as possible. A typical *upper body* plyometric exercise is to have a partner throw a medicine ball to you, then you throw it back as quickly as possible, stepping forward alternately with your right and left leg.

> *Plyometrics provide an overload to the musculature in a way which is different from weight training. Body weight accelerated by gravity provides a force and velocity which exceeds that of machine or free weights and also simulates actions present in many jumping, sprinting and throwing activities. This specificity in training is a necessary component for teaching the neuromuscular apparatus to respond more quickly and forcefully.*
>
> Donald A. Chu, Ph.D.*

Plyometrics have been used very effectively by track and field athletes, especially sprinters, jumpers and throwers. Sprinters are able to explode out of the starting blocks, jumpers have been able to prevent collapse of the takeoff leg when jumping and throwers have strengthened the pushing force of the legs as the throw is made. Plyometrics have also improved upper arm speed and strength: discus throwers, shot putters, javelin throwers, as well as baseball pitchers, basketball players and volleyball players are now using plyometric drills.

Warning: Plyometrics can be dangerous if the athlete does not have sufficient strength to withstand the forces generated. The sudden change from a loaded eccentric contraction to a quick near-maximal concentric contraction involves precise coordination and timing, as well as a high level of fitness; if not, injuries can easily result. For the high-intensity jumps (box jumps, one-leg hops, etc.), many trainers recommend that athletes first be able to do a full squat with 1½ to 2 times their body weight as a strength base.

Another key element in plyometric jumping is proper technique in foot placement: the athlete should land on the full foot to cushion the shock of landing and then roll forward and push off on the ball of the foot. Landing on the heel or ball of the foot transfers the impact to the knee and ankle joints rather than allowing the muscles (which are more elastic) to absorb the shock of landing.

For a full range of plyometric exercises and further information, see *Plyometrics for Fitness and Peak Performance* by Donald A. Chu, Ph.D. and Raymond Signier (Doubleday & Co., Inc., NY, 1986) and *Bounding to the Top* by Frank Costello (Track & Field News, Los Altos, CA, 1984).

Periodization

Periodization is a system of training that has been used in the Soviet Union for many years and is now being used increasingly in the United States, as well as other countries. It is based on the premise that maximum strength gains are made possible by four different training cycles or *periods*. The athlete starts with light weights and high repetitions, progresses to medium weights with medium repetitions, then to heavy weights with few repetitions and then takes one to two weeks of rest before starting the cycle again.

The theory is based upon the discovery that constant heavy-duty training does not lead to maximum progress. In fact, keeping up too high a level of intensity without adequate rest often leads to diminished performance, burn-out, or injury. Periodization allows the body to gradually adapt to the stress of exercise. Athletes have found that they can peak—reach maximum performance level—at a pre-designated time (usually the day of a competition).

*National Strength & Conditioning Association Journal, June/July, 1986.

There is an excellent chapter on periodization in *Lift Your Way to Youthful Fitness* by Jan and Terry Todd (Little, Brown and Company, 1985). The following chart is reprinted from that book:

Period	Phase	Description	Duration	Sets and Repetitions
One	HYPERTROPHY	High volume (High repetitions) Low intensity (Light weights)	4 weeks	1 set of 10 with warm-up weight 1 set of 10 with intermediate weight 3 sets of 10 with target weight
Two	BASIC STRENGTH	Moderate volume (Moderate repetitions) Medium intensity (medium weights)	4 weeks	1 set of 10 with warm-up weight 1 set of 5 with intermediate weight 3 sets of 5 with target weight 1 set of 10 with 70% of target weight*
Three	POWER**	Low volume (Low repetitions) High intensity (Heavy weights)	2 weeks	1 set of 10 with warm-up weight 1 set of 3 with light intermediate weight 1 set of 3 with intermediate weight 3 sets of 3 at target weight 1 set of 10 with 70% of target weight*
Four	REJUVENATION (Active Rest)***	Very low volume (Few repetitions; light forms of other exercise) Very low intensity (Very light weights or no weight training)	1 to 2 weeks	Do no organized weight work. Experiment with new exercises: cycle, play racquetball, swim, etc. Do not try to keep making gains.

*These single sets with 70%—sometimes called "down sets"—help to maintain the gains in lean body weight made during Hypertrophy.
**If you are not interested in the highest performance or maximum strength, you can skip the power phase and stay on a three-phase program. This is easier and involves less wear and tear.
***After the "Active Rest," begin the cycle again with Hypertrophy.

Some Principles of Exercise Physiology

Exercise physiology is the study of how the body functions during exercise. In recent years an enormous amount of research has taken place and more discoveries are made each year about the various effects of exercise on body parts, the type of exercise that produces specific results, and the various ways in which muscles adapt to different demands placed upon them. Here we make very brief mention of a few of the principles at work when muscles are stressed by weight training.

Specificity Principle. Muscles will adapt specifically to the type of stress imposed upon them. If you do a lot of distance running you will improve your cardiorespiratory endurance but do little to improve your skeletal-muscular strength. On the other hand, pure strength training with weights will yield strength gains but little cardiorespiratory improvement. Thus you must design your training program to fit the requirements of your sport and goals.

All or None Principle. Muscle fiber contracts on an "all or nothing" basis. If you work your biceps, say, against light resistance, the movement is not produced by a small amount of work on the part of the fibers in the biceps muscle. **R**ather, only a few fibers are working—to their fullest—and the other fibers are not involved. As you *increase* resistance, you *recruit* more and more fibers. To get maximum results, you continue adding resistance to the point where most or all the fibers have been recruited.

Use and Disuse Principle. When muscles are systematically overloaded they will respond by adapting to the stress: they will increase in size (hypertrophy) and strength. Conversely, if training ceases, the muscles will react to the lack of stress or stimulus by decreasing in size (atrophy) and strength, and losing tone. This is why people who have broken a bone are often shocked at the loss of muscle size in a limb when the cast is removed.

Individuality Principle. Individuals respond differently to the same exercise programs. There are many individual factors that will affect *your* response to training: heredity, nutrition, fitness level, motivation, health habits (rest and sleep), hormone and enzyme levels and environmental influences.

Agonist/Antagonist. The *agonist* is the muscle directly engaged in contraction. The *antagonist* is the muscle that has to relax at the same time (that the agonist contracts). When a doctor taps your knee with a rubber hammer, your knee jerks: the agonist (quadriceps) tightens and contracts while the antagonist (hamstring) stretches. When you bend your elbow and make a muscle in your arm, the biceps is the agonist, the triceps the antagonist.

In sports, the balancing of the contracting (shortening) agonist muscles and the controlled lengthening of the antagonist is crucial to smooth performance. Thus it is important to strengthen opposing muscle groups in your workouts (chest/upper back, quadriceps/hamstrings, etc.).

Concentric/Eccentric Contractions. A *concentric* muscular contraction is when the muscle contracts and shortens. Thus when you curl a dumbbell upwards, your biceps muscle shortens as it develops tension to overcome the resistance and contracts concentrically.

An *eccentric* muscular contraction is when the muscle lengthens while developing tension. When you slowly curl that same dumbbell downwards, the external resistance forces the muscle to lengthen and contract eccentrically.

In lifting weights, concentric muscular contractions generally occur when you lift the weights up, eccentric muscular contractions generally occur when you let the weights down. □

CARDIOVASCULAR TRAINING

A merry heart goes all day.
Shakespeare, *The Winter's Tale*

The heart is a muscular pump, about the size of your fist. It beats non-stop every minute of every day, sending blood throughout the circulatory system. In a typical day some 2000 gallons of blood will pass through the heart. Like any muscle, the heart needs exercise or it will deteriorate.

In the past, bodybuilders and power lifters often built strength and muscle while neglecting the body's most important muscle—the heart. Conversely, many endurance runners have often concentrated solely on cardiovascular endurance, with little regard for upper body strength.

These days that's all changing. A more enlightened attitude, along with the unprecedented interest in fitness has led athletes in all sports to recognize the value of *total conditioning.* Research and sports physiology have proven the value of all-around training. It's becoming much less common for the runner to only run, the swimmer to only swim, the lifter to only lift. In many ways the age of specialized, one-track training is over. We now know better.

If your goal is to be in the best possible condition, why work hard on muscular and strength development and neglect the heart and vascular system? You might *look* great on the outside, but inside the motor and pumping system that keeps the body healthy and alive can be suffering from neglect. A combination of weight training and cardiovascular endurance training is ideal.

The leading cause of death in America today is heart disease, and the most effective way to avoid this is by good nutrition and a cardiovascular exercise program. The cardio - vascular program should involve large muscle groups and the exercises should have two characteristics:

1. They should be done at a relatively low intensity, so you can keep exercising for 30-60 minutes at a time;
2. They should be *rhythmical,* meaning that there is a brief rest period for the main muscle group when another muscle group takes over.

The aerobic exercises should be performed at least three days a week for a desirable training effect to occur.

Consult Your Doctor

Before beginning a strenuous cardiovascular exercise program, check with your doctor, especially if you are over 35, overweight, under stress or have not exercised for a while.

Your exam should consist of a complete medical history, resting and stress *electrocardiogram,* blood analysis, urinalysis, chest x-ray, *pulmonary* function evaluation, and a coronary risk profile. These tests should provide your physician with the necessary data to evaluate your current state of health.

Risk Factor Questionnaire

If the answer to any of the following questions is "yes," be especially sure to see your doctor before beginning any exercise program.

	yes	*no*
1. Have you been sedentary for several years or are you more than 20 pounds overweight?	_____	_____
2. Are you ever extremely out of breath?	_____	_____
3. Do you smoke or have any history of lung disorder?	_____	_____
4. Do you take any prescribed medication regularly?	_____	_____
5. Have you ever had a heart attack or has your doctor said you have heart trouble, or a heart murmur?	_____	_____
6. Do you have frequent pains or pressure—in the left or mid-chest area, left neck, shoulder or arm—during or after exercise?	_____	_____
7. Do you often feel faint or have spells of severe dizziness?	_____	_____
8. Did your doctor ever say your blood pressure was too high or is not under control? Do you have high cholesterol?	_____	_____
9. Has your doctor said you have bone or joint problems such as arthritis?	_____	_____
10. Are you 35 or over and not accustomed to vigorous exercise?	_____	_____
11. Do you have a family history of premature coronary artery disease (heart attack or chest pain prior to age 50)?	_____	_____
12. Do you have a medical condition not mentioned here which might need special attention in an exercise program (for example, insulin-dependent diabetes)?	_____	_____

Aerobic/Anaerobic

Humans are able to move because of muscular contraction. Muscles pull on bones and cause our limbs and bodies to move, walk, run, swim, write, etc. The muscles use energy to contract in two ways: aerobically and anaerobically.

Aerobic: "with oxygen." *Aerobic exercises* are those where the demands of muscles for oxygen are met by the circulation of oxygen in the blood. The oxygen is supplied by the heart and lungs in an amount required by the activity. Typical aerobic exercises are distance running, bicycling, cross-country skiing and swimming—those that use large muscle groups.

These activities, although strenuous, are rhythmical and performed at less than all-out intensity. During exercise, there is a brief rest period for the main working muscle group (during which another muscle group does the work) and the blood stream brings nutrients to the muscle cells and removes metabolic wastes. This allows the movement to continue for a long period of time.

Anaerobic: "without oxygen." *Anaerobic activities* are those where the oxygen demands of the muscles are so high that the circulatory system cannot supply adequate oxygen. The muscles can continue to function (for a short time) by utilizing chemical processes that free oxygen within the muscle itself. "All-out" sports like sprinting, arm-wrestling, shot-putting and weightlifting are anaerobic exercises.

Here's how this works: the oxygen a sprinter inhales at the beginning of a 100-meter run does not get to the muscle cells until after the race is over. The sprinter uses anaerobic metabolism (the oxygen capacity within the muscles) to run the race. After the race the sprinters are gasping for air, chests heaving. They are replacing the "oxygen debt" of the muscles. Oxygen helps remove lactic acid and other products of muscular contraction from the muscle, and replenishes energy stores in the muscle.

Relative Amounts of Aerobic vs. Anaerobic Fitness Required in Different Sports

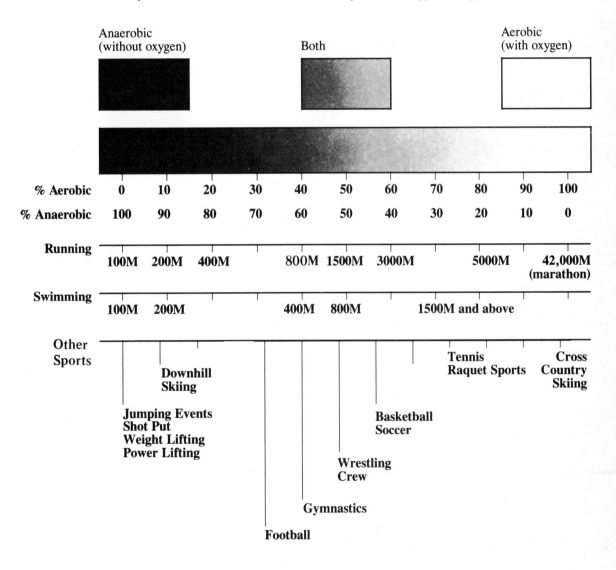

In the running and swimming events, researchers generally agree that at around three minutes (until about seven or eight minutes) there are relatively equal requirements in both the aerobic and anaerobic pathways for muscle energetics. From Aerobic Weight Training, *by Fred C. Hatfield, Ph.D. (1985, Contemporary Books, Inc.)*

Note that the strength events such as shot-putting and weightlifting (at the left) are exclusively anaerobic and can be trained for by using a weight program designed to build strength. At the right end of the chart are endurance sports such as marathon running and cross-country skiing where training involves aerobic *and* muscular endurance training. *However, most sports are in between these two extremes and involve both aerobic and anaerobic conditioning. A high level of fitness in both is the ideal.*

Monitoring Your Pulse

The cardiovascular training effect occurs when you are working your heart muscle at 70-85% of its maximum rate. (Maximum is the fastest your heart can beat and still efficiently pump blood to your body.) Here is a table showing that range: *

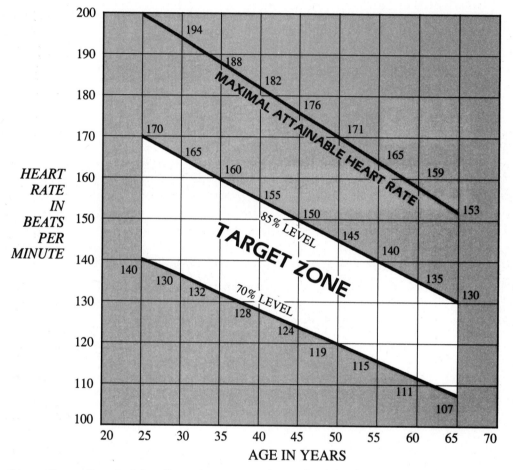

*According to the principles of exercise programming set forth by the American Heart Association and the President's Council on Physical Fitness and Sports. Source: Universal Workout Record, Universal Gym Equipment, Inc., Cedar Rapids, Iowa.

Summary of Cardiovascular Principles

Pulse rate: 70-85% of maximum
Days per week: Minimum of three
Minutes per day: 30-60 continuous

Checking Your Pulse—How to Do It:

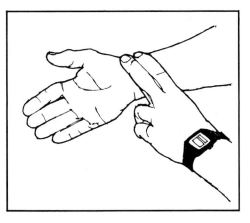

Place two fingers on your wrist as shown. Count the beats for 15 seconds and multiply by four to get your pulse rate.

Types of Cardiovascular Activities

There are two ways to get your cardiovascular training:

1. *Outside the gym.* Running, hiking, walking, swimming, cycling, cross-country skiing, rowing, and skipping rope are all popular cardiovascular activities. (Exercises such as bowling or golf do not raise your heart beat sufficiently to qualify. An ideal overall fitness program would include a weight training schedule supplemented by one of these activities for 30-60 minutes, three times a week.
2. *Inside the gym.* You can get your cardiovascular training *in* the gym if you keep the intensity level high enough for your pulse to stay within the target zone. One way to do this is to set up a circuit like this:

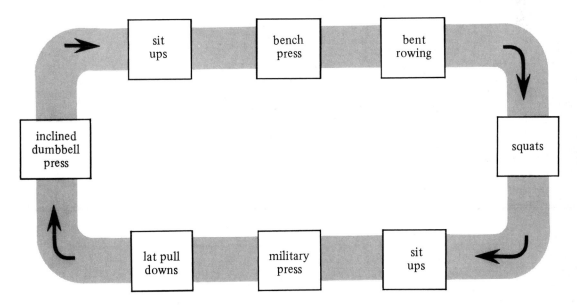

Do one exercise and move on immediately to the next exercise. *No resting!* Check your pulse to be sure you're in the target zone. (After doing this a while you'll know by your breathing if you're in the zone and you won't have to keep stopping to take your pulse.)

Aerobic conditioning is an integral part of total fitness. If you use weight training for muscle mass, strength, muscular endurance, or bodybuilding—activities that, because of their intensity level, are anaerobic in nature—it is advisable to supplement your program with some type of aerobic training. You'll not only build up your heart, lungs and circulatory systems but avoid overtraining and mental staleness, feel better and probably live longer.

Summary

Aerobic: with oxygen. Think of "air" = aerobic. Running, swimming, cycling for a long time.

Anaerobic: without oxygen. The opposite of aerobic. "Out-of-breath" activities, sudden bursts, the 100-meter dash, shot-putting, weightlifting.

Benefits of an Aerobic Program

- Increased ability of the heart and blood vessels to supply oxygen to the body
- Increased blood volume
- Increased lung capacity: ability to transport oxygen into the blood and remove carbon dioxide from the blood
- Better stamina, longer duration of effort before exhaustion
- Decrease in body fat
- Reduced stress and tension □

POWER OF POSITIVE LIFTING

Russian Revelation

In 1979, Dr. Charles Garfield, a good friend of mine and weight lifter, met with a group of Soviet sports psychologists and physiologists in Milan. They told him about the phenomenal effects of intense mental training on athletic performance. After spending several days with the Soviet researchers, Garfield had heard enough theory. He wanted to see results.

At a gym, the Soviets quizzed Garfield. "How long since you've done any serious training?" they asked. "Eight years." "What was your maximum bench press in your prime?" "365 pounds." "In recent years what is the most you've pressed?" "280 pounds."

It intrigued the Soviets that Garfield had once pressed 365. "How long would you have to train to make that lift again?" they asked. "Nine to twelve months," he said. The Soviet doctors then asked him, "Would you attempt a 300-pound lift right now?" Garfield reluctantly agreed to try. Spurred and encouraged by the Russians, and much to his surprise, Garfield (barely) made the lift.

Then the Soviet doctors went to work. They guided him into a state of deep relaxation for 40 minutes. Then they added 65 pounds to the 300. They had him visualize approaching the bar, lying on the bench and confidently making the lift. They told him to imagine each phase of the lift: the sound of the jangling weights, his breathing, the noises of exertion he ordinarily made when lifting.

Garfield got nervous, certain he couldn't do it. He began to worry about even pressing 300 again. But the Soviets calmly told him to visualize lifting the 365. They had him look closely at his hands, the weights, and said to imagine how his muscles would feel after he succeeded. As they talked him through the whole process again, the series of images, and then the total picture, began to clarify in Garfield's mind. "The imagery now imprinted in my mind began to guide my physical movements... The world around me seemed to fade, giving way to self-confidence, belief in myself and then to deliberate action.

"I lifted the weights!"*

Garfield had learned an important lesson in the power of mental training, concentration and visualization. It's a lesson that more and more athletes are using to their advantage.

Sports Psychology

Stress is real. Physiologically, the pulse quickens, the breathing rate changes. A relief pitcher in a tight spot feels it. A sprinter in the starting blocks feels it. A bodybuilder feels it before posing. It's a mistake to deny stress and the energy it creates. All of us have "choked"—tensed up under pressure. It may not have been in sports, but there have been times when the "heat" of a stressful situation has shot you down.

When this happens, it means the anxiety is out of control. You lose concentration and can't direct your attention. You tense up. It doesn't have to be that way. You can use stress to your advantage.

Stress keeps you alert; it prods you into being more productive. It's a challenge to control your responses to stressful situations, but it's a challenge you can win.

In sports, wholeness is essential. The most physically skilled competitor who ties up mentally will be unsuccessful. Until very recently, the mind/body integration and awareness so crucial for athletic success has been ignored in training for most sports. Now, taking a cue from the Soviets and East Germans, who pioneered the emphasis on holistic training, athletes work on the mental aspect of training as well as the physical.

*Peak Performance, Charles A. Garfield, Ph.D., with Hal Zinna Bennett. Jeremy B. Tarcher, Inc. 1984

Knowing that you can control your behavior and your response to stress gives you a great boost in confidence. There are strategies and skills you can learn which help keep your thoughts positive and constructive, dissipate needless tension, and redirect your attention when you do have a mental lapse. Let's get more specific.

Accentuate the Positive

The key to success in anything is to *rehearse success rather than rehearse failure.* All athletes must contend with negative thinking. It can be caused by previous negative experiences, the negative thoughts of others or your own self-doubts.

A friend of mine, Dan, played basketball for a U.S. Navy team. In one game, Dan was at the foul line with only a few seconds left to play. His team trailed by a point. If he made the two free throws they would win. To increase pressure on Dan, the opposing coach called a time-out.

During the time-out, Dan started "rehearsing failure," thinking what a goat he'd be if he missed. Dan's coach saw the state he was in. "Look, Dan," he said, "You're the best free-throw shooter on the team. There's no one I'd rather have shooting. Make the shots, be a hero and let's go home." The coach successfully redirected Dan's negative energy into a positive pattern and Dan made both shots.

Here's a simple way to practice accentuating the positive: Keep your workouts upbeat. Positive thinking is not only for competitions. Work on positive thoughts the same way you work on your body. All the time.

Think positive thoughts in practice. "The world looks good. I'm glad I'm training today. I feel great." Avoid thoughts like, "Things keep piling up around me." Or, "I'll never get things done properly." Remember that your training session is probably the only time you'll have all day that's just for you. You want it to be as pleasant, positive and productive as possible.

The Athletes' Guide to Sports Psychology (Leisure Press, 1984) deals with "mental skills for physical people." It has a long list of negative thoughts and their positive counterparts. Here are a few:

Negative Thoughts	Change to Positive Thoughts
I can't.	I can do it. I have done it many times before.
I am tired, I can't go on.	It is almost over, I know I can finish. The difficult part has passed.
I am getting worse instead of better.	I need to set daily goals and evaluate my progress on a regular basis.
The heat is so bad I cannot do anything.	The heat creates a greater challenge.
I am really nervous and anxious.	The last time I felt this way I performed my best.
I am afraid that I will make a fool of myself.	Unless I face the challenge and take the risk, I'll never know what I can accomplish.
I don't want to fail.	What is absolutely the worst thing that could happen to me? I could lose. If so, I will work harder to try to prevent that.

I don't think I am prepared.........	I have practiced and trained hard for this performance so I am prepared to do well.
I lost again. I'll never be a winner....	I can learn from losing. I need to talk with a coach to get some help regarding those things I need to improve.
It is not fair. I work just as hard as _____ but I don't do as well........	I may have to work harder than some to accomplish the same level. I am willing to work as hard as I have to because I want to succeed.
I never seem to be able to do this.....	This time I am going to think through and mentally prepare so that I can do it.

Concentration

In July, 1985, John Howard set the world land speed record for bicycles of 152 mph (drafting behind a race car). "I was very absorbed," said Howard. "My main concentration was on what was on the road in front. A helicopter was 10 feet above me, and I have no recollection of it. An atomic bomb could have exploded 1000 yards away and I wouldn't have known."*

Top performance occurs when you *focus* on a goal, ignoring the distractions on the sidelines. You narrow the band of attention to the task at hand: hitting the pitch, catching the pass, or lifting the weight. It's like tuning in a radio station; you want to eliminate the static.

Note: You don't need to concentrate intensely *all* the time. You can burn out mentally just as you can physically. A runner does not concentrate on form every time he trains. Sometimes he just runs for the joy of it. Likewise in lifting, you don't need to use visualization for each rep of each set. Save it for the last few reps of your key exercises. To maintain the power of intense concentration, you must do it at selected times, not every time you work out. Once you develop the knack, you save it for those special times. When you need it, it will be there.

Imagery

Imagery or visualization is the technique that helped Charlie Garfield lift 365 pounds. It's used by many athletes today and can help you achieve your goals.

I used my own version of imagery in 1971 when preparing for the Mr. Universe contest. I knew that Arnold Schwarzenegger would be my main competition, so I got the best possible photos of Arnold and taped them to my bathroom mirror. As I shaved each morning, here was Arnold in peak condition looking at me. Nose to nose with him, I'd tell myself, "I'm going to beat this guy."

I carried these thoughts with me everywhere. At meals, I'd tell myself that the food I ate was making me stronger, leaner, less prone to injury. And that it would help me beat Arnold. When I went to sleep, I'd concentrate on the sleep making me a stronger, better person and athlete. And that this deep relaxing sleep would help me beat Arnold.

In the end, Arnold withdrew from the competition. But I was ready and won the title.

*Esquire, May 1986

Herschel Walker, the great running back, uses visualization in his training and in a 1982 interview in *Sports Illustrated* with Terry Todd, talked about the importance of mental imagery: "My mind's like a general and my body's like an Army. I keep the body in shape and it does what I tell it to do. I sometimes even feel myself almost lifting up out of my body and looking down on myself while I run sprints. I'll be coaching myself from up above. 'Come on, Herschel . . . pick up those knees. Pump your arms!'"

And more recently, Bruce Morris of Marshall University in Hungtington, West Virginia, made the longest field goal in college basketball history—89'-10". Morris said, "All I could see was the rim, the basket, and the backboard. It seemed real close . . . it didn't seem that far away when I did it."* □

Esquire, May, 1986

SPORTS TRAINING PROGRAMS

SPORTS TRAINING PROGRAMS

The following 91 pages contain strength training programs for 21 different sports plus a program for the all-around athlete. Our advisors in developing these routines are 24 of the best coaches, trainers and athletes in the country.

We have analyzed the demands of each sport and selected exercises aimed at increasing strength, improving performance and preventing injuries. The workloads (sets and repetitions) have been geared to the requirements of each sport and to the different seasons where applicable (off-season, pre-season, in-season). The poundages used will vary according to the individual athlete (see "How much weight?" below). The exercises in the programs are shown with small drawings for quick and easy reference in the gym.

Note: Weight training is not an exact science. Although certain techniques and principles have been tested and analyzed in recent years, no two trainers agree on *all* aspects of any training program. These programs are not the *only* way to train for each sport. But they are sound and they will work. They are adaptable to all ages, for both sexes, and for athletes of varying abilities from high school to professional caliber.

General Instructions for Programs

- *Principles and techniques:* Read "Getting Started," pp. 14-17 and "How to Lift," pp. 18-19.

- *Instructions:* If you do not already know how to perform an exercise properly, use the page number listed under each exercise to look up the instructions.
  Not for beginners: Before starting any of these sports programs you should first have trained with one or more of the "General Conditioning" programs (pp. 20-25) or the "Beginning Bodybuilding" programs (pp. 35-37) for at least three months. *Or* have achieved a comparable level of fitness by other means. Also, consult with your coach or trainer, if you have one.

- *How much weight?:* We do not show poundages because everyone differs in strength. Choose poundages so you can complete all the reps in all the sets indicated. The last rep should be fairly difficult but possible.
  Experiment with poundages. Don't make it so easy on yourself you don't get a training effect. Don't make it so hard on yourself you burn out or get injured.

- *When to increase weights?:* Once you are doing all the reps easily, increase weight so last rep is again difficult.

- *Change things around:* Variety is the spice of continued interest in training. If you get bored, change to different exercises that work the same body parts. If there is any pain, switch to exercises that work the same body part, but with no pain.

- *Order of exercises:* Follow the order indicated.

- *Optionals:* Include these to strengthen weaknesses or for a longer training session. Do in order indicated, between regular exercises.

- *Home gym:* You can do all these programs at home with a simple set of free weights. When an exercise using a machine is shown, substitute a free weight exercise that works the same body part. For example, you could do a barbell squat instead of a leg press on a Universal machine, etc.

All-Around Athlete—Gary T. Moran, Ph.D., Human Anatomy and Kinesiology; triathlete . . . . p. 84

Aerobic Dance—Robin Pound, M.S., Pac-10 Strength and Conditioning Coach . . . . p. 86

Baseball—Barry Weinberg, Head Trainer, Oakland A's . . . . p. 88

Basketball—Kermit Washington, National Basketball Association All-Star 1980-1981; Fitness Consultant, Stanford University . . . . p. 92

Boxing—Roosevelt Sanders, Assistant Olympic Boxing Coach, 1984 . . . . p. 97

Cycling—John Howard, World Speed Record Holder (bicycle)—152.284mph; 7-time U.S. National Cycling Champion, 3-time Olympian . . . . p. 100

Football—Bill Starr, former Strength Coach—Baltimore Colts, Houston Oilers, University of Maryland, University of Hawaii; Author of *The Strongest Shall Survive* . . . . p. 104

Golf—Gary Wiren, Ph.D., one of only 25 master professionals in the U.S.; Master Teacher at the Boca Raton Hotel and Club . . . . p. 112

Gymnastics—Don Peters, Coach, 1984 Women's Olympic Gymnastics Team (gold medalists) . . . . p. 116

Ice Hockey—Bob Bourne, Left Wing, New York Islanders (Stanley Cup Champions, 1980-1983) . . . . p. 120

Powerlifting—Jan Todd, Member of the International Powerlifting Hall of Fame; Women's World Record Holder—Squat (545½ pounds); Head Coach, Longhorn Powerlifting Team, University of Texas at Austin . . . . p. 124

Rowing—Robin Pound, M.S. . . . . p. 130

Running—Gary T. Moran, Ph.D. . . . . p. 134

Skiing (Cross-Country)—Steven Gaskill, Nordic Technical Director, U.S. Ski Team; Peter Ashley, Head Women's Coach, U.S. Ski Team; Torbjorn Karlsen, Assistant Women's Coach, U.S. Ski Team . . . . p. 138

Skiing (Downhill)—John McMurtry, Head Technical Coach, U.S. Olympic Women's Alpine Skiing Team; John Atkins, Head Conditioning Coach, U.S. Olympic Women's Alpine Skiing Team; Topper Hagerman, Ph.D., Head Conditioning Trainer, U.S. Olympic Men's Alpine Skiing Team . . . . p. 142

Soccer—Horst Richardson, Head Coach, Colorado College, 2-time Far West Coach of the Year . . . . p. 146

Swimming—Doc Counsilman, Ph.D., Head Coach, Indiana University—6 NCAA titles, 23 Big Ten Conference titles; Head Coach, U.S. Olympic Men's Swim Team 1964, 1976 . . . . p. 149

Tennis—Bill Wright, Head Coach, University of Arizona, NCAA Coach of the Year, 1978 . . . . p. 153

Track and Field—Sam Adams, Head Coach, University of California at Santa Barbara; Coach, U.S. Olympic Decathletes, 1984 . . . . p. 156

Triathlon—Gary T. Moran, Ph.D. . . . . p. 165

Volleyball—Doug Beal, Ph.D., Coach, Men's Olympic Volleyball Team, 1984 (gold medalists); National Team Director, U.S. Volleyball Association . . . . p. 169

Wrestling—Joe Seay, Head Coach, Oklahoma State University; Coach, U.S. World Team, 1985; Jerry Palmieri, Head Assistant Strength and Conditioning Coach, Oklahoma State University . . . . p. 172

ALL-AROUND ATHLETE

By Gary T. Moran, Ph.D., Human Anatomy and Kinesiology; M.S., Exercise Physiology; Runner and Triathlete.

Most athletes participate in more than one sport. A high school athlete may play football, basketball and baseball and/or track. A white-collar worker may run, play racquetball and lift weights. An all-around athlete is one who is prepared to meet the demands of any physical activity.

The All-Around Athlete program is an extension of the General Conditioning Programs on pp. 20-25. It is for anyone who wants to advance beyond the earlier programs, but is not primarily interested in either bodybuilding or one particular competitive sport.

This is a full-body program, designed to exercise all the muscles and to develop both strength and muscular endurance. As a complement to this program, you should stretch and participate in aerobic training (swimming, running, aerobics classes), at least 3 days per week on non-weight training days and continue with your sport-specific training, i.e. technique, agility, etc.

For greater concentration on a specific sport, refer to the program for that sport.

Aims: Overall body strength.

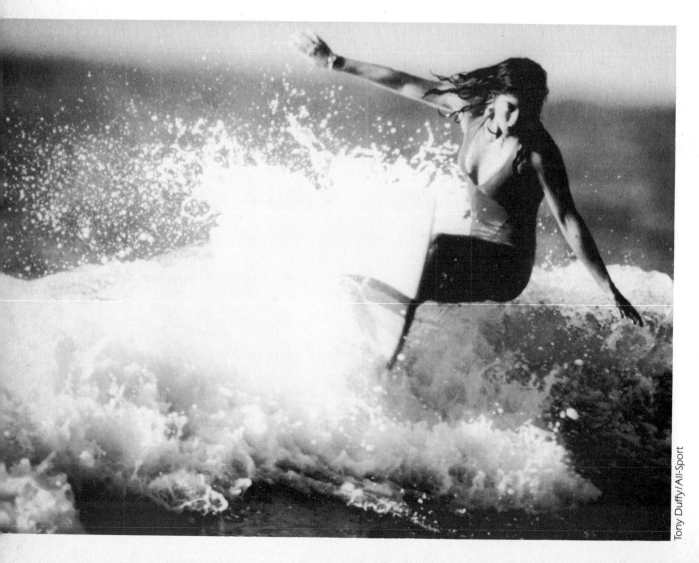

Tony Duffy/All-Sport

All-Around Athlete Program

Do the optional exercises that are most required by the sports you participate in or that strengthen weaknesses.

Days per week: 3, with 1 day rest between workouts.

Split routine: As an option, do exercises 1-7, M-W-F; exercises 8-12, T-Th-Sa.

Additional exercises: See "Track and Field," pp. 156-64.

exercises	sets	reps	exercises	sets	reps
1 *p.190 top*	2-3	15 to 40 per set	**7** *p.220 bottom*	3	10-10-8
2 *p.244 top*	3-5	12-10 (10) -8 (8)	**8** *p.284 bottom*	3	12-10-10
3 *p.205 top*	3-5	12-10 (10) -8 (8)	**Optional** *p.297 bottom*	2	10-10
4 *p.273 bottom*	3	12-10-8	**9** *p.293 middle*	3	12-10-8
5 *p.202 middle*	3	12-10-8	**10** *p.292 bottom*	3	12-10-8
Optional *p.277 middle*	2	10-10	**11** *p.290 middle*	2	10-10
Optional *p.253 bottom*	2	10-10	**Optional** *p.239 top*	2	10-10
6 *p.306 middle*	3	10-10-8	**12** *p.194 middle*	1-2	15 to 30 per set

GETTING STRONGER ©1986 Bill Pearl & Shelter Publications, Inc.

AEROBIC DANCE

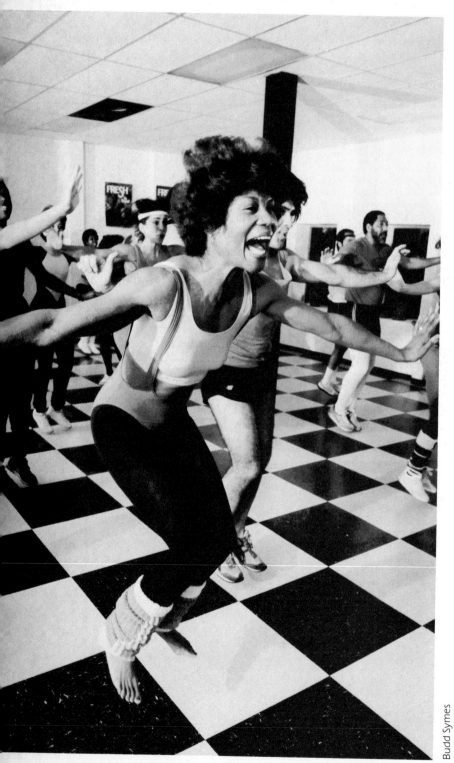

Budd Symes

By Robin Pound, M.S., Exercise Physiology and Anatomy; PAC–10 Strength and Conditioning Coach.

Aerobic dance is one of the best exercises for cardiovascular fitness. The aerobic dance weight training program is designed to increase strength and maintain balance in the major muscle groups. This allows you to perform the exercises with greater ease and less chance of injury. A year-round flexibility program should also be followed to reduce risk of injury.

Aims: A combination of strength and endurance, with an emphasis on strength. To emphasize endurance more than strength, use lighter weights and raise the number of repetitions per set.

Aerobic Dance Year-Round Program

There is only one program for aerobic dance because it is a year-round activity.

Days per week: 2, with at least 1 day rest and not more than 3 days rest between workouts.

Supersets: Do the first set of exercise 1(a), then immediately do the first set of exercise 1(b). Rest 1-2 minutes, then go on to second sets of 1(a), 1(b). Follow this format for the prescribed number of sets and reps.

exercises	sets	reps	exercises	sets	reps
1 (a) p.244 top	3	12-10-8	**5** (a) p.298 bottom	3	12 to 15 per set
(b) p.214 top	3	12-10-8	(b) p.299 top	3	12 to 15 per set
2 (a) p.282 top	3	12-10-8	**6** (a) p.190 middle	4	20 to 30 per set
(b) p.275 bottom	3	12-10-8	(b) p.216 middle	4	Max. 15 per set, then add weight
3 (a) p.225 middle	3	12-10-8			
(b) p.300 bottom	3	12-10-8 each arm			
4 (a) p.294 bottom	3	12-10-8			
(b) p.292 bottom	3	12-10-8			

Additional exercises:
1. Dumbbells may be substituted
2. Machines may be substituted
3. Chins
4. Good mornings
5. Lunges
6. Step-ups
7. Rotary torso work
8. Shoulder raises and flys
9. Bar dips

Exercise options
1. Circuit training instead of supersets
2. Strength training 3x/week instead of 2
3. Adjust workout for desired goals:
   - more weight, fewer reps = more strength
   - less weight, more reps = more muscular endurance

Problem areas
1. Use a year-round flexibility program as a complement to weight training.
2. Good shoes, a cushioned surface and close attention to joint soreness (knees, ankles, hips, etc.) can minimize aerobic dance injuries resulting from excessive impact.
3. Be careful of ballistic (jerking) exercise actions; do not go beyond the normal range of motion.
4. Carefully monitor your heart rate; stay within target zone. Work out at your own pace.
5. Be aware of lower back pain.
6. Modify movements to your own body's level of fitness and flexibility.□

BASEBALL

Steven E. Sutton/duomo

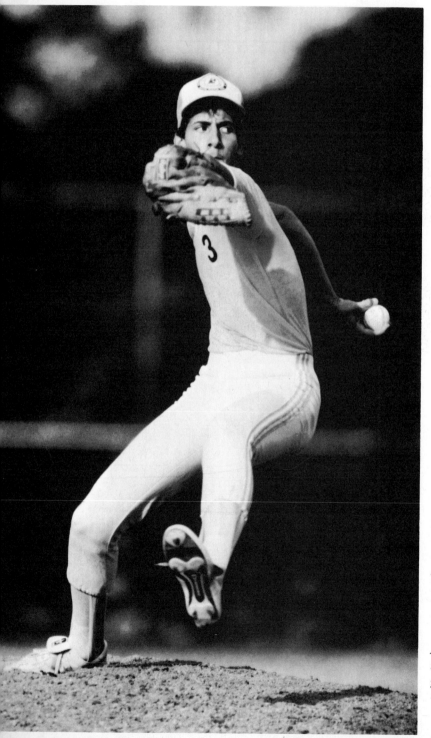

By Barry Weinberg, *Head Trainer,*
Oakland A's.

We use weight training for injury prevention, rehabilitation of injuries and for
strengthening individual weaknesses. We
try to isolate certain muscles specific to
the throwing motion and strengthen them
to prevent arm injuries.

A combination of various forms of
exercises works best: isometrics, isotonic
and isokinetic, plyometrics, active resis-
tive, and especially flexibility/stretching
exercises are all important in developing
a well-balanced program.

Players at different positions need
to emphasize different elements of the
program, and different body parts.

Pitchers: Cardiovascular endurance, lower
body leg strength and endurance. General
flexibility, strength and endurance emphasizing shoulders and elbows.

Catchers: Emphasize leg strength and
flexibility, agility. Hand and wrist
strength, abdominal strength.

Infielders and outfielders: Leg flexibility, general flexibility. Hand and wrist
strength, upper body strength and
endurance.

In addition to the exercises listed in
the programs, I recommend exercises that
emphasize the rotator cuff complex, consisting of internal and external shoulder
rotation—front, rear and side elevation
and a mid-range elevation isolating the
supraspinatus. Especially effective are
lightweight shoulder exercises stimulating
the small muscles (rotator cuff) essential
to the throwing motion.

Aims: Strengthen all major muscle groups
and achieve proper balance among the
groups.

Baseball Off-Season Program

This program is designed to strengthen and balance all major muscle groups of the body. Consult your coach or trainer about varying the exercises in the program to strengthen your particular weaknesses and/or correct muscle imbalance.

Days per week: 3, with 1 day rest between workouts.

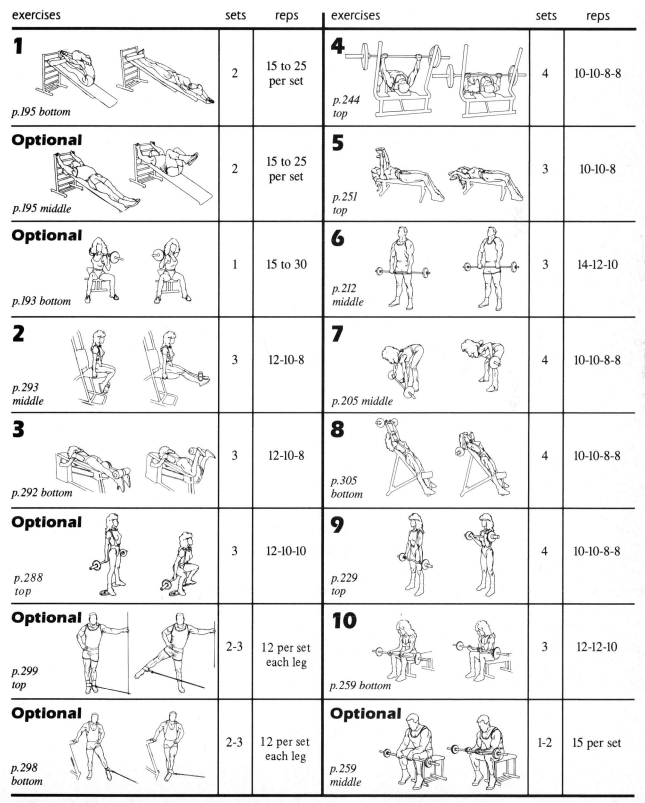

exercises	sets	reps	exercises	sets	reps
1 p.195 bottom	2	15 to 25 per set	**4** p.244 top	4	10-10-8-8
Optional p.195 middle	2	15 to 25 per set	**5** p.251 top	3	10-10-8
Optional p.193 bottom	1	15 to 30	**6** p.212 middle	3	14-12-10
2 p.293 middle	3	12-10-8	**7** p.205 middle	4	10-10-8-8
3 p.292 bottom	3	12-10-8	**8** p.305 bottom	4	10-10-8-8
Optional p.288 top	3	12-10-10	**9** p.229 top	4	10-10-8-8
Optional p.299 top	2-3	12 per set each leg	**10** p.259 bottom	3	12-12-10
Optional p.298 bottom	2-3	12 per set each leg	**Optional** p.259 middle	1-2	15 per set

GETTING STRONGER ©1986 Bill Pearl & Shelter Publications, Inc.

Baseball Pre-Season Program

This program is designed to build more strength. Start this program 4-6 weeks before the season. This is also the time to start incorporating baseball-specific exercises in the gym or out on the field. Get your body ready for baseball skills again.

Days per week: 3, with 1 day rest between workouts.

exercises	sets	reps	exercises	sets	reps
1 p.190 top	2	20 to 50 per set	**4** p.214 top	4	12-10-8-6
Optional p.201 bottom	2	20 to 50 per set each leg	**5** p.273 bottom	4	12-10-8-6
Optional p.193 bottom	1	30	**6** p.216 middle	2	Max. 15 per set, then add weight
2 p.284 top	4	12-10-8-6	**7** p.306 middle	4	12-10-8-6
Optional p.293 middle	2	15-15	**Optional** p.253 bottom	2	Max. 12 per set, then add weight
Optional p.292 bottom	2	15-15	**8** p.218 middle	4	12-10-8-6
Optional p.290 middle	2	10-8	**Optional** p.258 bottom	2-3	12-10 (8) each wrist
3 p.248 top	4	12-10-8-6	**Optional** p.259 top	2-3	12-10 (8) each wrist

Baseball In-Season Program

This program is designed to maintain strength levels acquired during the off- and pre-season programs. Abdominal, rotational and light weight work are essential parts of any in-season program. Pitchers should concentrate on light weight shoulder work (see various deltoid raises in "Shoulders" section).

Days per week: 2, with 1-2 days rest between workouts.

exercises		sets	reps	exercises		sets	reps
1 p.190 middle		1	20 to 50	**Optional** p.277 middle		2	10-10
Optional p.192 middle		1	15 to 20	**4** p.202 middle		2	10-8
2 p.296 bottom		2	10-8	**5** p.258 bottom		2	12-10 each wrist
Optional p.297 bottom		1-2	10 to 15 per set each leg	**6** p.259 top		2	12-10 each wrist
3 Light p.245 top		2	10-8	**Optional** p.263 top		1-2	Raise to top

Additional exercises:

1. Machines may be substituted
2. Dumbbells may be substituted
3. Step-ups with weights
4. Lunges with weights
5. Rotary torso work
6. Dead lift
7. Power cleans or high pulls
8. See "Forearms" pages for different wrist curl exercises
9. Seated dumbbell triceps curl
10. Standing one-arm triceps curl
11. Good mornings
12. Dumbbell rotator cuff work: dumbbell raises (posterior, anterior, medial), internal or external rotation

Exercise options:

1. Circuit training in the weight room
2. "On the field" conditioning circuit: sprints, agility, etc.
3. Plyometric exercises: upper or lower body
4. Weighted bats or fan bats

Problem areas:

1. A year-round stretching program to improve flexibility
2. Rotator cuff: see 4 or 5, above
3. Pay special attention to position, extra specific conditioning:
   - Rotator cuff work
   - Torso rotational strength work
   - Shoulder and arm flexibility, strength and endurance □

GETTING STRONGER ©1986 Bill Pearl & Shelter Publications, Inc.

BASKETBALL

By Kermit Washington, *Fitness Consultant at Stanford University, National Basketball Association All Star, 1980-81. First-Team Collegiate All-American, 1973.*

When most things are equal between two athletes, the stronger athlete will win out. Weight training is effective for gaining weight, strength, muscular endurance and stamina. It can also be used for injury rehabilitation and prevention. Personally, I credit weight training for relieving tendinitis in my knees, and prolonging my career by five years. More than anything though, weight training is a great way to gain confidence.

I started lifting when I entered college. I was 6'8" and weighed 160 pounds—too light to be an effective player. I needed weight for strength, endurance and stamina, but for confidence more than anything—because if I believed I could do something, I could do it. When I looked in the mirror after six months of lifting and saw a strong body, I felt like a strong person.

Basketball players first need ability performing basic basketball skills. Once those skills are acquired, players need the strength and power of a football player and the muscular endurance of a distance runner.

Since basketball players must have explosiveness and must *not* have aching joints, the athlete does not need to use heavy weights. Cutting back the time between sets is more important than increasing weight. Moderation is an important practice. I feel that if I had learned moderation at an earlier age, my career would have lasted more than nine seasons.

A solid flexibility program is also essential for minimizing the chance of injury.

Aims: Strengthen all major muscle groups and maintain muscle balance.

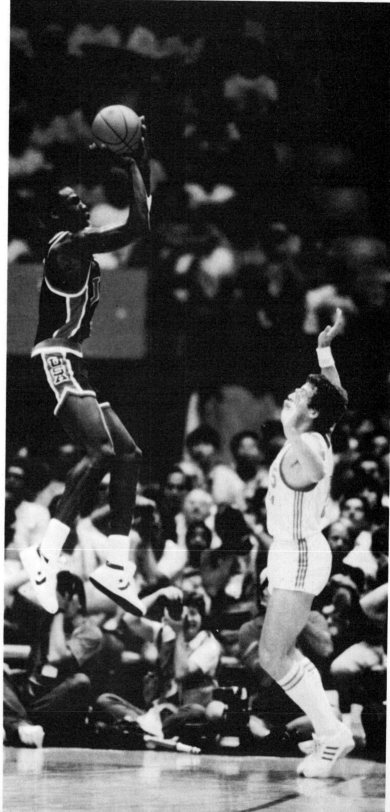

Dan Helms/duomo

Basketball Off-Season Program

This program is designed to strengthen the entire body, create body strength and balance, and correct weaknesses. The program will last 4-6 weeks and is designed to create a good base from which to establish a strength-building cycle that extends into the pre-season program. Consult your coach or trainer about varying the exercises to strengthen your particular weaknesses or correct muscle imbalance.

Days per week: 3, with 1 day rest between workouts.

exercises	sets	reps	exercises	sets	reps
1 p.244 top	4	12-10-10-8	**9** p.293 middle	3	10-10-8
2 p.205 top	4	12-10-10-8	**10** p.292 bottom	3	10-10-8
3 p.278 top	3	10-10-8	**11** p.238 top	2	15 to 25 per set
4 p.202 middle	3	10-10-8	**12** p.216 middle	2	Max. 15 per set, then add weight
5 p.249 bottom	3	10-10-8	**13** p.190 top	2	25 to 50 per set
6 p.218 bottom	3	10-10-8			
7 p.284 top	4	12-10-10-8			
8 p.289 middle	2	10-10 each leg			

GETTING STRONGER ©1986 Bill Pearl & Shelter Publications, Inc.

Basketball Pre-Season Program

This program lasts 6-8 weeks, or from the start of school in the fall to the beginning of the game schedule. It is designed to maximize strength gains. All strength work will be done with explosiveness in mind. At this time, players should also be involved in a general conditioning program with basketball-specific drills to prepare the athlete for practice and games.

Days per week: 3, with 1 day rest between workouts.

exercises	sets	reps	exercises	sets	reps
1 p.250 top	3	10-10-8	**8** p.284 bottom	3	10-10-8
2 p.204 middle	3	10-10-8 each arm	**Optional** p.297 bottom	2	10-10 each leg
3 p.273 top	2	10-8 each arm	**9** p.293 middle	3	10-10-8
4 p.210 top	2	Max. 12 per set, then add weight	**10** p.292 bottom	3	10-10-8
5 p.207 middle	2	10-10	**Optional** p.243 bottom	2	15 to 25 per set
6 p.303 top	3	10-8-8	**11** p.192 middle	2	15 to 25 per set
7 p.219 bottom	3	10-8-8 each arm	**12** p.190 middle	2	25 to 50 per set
Optional p.195 top	1-2	25 to 50 per set			

GETTING STRONGER ©1986 Bill Pearl & Shelter Publications, Inc.

Basketball In-Season Program

This program is designed to maintain strength levels acquired during the off-and pre-season programs.

Days per week: 2, with 1-2 days rest between workouts. Rest 2 days before games.

exercises		sets	reps	exercises		sets	reps
1 p.249 top		2	10-10	**Optional** p.293 middle		2	10-10
2 p.214 bottom		2	10-10	**Optional** p.292 bottom		2	10-10
3 p.277 middle		1	10	**Optional** p.216 middle		1	Max. 15, then add weight
4 p.253 bottom		1	Max. 15, then add weight	**8** p.194 middle		2	10 to 20 per set
5 p.306 middle		2	10-8	**Optional** p.193 bottom		1	30 to 40 per set each side
6 p.229 top		2	10-8				
7 p.296 bottom		2	10-10				
Optional p.289 middle		2	10-10 each leg				

GETTING STRONGER ©1986 Bill Pearl & Shelter Publications, Inc.

Additional exercises:

1. Dumbbells may be used instead of barbells
2. Machines may be substituted
3. Barbell dead lifts
4. Chins instead of pull-downs
5. Dumbbell lat rows
6. Standing calf raises
7. Lunges with weights
8. Nautilus shoulder flys
9. Dumbbell flys
10. Rotary torso work

Exercise options:

1. Circuit training: in weight room or on-the-court with basketball
2. Plyometric exercises, box or depth jumping, jump touches
3. Stadiums or stairs (running)

Problem areas:

1. A year-round stretching program to improve flexibility
2. Strong quadriceps help prevent knee injuries
3. Shoot year-round to maintain touch □

BOXING

By Roosevelt Sanders, Jr. *Assistant Olympic Boxing Coach, 1984, Assistant to the Executive Director, USA Amateur Boxing Federation.*

A boxer's punch gets its power from:

- leg extension and push-off
- trunk rotation
- arm action

Boxers need total body strength and endurance with proper muscle balance. More specifically, boxers need:

- shoulder strength to hold gloves up, chest and back strength to throw powerful punches and pull them back quicker
- torso strength for trunk rotation and absorption of punches
- leg strength for power of push-off on a punch, and the establishment of a strong base

In strengthening the athlete's upper body I recommend exercises for the trapezius, biceps, deltoids, pectorals, triceps and *latissimus dorsi.*

All boxers need to be flexible and in outstanding general condition. I recommend aerobic training and interval running as valuable additions to any training program.

It's important to note that strength training with weights, while designed to add strength, flexibility and endurance, should *not* be used in place of learning the fundamentals of amateur boxing.

Aims: Strength and endurance with a focus on balancing all major muscle groups.

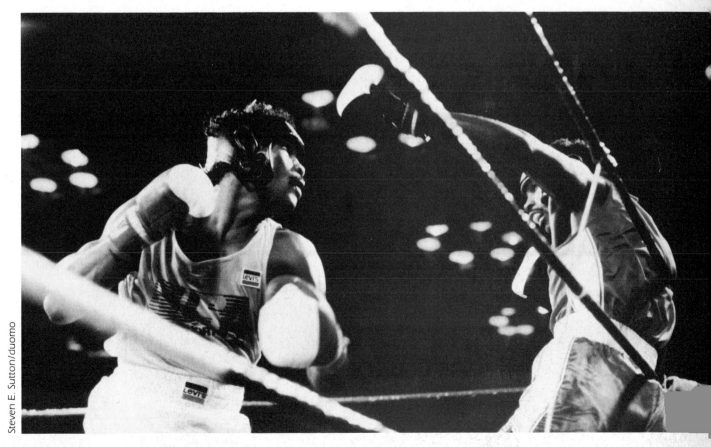

Steven E. Sutton/duomo

Boxing Year-Round Program

The program is done on an 8-12 week timetable. For more strength, do fewer repetitions and add more weight. For more muscular endurance, do more repetitions and use less weight. But remember that most of your endurance work will come in the ring.

Days per week: 3, with 1 day rest between workouts.

exercises	sets	reps	exercises	sets	reps
1 p.248 top	2-3	12-10 (8)	**Optional** p.291 top	1	15 to 30
2 p.202 top	2-3	12-10 (8)	**9** p.269 bottom	1	5 to 10
3 p.283 top	2-3	12-10 (8)	**Optional** p.259 bottom	2	15-15
4 p.214 top	2-3	12-10 (8)	**10** p.190 middle	1-2	15 to 30 per set
5 p.212 middle	2-3	12 per set	**Optional** p.196 middle	1-2	10 to 20 per set
6 p.244 top	2-3	12-10 (8)			
7 p.293 middle	2	15-15			
8 p.292 bottom	2	15-15			

Additional exercises

1. Lower back:
   - Weighted hyperextensions
   - Twisting hyperextensions
   - Good mornings
   - Stiff-legged dumbbell dead lifts
2. Rotary torso
3. Machines, barbells or dumbbells may be used
4. Lunges
5. Step-ups
6. Light dumbbell or hand weights for shadow boxing
7. Medicine ball torso work
8. Work neck in 4 directions
9. Abdominals and hip flexors
10. Dumbbell flys
11. Decline dumbbell flys
12. Standing dumbbell shoulder presses

Exercise options

1. Circuit strength training or circuit endurance training
2. Plyometrics for lower body; box and depth jumping, all jumps or bounds (with or without weights)
3. Conditioning:
   - High intensity — sprints, agility work
   - Distance work — running, swimming, aerobic dance, cycling

Problem areas

1. Year-round stretching for maximum flexibility.
2. Keep a close eye on joints — fingers, wrists, shoulders. Tape properly, don't overtrain, use proper technique.
3. This program will not slow you down: it will speed you up, and give you more power, strength and endurance.
4. Shoulders — This program will help you to hold hands up high longer.
5. Dead legs — This program will strengthen your legs for better support throughout a match, and help you to hold up under punishment or fatigue.
6. Mid-section — 5-7 days a week do:
   - Leg raises
   - Rotary sit-up or low back work
   - Crunches with and without fixed feet
7. Neck — 3-4 days a week do four-direction strengthening work. □

CYCLING

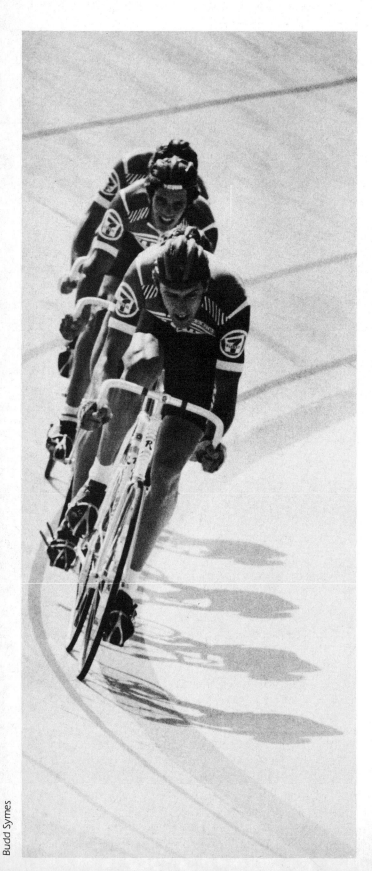

Budd Symes

By John Howard, 7-time U.S. National cycling champion, 3-time Olympian, Pan American Games gold medalist, Ironman Triathlon winner, 1981, 24-hour endurance record holder (514 mi.) and world cycle speed record holder (152.284 mph in 1985).

Weight training helps cyclists improve their muscular endurance and stamina. It is especially important to build strength in the quadriceps, hamstrings and lower back. A specific training program will depend upon what event you are training for:

• Speed or sprint training
• Endurance rides
• Combination of both

Sprint cyclists need a lot of sprint race training and explosive speed training to test the anaerobic threshold—the sort of stuff that hurts! They also need to balance other muscles with a general weight training program. Serious distance racers need to emphasize distance rides, for example one or two 3-4 hour rides a week. (Less serious riders can scale those figures back.)

The best way to improve your performance in cycling is to race as often as possible—every week if you can. Cardiovascular and muscular endurance training will be done on the bicycle to ensure maximum specificity of training. You should take both long overdistance training rides as well as shorter interval explosive sprint training. The amount and frequency of each type of training depends upon time of year, your event, upcoming races and your level of fitness.

Cycling is a great cardiovascular strength builder for all athletes. It is especially good for runners as it builds the very muscles that running neglects—the quadriceps.

Aims: Aims and goals vary according to the event you are training for, your personal strengths and weaknesses, and seasonal considerations. The programs shown here are for endurance cycling. If you are training for sprint racing, use more weight and do fewer reps. For example:

• Endurance: 14-12-10-8 reps
• Sprint: 8-6-4-2 reps

Cycling Off-Season Program

This will help develop strength and balance of major muscle groups, correct muscular imbalances, and emphasize thigh, leg, lower back and gluteal strength. The off-season program is more intensive than the in-season program.

Days per week: 3, with 1 day rest between workouts.

Supersets: Do the first set of exercise 1(a), then immediately do the first set of exercise 1(b). Rest 1-2 minutes, then go on to second sets of 1(a), 1(b). Follow this format for prescribed number of sets and reps.

exercises	sets	reps	exercises	sets	reps
1 (a) p.284 top	3	14-12-10	**4** (a) p.244 top	3	14-12-10
(b) p.293 middle	3	14-12-10	(b) p.203 top	3	14-12-10
(c) p.292 bottom	3	14-12-10	**5** (a) p.273 bottom	2	14-12
2 (a) p.299 top	2	14-12 each leg	(b) p.212 top	2	15-15
(b) p.298 bottom	2	14-12 each leg	**6** (a) p.225 middle	2	14-12
3 (a) p.238 top	1	10 to 15	(b) p.253 bottom	2	Max. 15 per set, then add weight
(b) p.237 bottom	1	20 to 25	**7** (a) p.216 middle	2	Max. 15 per set, then add weight
			(b) p.190 top	2	20 to 40 per set

Cycling In-Season Program

This is meant to maintain the strength gains of the off-season program.

Days per week: 2, with 1-2 days rest between workouts. Rest at least 2 days before competition.

Supersets: Do the first set of exercise 1(a), then immediately do the first set of exercise 1(b). Rest 1-2 minutes, then go on to second sets of 1(a), 1(b). Follow this format for prescribed number of sets and reps.

exercises	sets	reps	exercises	sets	reps
1 (a) p.296 bottom	2	14-12	**4** (a) p.248 bottom	2	14-12
(b) p.293 middle	2	14-12	(b) p.202 top	2	14-12
(c) p.292 bottom	2	14-12	**5** (a) p.273 middle	2	12-10 each arm
2 (a) p.299 top	1	14 each leg	(b) p.212 middle	2	15-15
(b) p.298 bottom	1	14 each leg	**6** (a) p.218 middle	1	12
3 (a) p.238 top	1	10 to 15	(b) p.253 bottom	1	Max. 12, then add weight
(b) p.238 bottom	1	20 to 25	**7** (a) p.216 middle	1-2	Max. 15 per set, then add weight
			(b) p.197 top	1-2	20 to 30 per set

Additional Exercises

1. Use dumbbells instead of barbells
2. Step-ups with weights
3. Lunges with weights
4. Seated lat rowing
5. Leg press
6. Chins instead of lat pull-downs
7. Upright rowing
8. Dumbbell dead lifts
9. Neck exercises
10. Rotary torso work
11. Wrist exercises

Exercise Options

1. Stretching (year-round)
2. Extra abdominal and lower back work year-round
3. Depth jumping
4. Box jumping
5. Running and jumping stadium steps
6. Circuit training
7. For variety use other exercises for same muscle groups one workout a week.

Problem Areas

1. Wrists and grip position
2. Neck fatigue
3. Lower back fatigue
4. Shoulder soreness and fatigue
5. Knees—may need to work on medial quads □

FOOTBALL

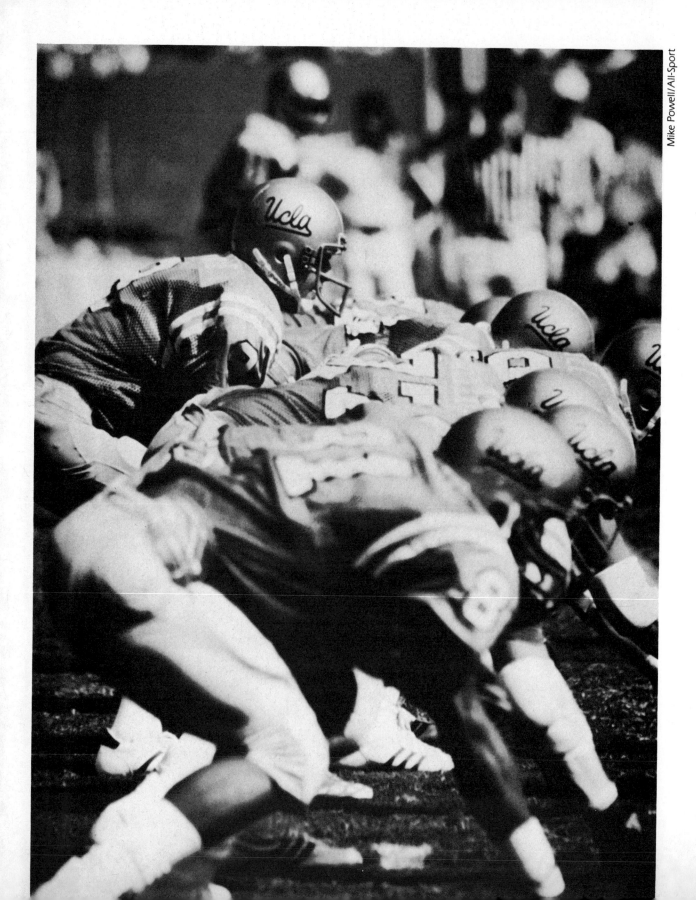

By Bill Starr, *former Strength Coach, Baltimore Colts, Houston Oilers, University of Hawaii, University of Maryland; Author,* The Strongest Shall Survive: Strength Training for Football *and* Defying Gravity.

My athletes participate in a weight training program primarily for strength. I feel that a stronger athlete is a better athlete, so my programs attempt to increase the total strength level of the entire body. I put most emphasis on certain major muscle groups: shoulder girdle, back, hips and legs. Yet *no* body parts are neglected. For example, hands and forearms are worked indirectly through the bench press (a "chest" exercise), by gripping the bar. Abdominals are worked during the warm-up and cool-down. You can use a solid strength base to increase endurance and to a lesser degree, flexibility and coordination.

There are different physical requirements for different positions, for example, defensive linemen and quarterbacks. But in terms of a strength program, I do not treat them differently. I start everyone with "The **Big Three**": power clean, squat and bench press. These movements incorporate the major muscle groups and are the basic exercises for all future and more advanced programs. A 250-pound lineman is going to be handling more weight than a 185-pound quarterback, so the concept of relativity is built in. Once the three primary exercises have been learned correctly, I slowly add other exercises.

The only times I give specific exercises to an athlete are:
• when the player has been injured and needs rehabilitation
• when a player has an obvious weakness in a specific area, and needs to increase strength at a faster pace in one particular body part.

I recommend a full session of stretching both before and after a weight session—and between sets if possible. When stretching, pay great attention to the leg biceps and shoulders.

I also recommend an aerobic program of running, biking or aerobics classes three times a week. Each aerobics day has a different emphasis:
• Tuesday: a short 20-minute fast run
• Thursday: a 40-minute run
• Saturday: one hour of aerobics

This puts an entirely different stress on the body each aerobics day.

Aims: To strengthen all the major muscle groups and to develop muscle balance.

Football Off-Season Program

This program is designed to build maximum strength and flexibility in all the major muscle groups. Begin off-season training right at the end of the football season, and continue until spring practice. And again, after spring ball up until summer practice and the actual season begins. Regardless of your weight training background, begin each new weight training season with "The Big Three" to ensure that all body parts receive equal emphasis.

Perform the exercises 3 times per week for the first six weeks, and use the heavy, light and medium system. The heavy day each week is test day. The light day (70% of max) is a form day—the day you should concentrate on honing your skill in each movement. This attention to form assists you in making faster gains. The medium day (85% of max) sets you up for the next heavy day. Light, medium and heavy refer to the total poundages for each day. They *do not* refer to the amount of effort you put forth. Always give 100% effort, and follow the prescribed order of exercises.

Before each session, do 10-15 minutes of stretching exercises and abdominal movements for the upper, lower and sides of the midsection. This helps eliminate the chance of injury. Your body will respond more favorably when warmed-up properly.

In addition to "The Big Three" and the abdominal movements, perform 2 sets of leg extensions and 2 sets of leg curls in supersets fashion, i.e., one following the other with no rest between sets. This additional high rep work is a preventive measure for the knees.

Wrap up the workout with another 10-15 minutes of stretching, emphasizing the shoulder girdle and hamstrings.

Circuit Training: For the first couple of weeks on "The Big Three", work the three lifts in a circuit. This ensures that all major body parts are being worked equally. In other words, do a set of power cleans, then a set of bench presses, followed by a set of squats until all sets are performed. After a few weeks, begin doing all the sets of a single exercise in order before moving on to the next.

Monday (Heavy Day)

		sets	reps
p.207 bottom		5	5 per set
p.244 top		5	5 per set
p.284 top		5	5 per set

The heavy day sets the pace for the week. The rest of the week is based on the accomplishments of the heavy day. Increase the power clean and bench by 5 pounds each week, and the squat by 10. Do not increase the poundages unless you have successfully completed the prescribed number of reps the previous week.

Football Off-Season Program

Wednesday (Light Day)

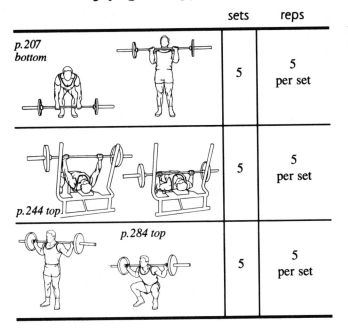

	sets	reps
p.207 bottom	5	5 per set
p.244 top	5	5 per set
p.284 top	5	5 per set

Use the weight of the third set of the heavy day as the top-end weight for the light day.

Friday (Medium Day)

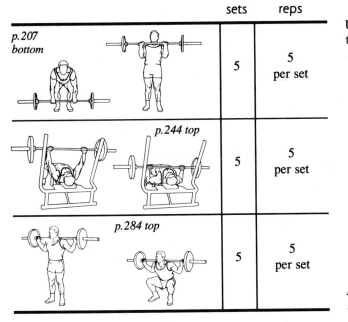

	sets	reps
p.207 bottom	5	5 per set
p.244 top	5	5 per set
p.284 top	5	5 per set

Use the weight of the fourth set of the heavy day as the top-end weight for the medium day.

Note: The exercises, sets and reps are the same on all three days, but the poundages vary.

Football Advanced Off-Season Program

Use this program until just before spring or summer practice. Then to get completely rested before the first day of practice, take a 3-4 day break that includes stretching, mental preparation, agility drills and sharpening of running stride. Stay on this program for 6 weeks, then add one more day of workouts and add exercises to increase the workload progressively. Follow this order of exercises. Use the same formula for choosing poundages as in the regular off-season. *Note:* Start light and increase poundages each set. In addition, stretch, do abdominal exercises, leg extensions and leg biceps each day.

exercises	sets	reps	exercises	sets	reps
Monday (Heavy Day)			**Wednesday (Light Day)**		
p.207 bottom	6	5-5-5-3-3-3	p.284 top	5	5-5-5-5-5
p.244 top	9	5-5-5-2-2-2-5-5-5	p.191 top	4	8-8-8-8
p.284 top	6	5-5-5-5-5-5	p.218 bottom	5	5-5-5-5-5
p.218 bottom	2	20-20 w/heavy weights	p.306 middle	2	20-20 w/heavy weights
Tuesday (Light Day)			**Friday (Medium Day)**		
p.207 bottom	5	5-5-5-5-5	p.284 top	6	5-5-5-3-3-3
p.279 bottom	6	5-5-5-5-5-5	p.212 middle	5	5-5-5-5-5
p.310 middle	3 / 3	5-5-5 / 3-3-3 w/weights	p.244 top	5	8-8-8-8-8
p.242 top (Change foot position ea. set: straight, inward, outward.)	3	30-30-30	p.244 bottom	2	8-8

GETTING STRONGER ©1986 Bill Pearl & Shelter Publications, Inc.

Football In-Season Program Week One

During two-a-days, lay off all weight work. Focus all your mental and physical energies on football, and football alone.

But as soon as a normal practice schedule begins, return to the weight room so that you can retain the strength you developed during the off-season.

Regardless of your strength level, work back into your weight program gradually. Football practice and games greatly increase physical and mental stress. So even if you were training at the most advanced level, work back into weight training.

Reorient yourself by once again using "The Big Three" as your basic foundation. It's beneficial to begin the in-season program by performing just one exercise per day during the first week back. Then increase steadily until you have achieved your off-season workload.

Note: Start light and increase your poundages each set.

Your top-end weight should be what you used on the "light" day during the off-season.

Each day, in addition to the one exercise, do 2 sets of 20 leg extensions and leg curls in supersets fashion. This helps protect the knees.

Remember to begin each session with stretching and abdominal exercises.

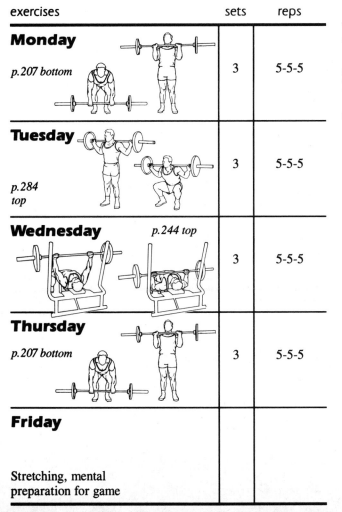

exercises	sets	reps
Monday p.207 bottom	3	5-5-5
Tuesday p.284 top	3	5-5-5
Wednesday p.244 top	3	5-5-5
Thursday p.207 bottom	3	5-5-5
Friday Stretching, mental preparation for game		

Football In-Season Program Week Two

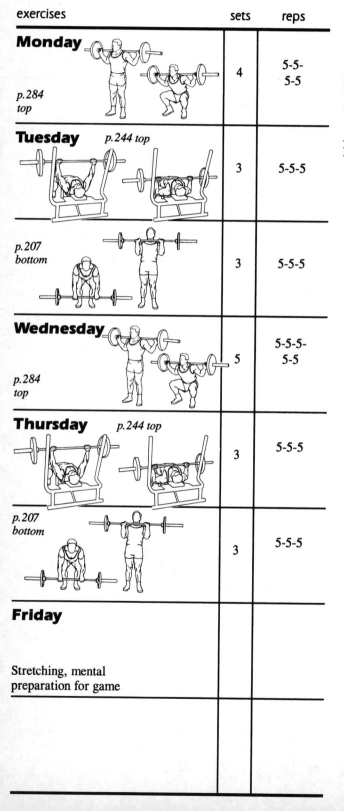

exercises	sets	reps
Monday p.284 top	4	5-5-5-5
Tuesday p.244 top	3	5-5-5
p.207 bottom	3	5-5-5
Wednesday p.284 top	5	5-5-5-5-5
Thursday p.244 top	3	5-5-5
p.207 bottom	3	5-5-5
Friday Stretching, mental preparation for game		

You may choose to stay with the Week One schedule for 2-3 weeks. That's O.K. It's better to move more slowly than too rapidly. As the season progresses, you will be adding more sets and more exercises. Within 2 months, you will be handling the same workload as during the off-season.

Remember: Stretch, do abdominals, leg extensions, leg curls every day.

Football In-Season Program Week Three

exercises	sets	reps
Monday 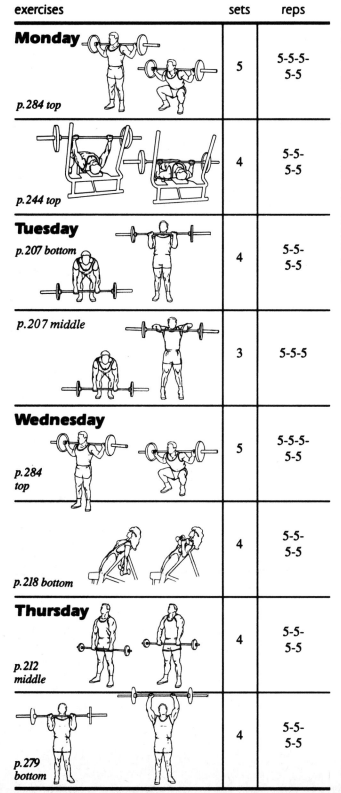 *p.284 top*	5	5-5-5-5-5
p.244 top	4	5-5-5-5
Tuesday *p.207 bottom*	4	5-5-5-5
p.207 middle	3	5-5-5
Wednesday *p.284 top*	5	5-5-5-5-5
p.218 bottom	4	5-5-5-5
Thursday *p.212 middle*	4	5-5-5-5
p.279 bottom	4	5-5-5-5

Continue to add sets and exercises in the following weeks. You may not reach the top-end weights you achieved during the off-season because of the stress of practice. But you should be doing all the exercises and handling close to the total workout.

Remember: Stretch, do abdominals, leg extensions, leg curls every day.

Getting stronger as the season progresses: By continually increasing the workload, you get stronger at the most critical part of the season, the end. You'll perform better and be more of an asset to your team. Even if your team isn't playing well, you'll attract attention for your strong play. College recruiters and pro scouts like a player who can still play hard in the fourth quarter and at the end of a long season, when the most important games are usually played.

Friday

Stretching, mental preparation for game □

GOLF

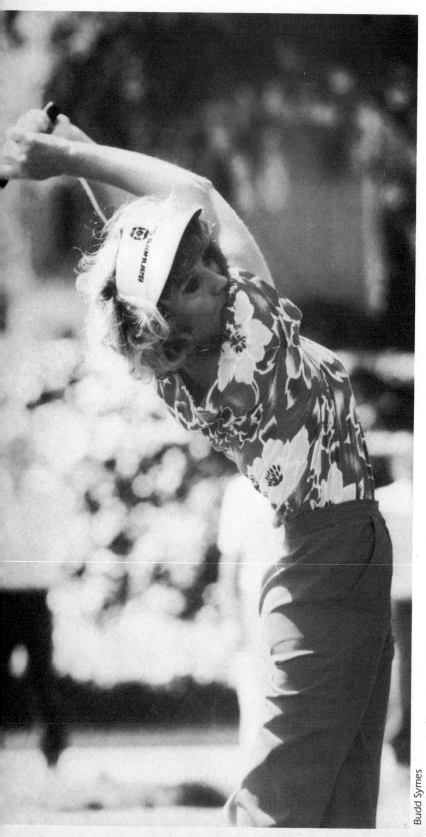

Budd Symes

By Gary Wiren, Ph.D., one of only 25 Master Professionals in the United States, Master Teacher at the Boca Raton Hotel and Club, featured on ESPN's "How to Play Your Best Golf."

Golfers can use weight training to increase strength, flexibility and muscular endurance. It helps develop balance for golfers with weak leg muscles. Getting stronger and more flexible also enhances techniques by allowing the athlete to assume advantageous biomechanical positions.

A golfer's technique reflects the natural selection process of choosing your own assets and finding a style to fit. Depending on this technique, golfers will vary in their strength emphasis. Generally, hands, forearms, trunk rotators and back are the most important areas of emphasis. Leg work is also important.

Strength in golf is of little use without flexibility. Most men with whom I work need more flexibility than strength work. The opposite is generally true for women. Golf is a rotary activity, so exercises emphasizing the rotary movements of the trunk and forearms are extremely important.

Other effective techniques for increasing strength for golf could include a program of calisthenics and the swinging of a weighted club (both for strength and flexibility). An innovative new technique in golf training is the use of deep muscle electronic therapy.

Golf is not a leader in the world of weight training for improvement in performance. The acceptance of improving strength and flexibility through weight training is relatively new to the sport, and an important breakthrough.

Aims: Strengthen all major muscle groups and develop proper muscle balance.

Golf Off-Season Program

The off-season program is designed to strengthen all major muscle groups and to provide proper muscle balance.

Days per week: 3, with 1 day rest between workouts.

exercises		sets	reps	exercises		sets	reps
1 p.198 bottom		1	15 to 25 each side	**6** p.259 bottom		1-2	15 to 20 per set
Optional p.196 bottom		1	10 to 25	**7** p.259 middle		1-2	15 to 20 per set
2 p.193 bottom		1	20 to 50 each side	**8** p.296 bottom		2	15-15
Optional p.191 middle		1	15 to 30 each side				
Optional p.199 top		1	25 to 50 each leg				
3 p.216 middle		2	8 to 15 per set				
4 p.274 middle		2	10-10				
5 p.306 middle		2	10-10				

GETTING STRONGER ©1986 Bill Pearl & Shelter Publications, Inc.

Golf Pre-Season Program

The pre-season program is similar to the off-season program, but with different exercises for certain body parts. During this time, more time is spent golfing and working on specific golfing skills. Always remember to include some form of cardiovascular training.

Days per week: 2, with 1-2 days rest between workouts.

exercises	sets	reps	exercises	sets	reps
1 p.197 bottom	1	15 to 25	**6** p.297 bottom	1-2	10 to 15 per set each leg
2 p.191 bottom	1	20 to 30 each side	**7** p.259 bottom	1-2	15 to 20 per set
Optional p.193 top	1	10 to 20	**8** p.259 middle	1-2	15 to 20 per set
3 p.216 middle	1	10 to 20 each side			
Optional p.198 top	1	25 to 50 each leg			
Optional p.198 bottom	1	15 to 30 each leg			
4 p.281 middle	2	10-10 each arm			
5 p.301 top	2	10-10 each arm			

Golf In-Season Program

The in-season program is designed to maintain levels achieved during the off- and pre-season programs. In season, hip, wrist and forearm work can be optional.

Days per week: 2, with 1-2 days rest between workouts, and 2 days rest before competitions. Some golfers are more relaxed and swing more smoothly if they have a weight workout on a golfing day, or 1 day prior to golfing. Others need more time off before golfing. Find the schedule that works best for you.

exercises	sets	reps	exercises	sets	reps
1 p.216 middle	1-2	5 to 10 per set	**4** p.203 top	2	10-10
2 p.190 top	1	10 to 20	**Optional** p.248 bottom	1-2	10 (10)
3 p.193 bottom	1	15 to 30 each side	**5** p.307 bottom	2	10-10
Optional p.289 middle	1-2	10 per set each side	**6** p.263 top	1-2	Floor to top
Optional p.275 bottom	1-2	10 (10)			

Additional Exercises:

1. Machines may be substituted
2. Dumbbells may be substituted
3. Leg extensions
4. Step-ups with weights
5. Lunges with weights
6. Shoulder shrugs
7. Lateral dumbbell raises
8. Medicine ball exercises

Exercise Options:

1. Circuit training
2. Nautilus, pulleys or cable exercises
3. Weighted club exercises
4. Sport-specific resistance exercises that copy swing

Problem Areas:

1. A year-round flexibility program is very important.
2. Pay attention to individual strengths or weaknesses when devising programs.
3. Some type of cardiovascular conditioning should be done year-round: biking, swimming, aerobics, circuit training, running.□

GYMNASTICS

*By Don Peters. Head Coach, U.S.
National Women's Gymnastics Team;
Head Coach, 1984 Women's Olympic
Gymnastics Team (gold medalists).*

Very few gymnastics coaches use weights, and weight training is not a major part of our gymnastics program. I believe in the principle of *specificity*. You should work the specific muscles the same way they're used in your particular sport or event. We do a lot of gymnastics exercises using the body as the resistance.

We *will* use weight training to strengthen specific individual weaknesses. Women gymnasts have a lot of lower leg injuries because their events are mostly leg-oriented. Ankle injuries and stress fractures are common. The men have a lot of upper body injuries, often rotator cuff and shoulder girdle injuries. Increased strength through weight training leads to better body balance, better handling of stress and fewer injuries.

Our fitness exercises are geared to strength and flexibility. We don't worry much about endurance because the longest event only takes 90 seconds.

Aims: The three gymnastics programs are designed to strengthen the major muscle groups and correct muscle imbalances. After consulting with the coach and participating in strength testing, design the workout that's best for you. All workouts must be tailored to the individual.

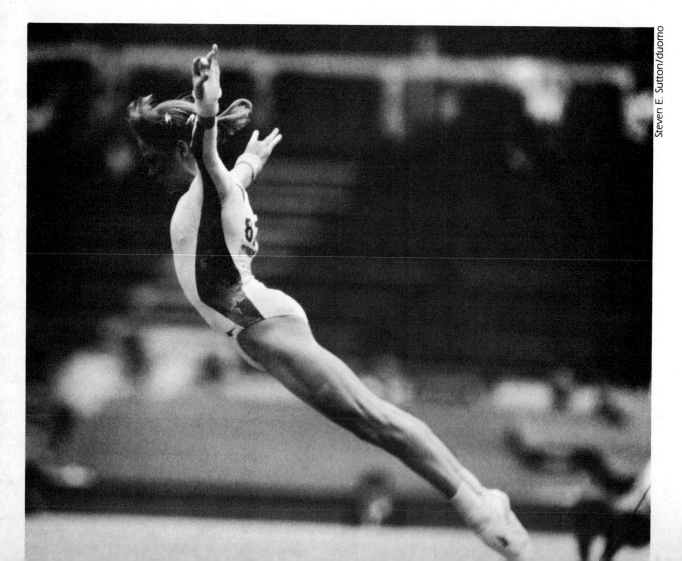

Steven E. Sutton/duomo

Gymnastics Off-Season Program

Use this program from spring to late summer. During the first month or two, use lighter weights and more repetitions. In late summer, use heavier weights and less repetitions. Remember the aims of the program—to strengthen the major muscle groups and correct muscle imbalances.

Days per week: 3, with 1 day rest between workouts.

exercises	sets	reps	exercises	sets	reps
1 p.244 top	4	12-10-10-8	**Optional** p.293 middle	3	15-15-15
2 p.202 top	4	12-10-10-8	**Optional** p.292 bottom	3	15-15-15
3 p.279 bottom	3	12-10-8	**7** p.299 top	2-3	12 per set each leg
4 p.192 top	3	12-10-8	**8** p.298 bottom	2-3	12 per set each leg
5 p.253 bottom	3	Max. 10 per set, then add weight	**9** p.243 bottom	3	15 to 20 per set
Optional p.306 middle	3	12-10-10	**10** p.201 middle	3	8 to 15 per set
Optional p.220 bottom	3	12-10-10	**Optional** p.198 bottom	1	25 to 50 each leg
6 p.296 top	4	12-10-10-8	**Optional** p.216 middle	1	Max. 15, per set, then add weight

GETTING STRONGER ©1986 Bill Pearl & Shelter Publications, Inc.

Gymnastics Pre-Season Program

Now that you've created better muscle balance and base strength levels, it is time to increase your strength. Use this program until the start of the season.

Days per week: 3, with 1 day rest between workouts.

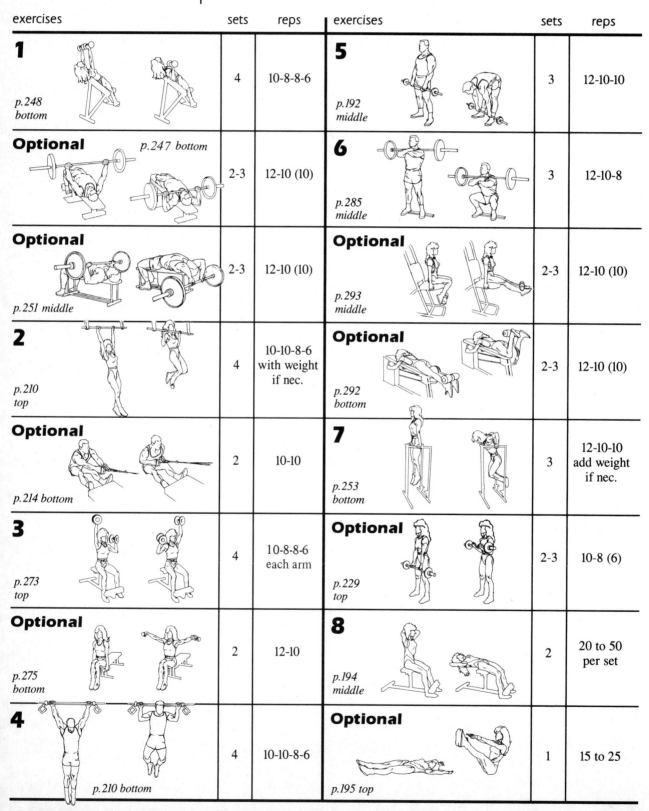

exercises	sets	reps	exercises	sets	reps
1 p.248 bottom	4	10-8-8-6	**5** p.192 middle	3	12-10-10
Optional p.247 bottom	2-3	12-10 (10)	**6** p.285 middle	3	12-10-8
Optional p.251 middle	2-3	12-10 (10)	**Optional** p.293 middle	2-3	12-10 (10)
2 p.210 top	4	10-10-8-6 with weight if nec.	**Optional** p.292 bottom	2-3	12-10 (10)
Optional p.214 bottom	2	10-10	**7** p.253 bottom	3	12-10-10 add weight if nec.
3 p.273 top	4	10-8-8-6 each arm	**Optional** p.229 top	2-3	10-8 (6)
Optional p.275 bottom	2	12-10	**8** p.194 middle	2	20 to 50 per set
4 p.210 bottom	4	10-10-8-6	**Optional** p.195 top	1	15 to 25

GETTING STRONGER ©1986 Bill Pearl & Shelter Publications, Inc.

Gymnastics In-Season Program

This program is designed to help you maintain strength levels achieved during the off- and pre-season programs. The number of exercises, sets and reps have been cut back to a maintenance level. In addition to this program, you will be doing specific gymnastics skills and movements, abdominal and flexibility work during practice. If additional hip and lower back exercises are necessary, add them to the program.

Days per week: 2, with 1-2 days rest between workouts and 2 days before competition.

exercises	sets	reps	exercises	sets	reps
1 p.279 bottom	2	10-8	**5** p.306 middle	2	12-10
2 p.248 top	1-2	10 (8)	**6** p.297 bottom	1-2	10 to 15 per set
3 p.210 top	2	12-10	**Optional** p.284 top	2	12-12
4 p.213 bottom	2	10-8	**7** p.190 middle	1	25 to 50
Optional p.216 middle	1	Max. 15, then add weight	**Optional** p.197 top	1-2	15 per set

Additional exercises
1. Dumbbells may be used instead of barbells
2. Machines may be substituted
3. Power cleans
4. Power high pulls
5. Seated lat rows
6. Incline bench press
7. Step-ups
8. Lunges
9. Good mornings
10. Extra abdominal exercises
11. Rotary torso work

Exercise options:
1. Specific gymnastic movements for exercises using body weight and strapped-on weight for added resistance
2. Plyometric exercises
3. Circuit training

Problem areas:
1. *Wrists:* Do wrist extensions and flexions, pronation-supination and adduction-abduction exercises.
2. *Ankles:* Work 4 ways; toe raises for plantar extension, dorsiflexion with straps or surgical tubing, inversion-eversion or angle board.
3. *Shoulders:* Do dumbbell exercises for rotator cuff conditioning, internal and external rotation as well as adduction.□

ICE HOCKEY

By Bob Bourne, Left Wing, New York
Islanders, Stanley Cup Champions,
1980, 1981, 1982, 1983.

The four most important areas to work on for
ice hockey are:
1. Muscular endurance in legs, thighs and hips
2. Strengthening of the lower back for the
   unnatural position required in skating
3. Shoulder strengthening and conditioning
4. Chest strengthening in order to command
   position all over the ice
I recommend a lot of shoulder and leg exercises
for hockey players. Any exercises that
strengthen weaknesses in knees and shoulders
can cut down on injuries. You should also
strengthen the abdominal muscles, as this
will help prevent lower back pain.

Stretching exercises and calisthenics are also
critical in injury prevention. If you are not
warm and loose there is a high risk of injury.

Currently we use a summer (off-season)
program of stretching five times a week, weight
training three times a week, aerobics two times
a week and anaerobics once a week.

Aims: To increase strength levels and create
proper muscle balance. The lower body, lower
back and torso, chest and shoulders are given
special emphasis for strength and endurance.

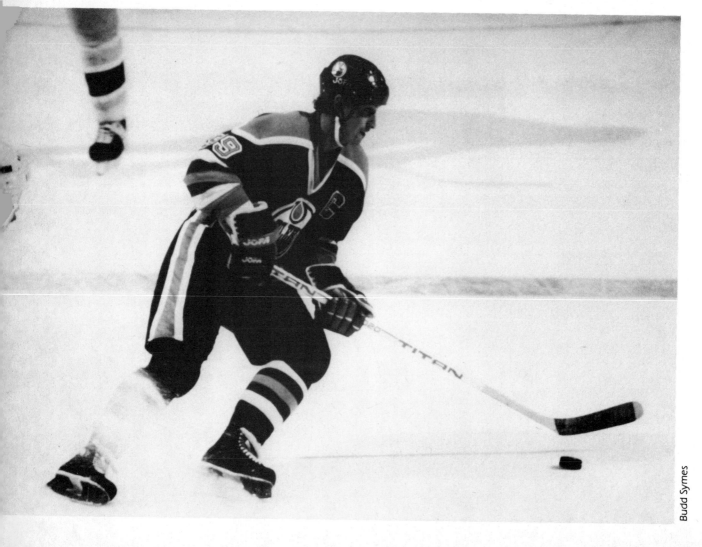

Budd Symes

Ice Hockey Off-Season Program

Use this program from 2-3 weeks after the season to 4-8 weeks before the start of the next season. It is intended to strengthen and balance all the major muscle groups in the body. There is special emphasis on the lower body, lower back and torso, knees, chest and shoulder strength and endurance.

Days per week: 3, with 1 day rest between workouts.

exercises	sets	reps	exercises	sets	reps
1 p.293 middle	3	15-15-15	**Optional** p.192 middle	2	10-8
2 p.292 bottom	3	10-10-10	**7** p.300 top	3	10-8-8
3 p.290 top	2	10-10 each side	**8** p.218 bottom	3	10-8-8
4 p.248 bottom	3	10-8-8	**9** p.190 top	1-2	15 to 30 per set
Optional p.248 top	3	10-8-8	**10** p.193 top	1	25 to 50 each side
5 p.279 bottom	3	10-8-8	**11** p.196 middle	1	15 to 50
Optional p.274 top	3	10-8-8	**Optional** p.199 bottom	1	25 to 50 each leg
6 p.203 top	3	12-12-12	**Optional** p.198 bottom	1	25 to 50 each leg

GETTING STRONGER ©1986 Bill Pearl & Shelter Publications, Inc.

Ice Hockey Pre-Season Program

This program is for the final 4-8 weeks before the season starts. You are going for maximum strength gains and specific conditioning for hockey.

Days per week: 3, with 1 day rest between workouts.

exercises	sets	reps	exercises	sets	reps
1 p.289 middle	3	10-10-10 each side	**7** p.305 bottom	3	8-8-8
2 p.296 bottom	3	10-10-10	**8** p.225 middle	3	8-8-8
3 p.244 top	3	8-8-8	**Optional** p.259 bottom	2	20-20
Optional p.245 top	3	8-8-8	**9** p.194 top	1	25 to 50
4 p.275 bottom	3	8-8-8	**10** p.192 top	1	25 to 50
Optional p.280 top	3	8-8-8 each arm	**11** p.197 top	1	15 to 30
5 p.209 top	3	Max. 12 per set, then add weight	**Optional** p.199 top	1	25 to 50 each leg
6 p.216 middle	1-2	Max. 15 per set, then add weight	**Optional** p.238 top	3	20 to 25 per set

Ice Hockey In-Season Program

This program is designed to maintain strength levels built up during off- and pre-season programs.

Days per week: 2, with 1-2 days rest between workouts and at least 2 days before games.

exercises		sets	reps	exercises		sets	reps
1 *p.190 top*		1-2	25 to 100 per set	**6** *p.290 middle*		2-3	8-8 (8) each leg
2 *p.194 bottom*		1-2	10 to 20 per set	**7** *p.221 top*		2-3	8-8 (8)
3 *p.257 top*		2-3	5-5 (5)	**8** *p.259 bottom*		1-2	20 (20)
4 *p.279 bottom*		2-3	8-8 (6)	**9** *p.296 bottom*		2-3	15-15 (15)
5 *p.204 middle*		2-3	10-10 (8)	**10** *p.237 bottom*		2-3	20 to 25 per set

Additional exercises:

1. Machines may be substituted
2. Dumbbells may be substituted
3. Bent arm pullover
4. Bar dips
5. Rotary torso exercises
6. Good mornings
7. Palms-down wrist curls
8. Bent-over cable rotators: simulate shot, lead with each shoulder, follow through with cable pulley as resistance

Exercise options:

1. Circuit training in weight room
2. Conditioning: sprints, agility runs, stadiums, bicycle, jump rope, etc.
3. Make sure you get a little of both:
   (1) short, high intensity anaerobic and
   (2) longer distance, lower intensity aerobic workout for conditioning.

Problem areas:

1. Lower back: Strengthen and make more flexible with this program.
2. Stretch year-round for improved flexibility.
3. Strengthen legs to help protect the knees.
4. Strengthen shoulders to help prevent injury. □

POWERLIFTING

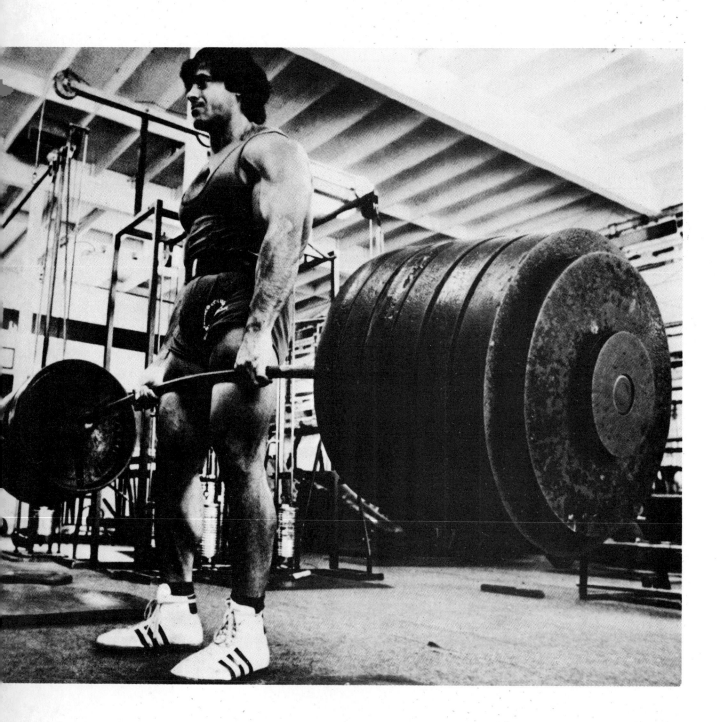

By Jan Todd, *Head Coach, Longhorn Power-lifting Team, University of Texas at Austin; Co-author,* Lift Your Way to Youthful Fitness; *Coach, U.S. Women's Powerlifting Team, 1981 & 1985 World Champions; Coach, U.S. Men's Powerlifting Team, 1981 & 1984 World Champions; Member International Powerlifting Hall of Fame; Women's World Record Holder, Squat (545½ pounds).*

Powerlifting requires simple brute strength. It does not require great endurance, flexibility or quickness of motion. To be a good powerlifter, you need to be relatively coordinated, have a good sense of balance and be able to exert great strength by pushing or pulling.

A good powerlifting program is built around three principles:
1. The first part of the program should create a state of hypertrophy (muscular enlargement).
2. Training weights should come near, *but not exceed*, your limit. Psychologically, it is important to succeed! Never "max out" until the day of competition.
3. Pay careful attention to technique. Bad habits must be corrected in the early stages of lifting.

Powerlifting contests involve three lifts: squat, deadlift and bench press. Most contests are won by squats and deadlifts. These lifts depend on lower back, hip and leg strength. The bench press is a test of chest, arm and shoulder strength. Despite the specific nature of the lifts, you need to strengthen your entire body.

Powerlifters do not need the flexibility of a gymnast, but a certain degree of flexibility is necessary. Stretching should be done after some sort of warmup, and the stretches should move the joints in a slow, controlled manner through their full range of motion.

Partial squats and partial deadlifts are also integral parts of my training. I do them during the final eight weeks of my training cycles and try to increase the poundages weekly. I always do partial squats immediately following heavy squat workouts, and use 100 pounds more than in the full squat. I do partial deadlifts on the same day as the heavy squats, and set the bar just below the middle of my knees. They are not included in the exercise programs on the following pages because they are generally used only by advanced lifters. Train for at least one cycle before adding them to your program.

The most important innovation in power-lifting in the past 20 years has been the use of *periodization*, involving four distinct phases. This method acts as a safeguard against overtraining while allowing you to peak for competitions.
1. *Hypertrophy:* High repetitions (10-20 reps per set) with relatively light weights for 4-5 weeks
2. *Strength-power:* Medium repetitions (5-8 reps per set) with heavier weights for 4 weeks
3. *Peaking:* Low repetitions (2-3 reps per set) with heavy weights for 3 weeks, culminating in a competition.
4. *Active rest:* Rest and non-lifting activities (cycling, running) for 1-2 weeks. After the "active rest", begin hypertrophy again at a slightly higher level than your first cycle.

In periodization, each exercise is worked "heavy" once a week—meaning that you do 3 sets of the correct number of reps (called "target sets") with as heavy a weight as you can correctly use for the full number of reps—and "light" once a week using 85% of the weight used for the "target sets" of the previous workout.

Aims: To develop strength

Powerlifting Monday Program

This program follows the periodization cycle:
1. *First 4 weeks:* Hypertrophy—high reps, relatively light weights
2. *Next 4 weeks:* Strength/power—medium reps, heavier weights
3. *Next 3 weeks:* Peaking—low reps, heavy weights
4. *Final phase:* 1-2 weeks of active rest (no lifting). Cycle, swim, run, etc. After this phase, begin hypertrophy again at a slightly higher level than when you started your first cycle.

exercises	4 weeks		4 weeks		3 weeks	
	sets	reps	sets	reps	sets	reps
1 p.206 middle — Heavy	5	10 per set	5	10-5-5-5-5	5	10-3-3-3-3
2 p.284 top — 85%*	5	10 per set	5	10-5-5-5-5	5	10-3-3-3-3
3 p.294 bottom — 85%*	5	10 per set	5	10-5-5-5-5	5	10-3-3-3-3
4 p.292 bottom — 85%*	5	10 per set	5	10-5-5-5-5	5	10-3-3-3-3
5 p.293 middle — 85%*	5	10 per set	5	10-5-5-5-5	5	10-3-3-3-3
6 p.190 middle	5	20 to 25 per set	5	25 to 40 per set	5	40 to 50 per set

*85% of target weight used on previous Thursday

GETTING STRONGER ©1986 Bill Pearl & Shelter Publications, Inc.

Powerlifting Tuesday Program

This program follows the periodization cycle:

1. *First 4 weeks:* Hypertrophy—high reps, relatively light weights
2. *Next 4 weeks:* Strength/power—medium reps, heavier weights
3. *Next 3 weeks:* Peaking—low reps, heavy weights
4. *Final phase:* 1-2 weeks of active rest (no lifting). Cycle, swim, run, etc. After this phase, begin hypertrophy again at a slightly higher level than when you started your first cycle.

exercises	4 weeks		4 weeks		3 weeks	
	sets	reps	sets	reps	sets	reps
1 Heavy p.244 top	5	10 per set	5	10-5-5-5-5	5	10-3-3-3-3
2 Heavy p.245 top	5	10 per set	5	10-5-5-5-5	5	10-3-3-3-3
3 Heavy p.244 bottom	5	10 per set	5	10-5-5-5-5	5	10-3-3-3-3
4 p.202 middle 85%*	5	10 per set	5	10-5-5-5-5	5	10-3-3-3-3
5 p.203 bottom 85%*	5	10 per set each arm	5	10-5-5-5-5 each arm	5	10-3-3-3-3 each arm
6 p.229 top 85%*	5	10 per set	5	10-5-5-5-5	5	10-5-5-5-5
7 p.190 middle	5	20 to 25 per set	5	25 to 40 per set	5	40 to 50 per set
8 p.196 top	5	20 to 25 per set	5	25 to 40 per set	5	40 to 50 per set

GETTING STRONGER ©1986 Bill Pearl & Shelter Publications, Inc.   *85% of target weight from previous Tuesday

Powerlifting Thursday Program

This program follows the periodization cycle:

1. *First 4 weeks:* Hypertrophy—high reps, relatively light weights
2. *Next 4 weeks:* Strength/power—medium reps, heavier weights
3. *Next 3 weeks:* Peaking—low reps, heavy weights
4. *Final phase:* 1-2 weeks of active rest (no lifting). Cycle, swim, run, etc. After this phase, begin hypertrophy again at a slightly higher level than when you started your first cycle.

exercises	4 weeks		4 weeks		3 weeks	
	sets	reps	sets	reps	sets	reps
1 p.284 top 85%*	5	10 per set	5	10-5-5-5-5	5	10-3-3-3-3
2 p.206 middle Heavy	5	10 per set (light weights)	5	10-5-5-5-5	5	10-3-3-3-3
3 p.294 bottom Heavy	5	10 per set	5	10-5-5-5-5	5	10-3-3-3-3
4 p.292 bottom Heavy	5	10 per set	5	10-5-5-5-5	5	10-3-3-3-3
5 p.293 middle Heavy	5	10 per set	5	10-5-5-5-5	5	10-3-3-3-3
6 p.190 middle	5	20 to 25 per set	5	25 to 40 per set	5	40 to 50 per set

*85% of target weight from previous Monday

GETTING STRONGER ©1986 Bill Pearl & Shelter Publications, Inc.

Powerlifting Friday Program

This program follows the periodization cycle:

1. *First 4 weeks:* Hypertrophy–high reps, relatively light weights
2. *Next 4 weeks:* Strength/power–medium reps, heavier weights
3. *Next 3 weeks:* Peaking–low reps, heavy weights
4. *Final phase:* 1-2 weeks of active rest (no lifting). Cycle, swim, run, etc. After this phase, begin hypertrophy again at a slightly higher level than when you started your first cycle.

exercises	4 weeks		4 weeks		3 weeks	
	sets	reps	sets	reps	sets	reps
1 p.202 middle — Heavy	5	10 per set	5	10-5-5-5-5	5	10-3-3-3-3
2 p.203 bottom — Heavy	5	10 per set per arm	5	10-5-5-5-5 each arm	5	10-3-3-3-3 each arm
3 p.244 top — 85%*	5	10 per set	5	10-5-5-5-5	5	10-3-3-3-3
4 p.245 top — 85%*	5	10 per set	5	10-5-5-5-5	5	10-3-3-3-3
5 p.244 bottom — 85%*	5	10 per set	5	10-5-5-5-5	5	10-3-3-3-3
6 p.229 top — Heavy	5	10 per set	5	10-5-5-5-5	5	10-3-3-3-3
7 p.190 middle	5	20 to 25 per set	5	25 to 40 per set	5	40 to 50 per set
8 p.196 top	5	20 to 25 per set	5	25 to 40 per set	5	40 to 50 per set

GETTING STRONGER ©1986 Bill Pearl & Shelter Publications, Inc.   *85% of target weight from previous Tuesday

ROWING

By Robin Pound, M.S., *Exercise Physiology and Anatomy; PAC–10 Strength and Conditioning Coach.*

Crew is primarily an endurance event. Most of the muscular endurance work takes place during "on the water" training. However, strength is needed for starts, catching up or pulling away, and the finish. Crew athletes tend to have much stronger pulling muscles in the upper body than pushing muscles; hence muscle imbalance. This program is designed to create proper muscle balance and increase strength.

As with most sports, a thorough stretching and warmup program is advisable before strenuous workouts and competition.

Aims: To balance strength levels of the major muscle groups.

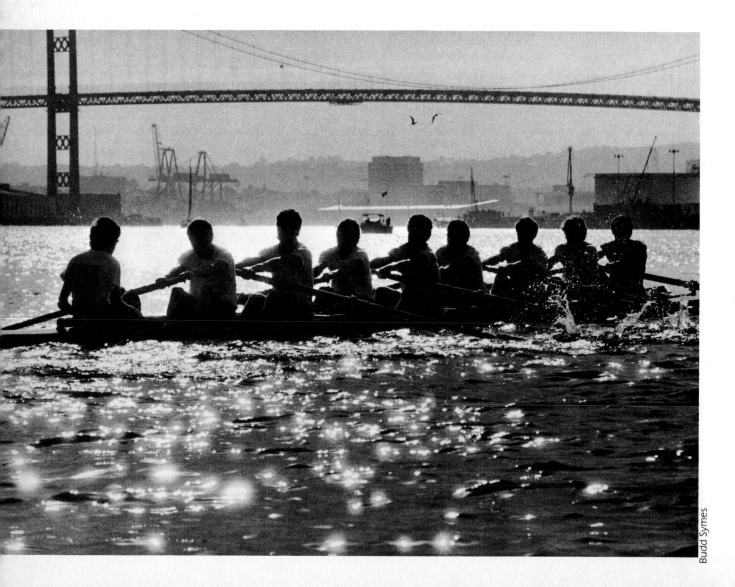

Budd Symes

Rowing Off-Season Program

This program will create proper body muscle balance and raise strength levels. Use it for 3-6 months depending on your program and location. This program runs until 4-6 weeks prior to the season.

Days per week: 2, with at least 2 days rest between workouts.

Supersets: Do the first set of exercise 1(a), then immediately do the first set of exercise 1(b). Rest 1-2 minutes, then go on to second sets of 1(a), 1(b). Follow this format for the prescribed number of sets and reps.

exercises	sets	reps	exercises	sets	reps
1 (a) p.190 middle	3	25 to 50 per set	**4** (a) p.284 top	3	10-8-8
(b) p.216 middle	3	Max. 15 per set then add weight	(b) p.292 bottom	3	10-8-8
2 (a) p.244 top	3	10-8-8	**5** (a) p.298 bottom	3	12-15 per set
(b) p.214 top	3	10-8-8	(b) p.299 top	3	12-15 per set
Optional (a) p.245 top	3	10-8-8	**Optional** (a) p.290 top	3	10-10-10
Optional (b) p.203 bottom	3	10-8-8 each arm	**Optional** (b) p.206 bottom	3	10-10-10
3 (a) p.207 bottom	3	5-5-5			
(b) p.225 middle	3	10-8-8			

Rowing Pre-Season Program

The pre-season goal is to peak strength gains before the first competition. Use this program for 4-6 weeks. You should do more "on the water" work than during the off-season.

Days per week: 3, with 1 day rest between workouts.

Supersets: Do the first set of exercise 1(a), then immediately do the first set of exercise 1(b). Rest 1-2 minutes, then go on to second sets of 1(a), 1(b). Follow this format for the prescribed number of sets and reps.

exercises	sets	reps	exercises	sets	reps
1 (a) p.195 middle	3	15 to 30 per set	**4** (a) p.284 top	3	8-6-4
(b) p.216 middle	3	Max. 15 per set then add weight	(b) p.292 bottom	3	10-8-6
2 (a) p.244 top	3	8-6-4	**5** (a) p.298 bottom	3	12-15 per set
(b) p.214 top	3	10-8-6	(b) p.299 top	3	12-15 per set
Optional (a) p.248 bottom	3	8-6-4	**Optional** (a) p.290 top	3	10-10-10
Optional (b) p.202 bottom	3	10-8-6 each arm	**Optional** (b) p.297 bottom	3	10-10-10
3 (a) p.207 bottom	3	5-3-3			
(b) p.225 middle	3	10-8-6			

Rowing In-Season Program

This program is designed to maintain muscle balance and strength levels attained in the off- and pre-season programs.

Days per week: 2, with 1-2 days rest between workouts and 2 days before competition.

Supersets: Do the first set of exercise 1(a), then immediately do the first set of exercise 1(b). Rest 1-2 minutes, then go on to second sets of 1(a), 1(b). Follow this format for the prescribed number of sets and reps.

exercises	sets	reps	exercises	sets	reps
1 (a) p.195 top	3	20-30 per set	**3** (b) p.203 bottom	3	10-8-6
(b) p.216 middle	3	Max. 15 per set then add weight	**4** (a) p.207 bottom	3	5-5-5
2 (a) p.244 top	3	8-6-6	(b) p.225 middle	3	10-8-6
(b) p.214 top	3	10-8-6	**5** (a) p.284 top	3	10-8-6
3 (a) p.253 bottom	3	Max. 15 per set then add weight	(b) p.292 bottom	3	10-8-10

Additional exercises:

1. Dumbbells may be used instead of barbells
2. Machines may be used
3. Lower or upper back machines—rows or pulls
4. Chins
5. Dumbbell shoulder flys
6. Upright rows
7. Barbell rows lying stomach down on high bench
8. T-bar rows
9. Shoulder press
10. Shoulder shrugs

Exercise options:

1. Circuit training in weight room for first 4 weeks (10-15 reps)
2. Rowing ergometer for sprints and technique work

Problem areas:

These programs will correct the muscle imbalances that can occur because of the large amount of "on water" training with pulling muscles of the upper body. Try to lift 2-3 times per week, but lift only on days that you do high intensity interval work on the water. Make sure to have 1-3 days of overdistance endurance work before you go back to the weights. This will ensure adequate recovery. The high intensity interval work should only be done twice a week with 2-3 days between workouts.□

RUNNING

By Gary T. Moran, Ph.D., Human Anatomy and Kinesiology; M.S., Exercise Physiology; Runner and Triathlete.

Distance runners can use weight training to strengthen the major muscle groups, and most importantly, to help prevent injuries. Strong and balanced muscles support the skeletal structure in proper biomechanical alignment, and absorb the contact shock and stress from the pounding that is involved in distance running.

I suggest the *split routine* (see instructions at the top of each program) as it takes less time each day and adds variety to your workout.

It's important to take care when integrating weight training into your running schedule. For example, you do not want to do a strenuous leg workout just before hill training or interval training, but rather after your run. Whenever possible, do your weight work several hours after your run.

Also, supplement your weight training and running with a stretching program.

Aims: To prevent injuries and to strengthen and balance the major muscle groups.

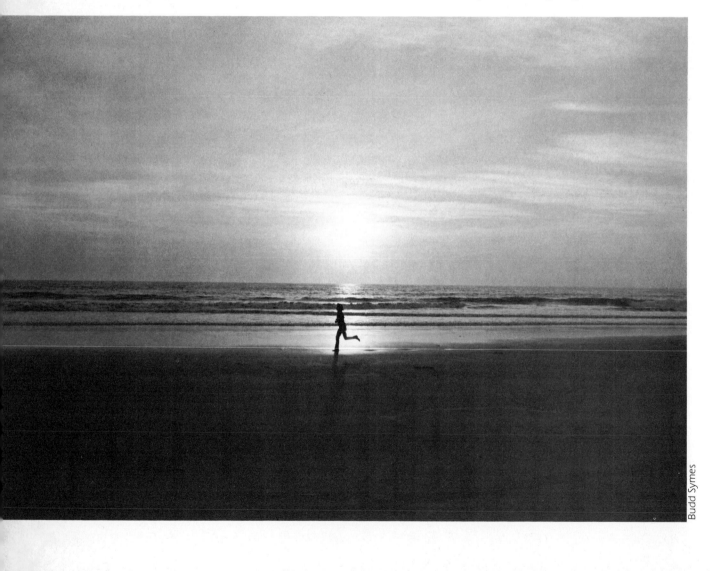

Budd Symes

Running (Distance) Off-Season Program

Use this program during the non-competitive portions of the year.

Days per week: You can do either a regular routine or a split routine:
(a) *Regular routine:* 3 days per week, with 1 day rest between workouts
(b) *Split routine:* M-W-F, exercises 1-4; T-Th-Sat, exercises 5-8

Supersets: Do the first set of exercise 1(a), then immediately do the first set of exercise 1(b). Rest 1-2 minutes, then go on to second sets of 1(a), 1(b). Follow this format for prescribed number of sets and reps.

exercises	sets	reps	exercises	sets	reps
1 (a) p.249 middle	3	10-8-8	(b) p.292 bottom	3	10-10-8
(b) p.214 bottom	3	10-8-8	**Optional** (a) p.298 middle	2	12-10 each leg
2 p.277 middle Use close grip	2	10-10	**Optional** (b) p.298 top	2	12-10 each leg
3 (a) p.307 bottom	3	10-10-8	**Optional** (a) p.298 bottom	2	12-10 each leg
(b) p.219 middle	3	10-10-8 each arm	**Optional** (b) p.299 top	2	12-10 each leg
4 p.190 top	2	15 to 40 per set	**Optional** p.297 bottom	2	10-10 each leg
5 p.284 bottom	3	10-10-8	**7** p.216 middle	1	10 to 15
6 (a) p.293 midd...	3	10-10-8	**8** p.195 top	2	10 to 25

GETTING STRONGER ©1986 Bill Pearl & Shelter Publications, Inc.

Running (Distance) In-Season Program

Use this program during the competitive season.

Days per week: You can do either a regular routine or a split routine:
(a) *Regular routine:* 2 days per week, with 2 or more days rest prior to race
(b) *Split routine:* M-W, exercises 1-3; T-Th, exercises 4-6, with 2 or more days rest prior to race

Supersets: Do the first set of exercises 1(a), then immediately do the first set of exercise 1(b). Rest 1-2 minutes, then go on to second sets of 1(a), 1(b). Follow this format for prescribed number of sets and reps.

exercises	sets	reps	exercises	sets	reps
1 (a) p.244 top	2	10-8	**Optional** (a) p.298 middle	1	10 each leg
(b) p.210 bottom	2	3-10 per set	**Optional** (b) p.298 top	1	10 each leg
2 p.279 bottom	1	12	**Optional** (a) p.298 bottom	1	10 each leg
3 (a) p.309 top	2	10-10	**Optional** (b) p.299 top	1	10 each leg
(b) p. 219 bottom	2	10-10 each arm	**Optional** p.290 top	1	10 each side
4 p.296 top	2	12-10	**5** p.297 bottom	1	10 each leg
Optional (a) p.292 bottom	1-2	12 (10)	**Optional** p.216 middle	1	10 to 15
Optional (b) p.293 middle	1-2	12 (10)	**6** p.190 middle	2	15 to 25 per set

GETTING STRONGER ©1986 Bill Pearl & Shelter Publications, Inc.

Additional exercises:

1. Dumbbells may be substituted for barbells
2. Machines may be substituted for free weights
3. Sit-ups with weights
4. Good mornings
5. Rotary torso work
6. Clean and jerk
7. Squats with weight held in front
8. Close grip bench press
9. Standing dumbbell press

Exercise options:

1. Circuit training in the weight room
2. Plyometrics: bounding
3. Medicine ball exercises
4. Conditioning: track intervals

Problem areas:

1. Stretch year-round for maximum flexibility and to prevent injuries.
2. Joints: ankles, knees, hip stress. Let joints adapt gradually to work load. □

SKIING (CROSS-COUNTRY)

By Steven Gaskill, *Nordic Technical Director, U.S. Ski Team;* **Peter Ashley**, *Head Women's Coach, U.S. Ski Team;* **Torbjorn Karlsen**, *Assistant Women's Coach, U.S. Ski Team.*

Cross-country skiing is a maximum endurance workout in itself. The best way to improve strength is through specific training. The intent of your strength training should be to duplicate the movement patterns, speed, load/resistance and working time period for that movement to be used in skiing. If you do this as specifically as possible, you will achieve a training response in the exact muscle fibers needed for overcoming a specific stress. Only those muscle cells/fibers needing training get trained.

The best results in specific training are achieved when you have a good base from general strength training (light load and heavy repetitions). We recommend 2-4 sessions a week of between 10 and 60 minutes depending on your level of fitness. Also, remember to gradually increase your training load, and to vary your exercises.

Aims: The three cross-country skiing programs are designed to strengthen all major muscle groups and to develop muscle balance.

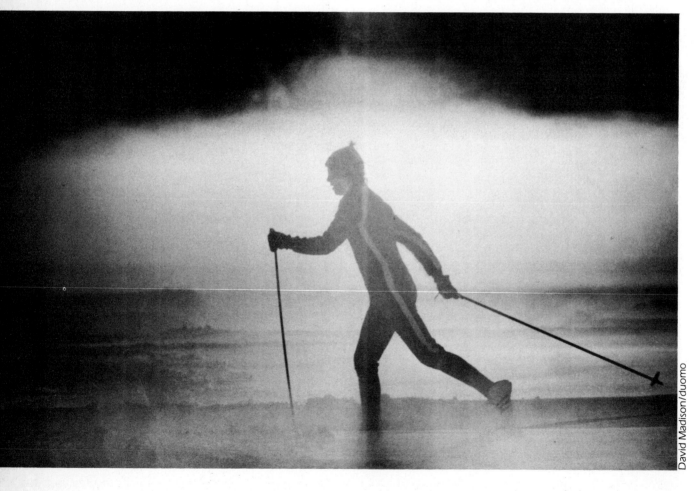

David Madison/duomo

Skiing (Cross-Country) Off-Season Program

This program is designed to build strength and balance for all major muscle groups. It is not a maximum strength program. Muscular endurance will come mostly from sport-specific exercises and skiing workouts. To alter the program for more endurance gains, lower the weight used, and do more reps.

Days per week: 3, with 1 day rest between workouts.

exercises	sets	reps	exercises	sets	reps
1 p.284 top	4	12-12-10-10	**Optional** p.244 top	2-3	12-10 (8)
Optional p.293 middle	1-2	15 per set	**5** p.277 middle	3	10-10-8
Optional p.292 bottom	1-2	15 per set	**6** p.251 top	3	10-10-8
2 p.298 middle	2	10-10 each leg	**7** p.306 middle	4	12-12-10-10
3 p.298 top	2	10-10 each leg	**Optional** p.219 middle	2-3	12-10 (8) each arm
Optional p.298 bottom	3	10-10-10 each leg	**8** p.200 top	1	20 to 50 each leg
4 p.214 top	4	12-12-10-10	**9** p.198 bottom	1	15 to 30 each leg
Optional p.203 top	2-3	12-10 (8)	**Optional** p.201 bottom	1	15 to 30 each leg

GETTING STRONGER ©1986 Bill Pearl & Shelter Publications, Inc.

Skiing (Cross-Country) Pre-Season Program

Begin this program 6 weeks prior to the season. It is designed to increase strength. Be sure to include a specific movement workout involving skiing or skiing movements and follow a yearly cycle that peaks you for the season, and includes both sprint or hill work and endurance skiing.

Days per week: 3, with 1 day rest between workouts. A specific movement workout counts as 1 workout day.

exercises	sets	reps	exercises	sets	reps
1 p.287 top	4	10-10-8-8	**Optional** p.211 bottom	2	Max. 10 per set, then add weight
Optional p.290 top	2	10-10 each side	**5** p.275 bottom	3	10-10-8
Optional p.293 middle	2	15-15	**Optional** p.274 top	2	10-8
Optional p.292 bottom	2	15-15	**6** p.249 top	4	10-10-8-8
2 p.298 middle	2	10-10 each leg	**7** p.253 bottom	3	Max. 15 per set, then add weight
3 p.298 top	2	10-10 each leg	**Optional** p.219 top	2	10-8 each arm
Optional p.242 top	2-3	15 to 20 per set	**8** p.201 middle	1-2	15 to 30 per set
4 p.202 top	3	10-8-8	**Optional** p.190 middle	1	25

Skiing (Cross-Country) In-Season Program

This program is designed to maintain strength levels achieved during the off- and pre-season programs. The three weekly workouts may be divided among weight training and specific movement training.

Days per week: 2 days weight training and 1 day specific movement workout or 1 day weight training and 2 days specific movement workout or 1 day of each—depending on your schedule. Rest 2 days before competition.

exercises	sets	reps	exercises	sets	reps
1 p.290 top	3	10-10-10 each side	**4** p.215 bottom	1-2	10 (8)
Optional p.289 middle	1-2	10 to 12 per set each side	**5** p.211 bottom	2	10-8
2 p.298 middle	2	10-10 each leg	**6** p.302 middle	2	10-10
3 p.298 top	2	10-10 each leg	**Optional** p.201 top	1-2	10 to 15 per set each leg
Optional p.244	2	10-10			

Additional exercises:
1. Machines may be substituted
2. Dumbbells may be substituted
3. Deadlift
4. Seated lat rows
5. Running arm motion with dumbbells
6. Poling motion (double or diagonal) with dumbbells
7. Dumbbell lat rows
8. Step-ups with weight
9. Good mornings
10. Stride jumps (with weight if needed)
11. Rotary torso work

Exercise options:
1. Roller skis
2. Circuit training in the weight room, gym or outdoors
3. A cross-country ergometer
4. Plyometric exercises
5. Conditioning: running, sprints, agility, hills, stairs, basketball, swimming, biking

Problem areas:

Use a year-round stretching program to maximize flexibility. □

SKIING (DOWNHILL)

By John McMurtry, M.A., Head Technical Coach 1980-1984, U.S. Women's Alpine Ski Team & U.S. Olympic Women's Alpine Ski Team; John Atkins, M.S., Head Conditioning Coach, U.S. Olympic Women's Alpine Ski Team; Topper Hagerman, Ph.D., Head Conditioning Coach and Team Exercise Physiologist, U.S. Olympic Men's Alpine Ski Team. In 1984 the U.S. won three gold and two silver medals in alpine skiing at the Winter Olympics in Sarajevo, Yugoslavia.

Our athletes use weight training to develop greater strength and endurance, and to improve overall athletic performance. Also, since alpine skiing is such a high-risk sport, we use weight training to help prevent injuries.

Alpine skiing requires total strength development of the legs, thighs, gluteals, hips, abdominals and lower back. Both power and muscular endurance are essential.

We also recommend a static stretching program using a partner for increased flexibility, and maintaining a good aerobic base through running or cycling. Football-type agility drills and martial arts workouts are also valuable training methods.

An innovative training tool is the S.P.O.R.T. CORD, an elastic stretch cord device. It is particularly valuable for strength and muscle endurance training. The 1/3 knee dips, lateral agility exercise and adductor/abductor exercise are excellent for skiers in training. For information write S.P.O.R.T., P.O. Box 731004, South Lake Tahoe, Calif. 95731.

Aims: To develop muscle balance, and to strengthen all major muscle groups. A stronger, better conditioned athlete is less susceptible to injury.

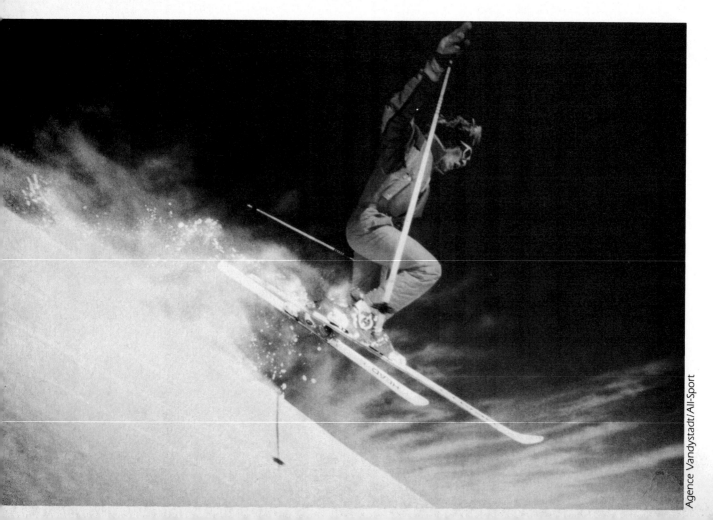

Agence Vandystadt/All-Sport

Skiing (Downhill) Off-Season Program

This program is designed to strengthen all major muscle groups, and create muscle balance. Follow this program until pre-season workouts begin.

Days per week: 3, with 1 day rest between workouts.

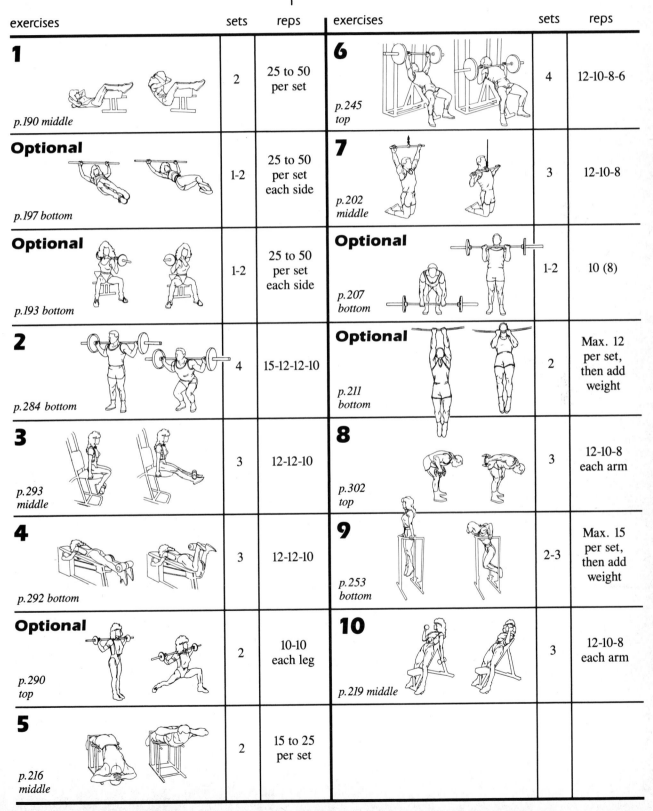

exercises	sets	reps	exercises	sets	reps
1 p.190 middle	2	25 to 50 per set	**6** p.245 top	4	12-10-8-6
Optional p.197 bottom	1-2	25 to 50 per set each side	**7** p.202 middle	3	12-10-8
Optional p.193 bottom	1-2	25 to 50 per set each side	**Optional** p.207 bottom	1-2	10 (8)
2 p.284 bottom	4	15-12-12-10	**Optional** p.211 bottom	2	Max. 12 per set, then add weight
3 p.293 middle	3	12-12-10	**8** p.302 top	3	12-10-8 each arm
4 p.292 bottom	3	12-12-10	**9** p.253 bottom	2-3	Max. 15 per set, then add weight
Optional p.290 top	2	10-10 each leg	**10** p.219 middle	3	12-10-8 each arm
5 p.216 middle	2	15 to 25 per set			

GETTING STRONGER ©1986 Bill Pearl & Shelter Publications, Inc.

Skiing (Downhill) Pre-Season Program

This program begins 4-6 weeks prior to the start of the season. It is designed to maximize strength gains in preparation for competition. You will also be skiing during this time.

Days per week: 3, with 1 day rest between workouts.

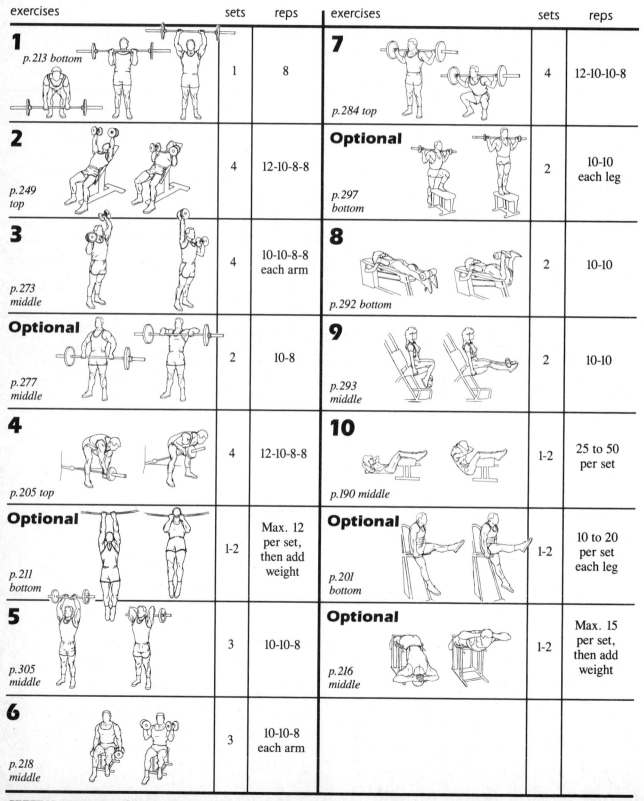

exercises	sets	reps	exercises	sets	reps
1 p.213 bottom	1	8	**7** p.284 top	4	12-10-10-8
2 p.249 top	4	12-10-8-8	**Optional** p.297 bottom	2	10-10 each leg
3 p.273 middle	4	10-10-8-8 each arm	**8** p.292 bottom	2	10-10
Optional p.277 middle	2	10-8	**9** p.293 middle	2	10-10
4 p.205 top	4	12-10-8-8	**10** p.190 middle	1-2	25 to 50 per set
Optional p.211 bottom	1-2	Max. 12 per set, then add weight	**Optional** p.201 bottom	1-2	10 to 20 per set each leg
5 p.305 middle	3	10-10-8	**Optional** p.216 middle	1-2	Max. 15 per set, then add weight
6 p.218 middle	3	10-10-8 each arm			

GETTING STRONGER ©1986 Bill Pearl & Shelter Publications, Inc.

Skiing (Downhill) In-Season Program

This program is designed to maintain strength levels achieved during the off- and pre-season programs. If you are traveling a lot, devise a workout that you can do in your room. If you have the time, include hip work, standing toe raises, leg flexions and extensions, and other exercise options in your program.

Days per week: 2, with 1-2 days rest between workouts and 2 days before competitions.

exercises	sets	reps	exercises	sets	reps
1 p.296 bottom	3	10-10-8	**Optional** p.249 top	2	10-8
Optional p.293 middle	2	10-10	**4** p.202 top	3	10-10-8
Optional p.292 bottom	2	10-10	**5** p.253 bottom	3	Max. 10 per set, then add weight
2 p.207 bottom	2	10-8	**6** p.201 bottom	1-2	15 to 25 per set each leg
3 p.216 middle	1-2	Max. 15 per set, then add weight			

Additional exercises:

1. Dumbbells may be substituted
2. Machines may be substituted
3. Deadlift
4. Dumbbell lat rows
5. Free-hand squats
6. Good mornings
7. Jump squats to tuck position
8. Rotary torso
9. Triceps press downs

Exercise options:

1. Circuit training in the weight room or outdoors
2. Plyometric exercises: depth jumping, box jumping, bounding, jump touches
3. Running: distance, sprints, agility, stadiums, hills
4. Other conditioning: swimming, basketball, racquetball
5. Dry-season skiing, roller skiing, artificial snow

Problem areas:

1. Pay attention to knee, ankle and hip joints; program will strengthen surrounding musculature.
2. Use a year-round total body flexibility program, static or PNF.
3. Torso work will condition and strengthen abdominals or low back.□

SOCCER

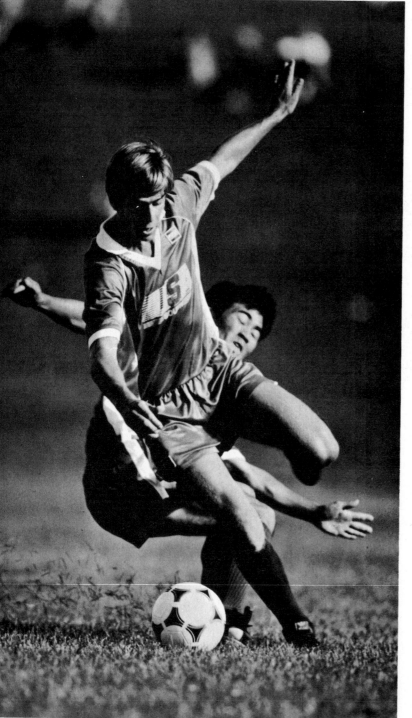

Steve E. Sutton/duomo

By Horst Richardson, Men's Varsity Soccer Coach, Colorado College, Colorado Springs, CO, Far West Coach of the Year, 1982-83

Soccer requires muscular endurance, a great deal of strength in the lower body and proper muscle balance throughout the entire body. Soccer players must be able to jump, accelerate with power, change direction quickly, and have high levels of coordination, agility and endurance. The knee joint must be protected from injury by strengthening surrounding muscle groups.

Flexibility, agility and stretching exercises are an important part of our routine. (We work with our college dance department on these skills.) On the field our players do stretching exercises using their own body weight or a partner's body as resistance.

Different players need to emphasize different muscle groups:
- *Goalkeepers:* Leg and thigh strength, upper body and shoulder strength, jumping ability
- *Strikers and stopper backs:* Leg and thigh strength for jumping, neck strength for head balls.
- *Outside fullbacks, wings and mid-fielders:* Legs and thighs for strength, muscular endurance and cardio-vascular endurance

Aims: Our soccer players use weight training to:
- Develop strength
- Develop local muscle endurance
- Prevent injuries
- Rehabilitate after injuries

Soccer Off-Season Program

This program is designed to create muscle balance and strength throughout the body and prepare you for the in-season program.

Days per week: 3, with 1 day rest between workouts.

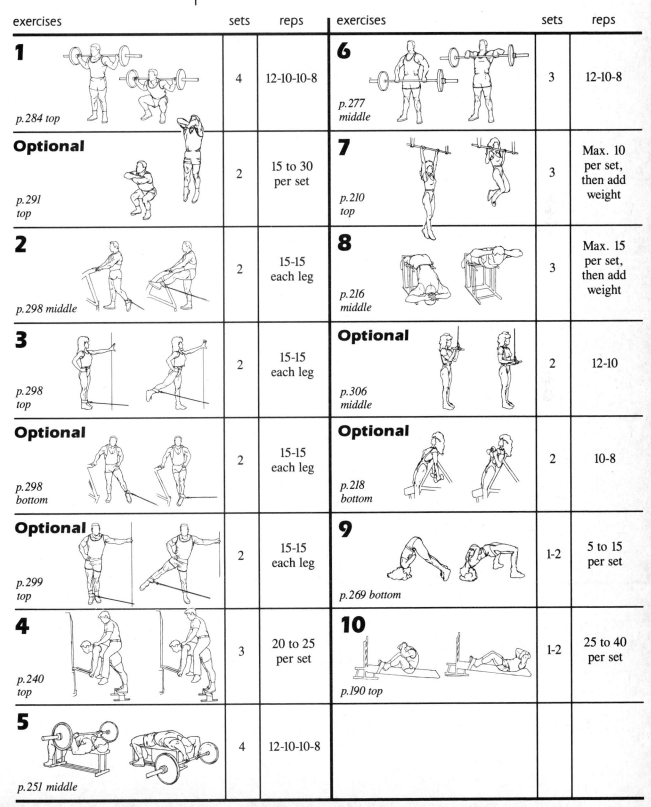

exercises	sets	reps	exercises	sets	reps
1 p.284 top	4	12-10-10-8	**6** p.277 middle	3	12-10-8
Optional p.291 top	2	15 to 30 per set	**7** p.210 top	3	Max. 10 per set, then add weight
2 p.298 middle	2	15-15 each leg	**8** p.216 middle	3	Max. 15 per set, then add weight
3 p.298 top	2	15-15 each leg	**Optional** p.306 middle	2	12-10
Optional p.298 bottom	2	15-15 each leg	**Optional** p.218 bottom	2	10-8
Optional p.299 top	2	15-15 each leg	**9** p.269 bottom	1-2	5 to 15 per set
4 p.240 top	3	20 to 25 per set	**10** p.190 top	1-2	25 to 40 per set
5 p.251 middle	4	12-10-10-8			

GETTING STRONGER ©1986 Bill Pearl & Shelter Publications, Inc.

Soccer In-Season Program

This program is designed to maintain muscle strength and balance levels built in the off-season.

Days per week: 2, with 1-2 days rest between each workout, and 2 days before a game.

exercises	sets	reps	exercises	sets	reps
1 p.296 bottom	3	12-12-10	**Optional** p.269 bottom	1-2	5 to 15 per set
2 p.243 bottom	3	20 to 25 per set	**5** p.293 middle	2	15-12
3 p.213 bottom	2	10-8	**6** p.292 bottom	2	15-12
4 p.251 top	2	12-10	**7** p.190 middle	1	25 to 50
Optional p.253 bottom	2	Max. 12 per set, then add weight			

Additional exercises:

1. Dumbbells may be substituted
2. Machines may be substituted
3. Ankle (inversion-eversion) work
4. Leg raises and hip flexor work with surgical tube or pulley
5. Step-ups with weight
6. Seated lat rows
7. Incline bench press
8. Lunges
9. Wide grip front lat pull-down
10. Free-hand squats
11. Seated free-hand neck resistance
12. Good mornings

Exercise options:

1. Circuit training in the weight room or on-the-field conditioning using soccer skills, agility, sprints, etc.
2. Plyometric exercises: depth jumping, box jumps, bounding
3. Running or hopping up stadium steps or stairs

Problem areas:

1. Overwork of lower body: pay attention to leg fatigue and pain; adjust workouts accordingly.
2. Stretch year-round for maximum flexibility.□

SWIMMING

By James E. "Doc" Counsilman, Ph.D., Coach, Indiana University (6 NCAA titles, 23 Big Ten Conference titles); Coach, Olympic Men's Swim Team 1964, 1976; swam the English Channel at age 58. Author of Science of Swimming *and* The Complete Book of Swimming.

My athletes use weight training to increase strength and explosive power. By increasing strength, they can also increase endurance. If you have to use every motor unit to pull your arm through the water at the desired speed to swim fast, you'll tire quickly. But if you can improve your strength to the point where you only need to use a portion of the motor units, you can alternate motor units and thereby improve your strength endurance.

All swimmers need strength, explosive power and endurance in the arm depressors, arm medial rotators, elbow extensors (mainly triceps), wrist flexors, leg and ankle extensors (for turns and starts), abdominals and back (for fixation of the hips) and the arm elevator muscles (deltoids). Breaststrokers also need to emphasize work on the leg adductors.

Swimmers must keep their elbows high on the pull, and therefore need strong arm rotator (medial) muscles. These are often the most neglected muscles for swimmers. But it is essential to strengthen the rotator cuff muscles by doing this arm rotator exercise:
- Lie on back, elbows on floor.
- Grasp barbell, hands just wider than shoulders, with bar just behind head, elbows bent.
- Keeping elbows bent, bring bar forward, not up, in semicircular motion until forearms are vertical to floor.

Since explosive power is so important to swimmers, we use a biokinetic swim bench that permits variable resistance and has acceleration programmed into it so the swimmer simulates the acceleration pattern of champion swimmers. I believe it improves explosive power because we do much of our exercising on the device at a fast speed.

My swimmers also do stretching exercises for the ankles and shoulders, and use an isokinetic leaper (60-120 jumps in sets of 30—keep back straight to avoid injury—3-5 days a week) to improve jumping ability for starts.

Aims: To strengthen all the major muscle groups and to develop proper muscle balance.

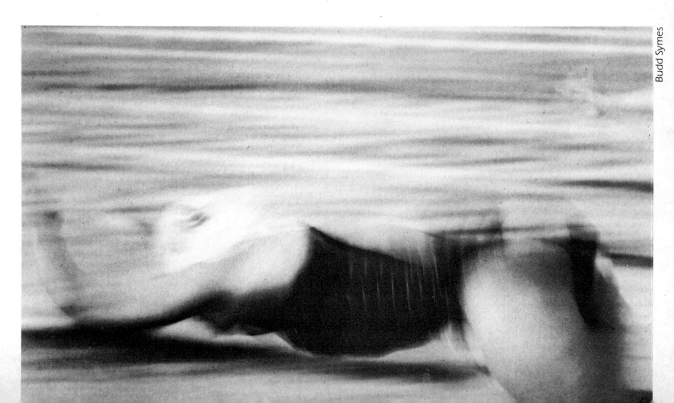

Budd Symes

Swimming Off-Season Program

This program is designed to increase strength and create proper muscle balance. The program should last from late spring to late summer, or until you begin the pre-season program.

Days per week: 3, with 1 day rest between workouts.

Supersets: Do the first set of exercise 1(a), then immediately do the first set of exercise 1(b). Rest 1-2 minutes, then go on to second set of 1(a), 1(b). Follow this format for the prescribed number of sets and reps.

exercises	sets	reps	exercises	sets	reps
1 (a) p.190 middle	1-2	25 to 50 per set	**4** (a) p.306 middle	3	12-10-8
(b) p.216 middle	1-2	15 to 25 per set	(b) p.229 top	3	10-8-8
2 (a) p.249 top	4	12-10-8-8	**5** (a) p.293 middle	3	15-15-15
(b) p.202 middle	4	12-10-8-8	(b) p.292 bottom	3	10-10-10
Optional (a) p.256 top	3	12-10-8	**6** (a) p.298 middle	2	15-10 per set each leg
Optional (b) p.274 top	3	12-10-8	(b) p.298 top	2	15-10 per set each leg
3 (a) p.275 bottom	3	12-10-8	**Optional** (a) p.199 bottom	1	25 to 50 each leg
(b) p.274 bottom	3	12-10-8	**Optional** (b) p.197 bottom	1	25 to 50 each leg

Swimming Pre-Season Program

This program is designed to build as much strength as possible heading into the season, and lasts 4-8 weeks.

If it is available to you, now is the time to utilize an isokinetic circuit one day each week as a substitute for weight training.

Days per week: 3, with 1 day rest between workouts.

Supersets: Do the first set of exercise 1(a), then immediately do the first set of exercise 1(b). Rest 1-2 minutes, then go on to second set of 1(a), 1(b). Follow this format for the prescribed number of sets and reps.

exercises	sets	reps	exercises	sets	reps
1 (a) p.194 top	1-2	20 to 50 per set	**4** (a) p.305 middle	3	10-8-8
(b) p.195 middle	1-2	15 to 35 per set	(b) p.222 top	3	10-8-8 each arm
2 (a) p.256 top	4	10-8-8-8	**5** (a) p.290 bottom	3	10-10-10 each leg
(b) p.277 middle	4	10-8-8-8	(b) p.298 middle	3	10-10-10
Optional (a) p.248 bottom	3	10-8-8	**6** (a) p.290 middle	3	10-10-10 each leg
Optional (b) p.203 middle	3	10-8-8	(b) p.291 bottom	3	20-25-30
3 (a) p.278 top	3	10-8-8	**Optional** (a) p.198 top	1	25 to 50 each leg
(b) p.279 middle	3	10-8-8	**Optional** (b) p.199 top	1	25 to 50 each leg

GETTING STRONGER ©1986 Bill Pearl & Shelter Publications, Inc.

Swimming In-Season

There are different philosophies about weight training during the season. Some programs cut their swimmers back to a maintenance program. The maintenance program is done twice a week with 1-2 days between workouts, and at least 2 days before competitions. The maintenance program cuts back on the number of exercises (3 sets of each, 6-10 reps). For an effective maintenance program, find the one exercise for each major muscle group that will work best for you during your in-season program. For example:

1. Dumbbell bench press (chest)
2. Upright rowing (shoulders)
3. Arm curls (biceps)
4. Squats (thighs)
5. Standing toe raises (calves)
6. Abdominal crunches (abdominals)

These exercises comprise one possible, effective in-season maintenance program.

Some coaches prefer that their swimmers use less weight and combine some basic exercises with a circuit program during the season. Other coaches prefer using a mixture of free weights and isokinetics, working toward *all* isokinetics by the end of the season.

Swimmers need to get together with their coaches to design the best program for them. But remember, make sure to do some type of strength training in-season. You need to maintain most of the strength gains of the off- and pre-season programs in order to maximize performance. Take at least 1 day off between workouts, and at least 2 days prior to competitions.

Additional exercises:

1. Biokinetic or isokinetic machines with pulleys so you can simulate exact stroke movement with resistance and feedback
2. Pulleys, cables or tubing to simulate stroke with resistance
3. Dumbbells may be substituted
4. Machines may be substituted
5. Dumbbell shoulder flys
6. Straight arm pull-overs
7. Standing wrist rolls
8. Seated wrist curls

Exercise options:

1. Circuit training in weight room or an isokinetic circuit
2. Out-of-water conditioning: basketball, agility circuit, interval sprints

Problem areas:

1. Stretch year-round for maximum flexibility.
2. Do flexibility and strengthening exercises for rotator cuff.
3. Do varied types of swimming year-round: distance, intervals, speed work. □

TENNIS

By Bill Wright, *Men's Tennis Coach, University of Arizona; formerly Coach at University of California at Berkeley; NCAA Coach of the Year, 1980; Pac-10 Conference Coach of the Year, 1982; author of* Aerobic Tennis. *The Cal Bears won the 1980 National Indoor Team Championship.*

All my athletes participate in a weight training program with three goals in mind:
1. Increased development of upper body and offhand strength
2. Overall endurance and explosiveness
3. Cardiovascular development with overloaded circuit training and aerobic dance classes

Different strokes require strength in different areas:
- *All shots*—strengthen the oblique or "twisting muscles," because all shots require twisting
- *Serving and overheads*—strengthen lower back
- *Volleying*—strengthen the forearms

You can never be too fit. My athletes do a wide variety of activities to get an edge on their opponents: throwing and catching a medicine ball, hopping and running stadium steps, short sprints, direction-changing sprints, aerobic dance classes.

Aims: To strengthen all major muscle groups, create proper muscle balance and prevent injuries.

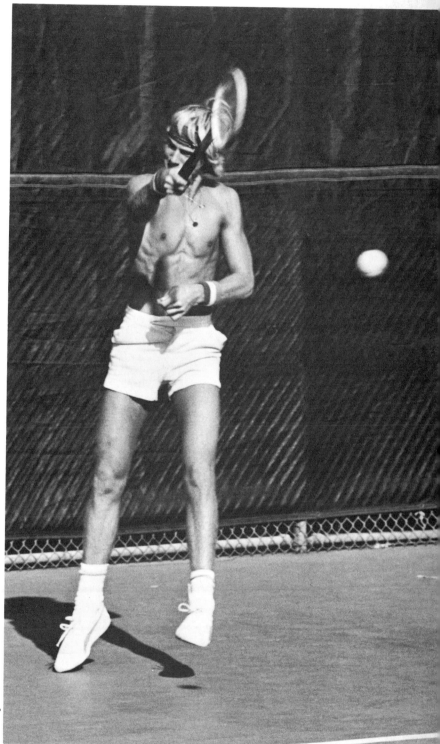

Budd Symes

Tennis Off-Season Program

Variations on this program can be made after consultation between coach and player and determination of the player's muscle balance and strength level. The off-season program may vary due to weather, location and facilities.

Days per week: 3, with 1 day rest between workouts.

Pre-Season: If time allows, you can follow a pre-season program for 4-6 weeks designed to focus on maximum strength gains. To do this, follow the off-season program, but increase the weights and decrease the reps. This is also the time to build up maximum cardiovascular endurance with on-court conditioning.

exercises	sets	reps	exercises	sets	reps
1 p.190 top	1-2	25 to 50 per set	**Optional** p.214 bottom	2	12-10
2 p.193 bottom	1	25 to 50 each side	**7** p.253 bottom	2-3	Max. 15 per set, then add weight
3 p.213 top	1-2	15 per set each side	**Optional** p.218 middle	1-2	10 per set
Optional p.216 middle	1-2	Max. 15 per set, then add weight	**8** p.259 bottom	2	15-20
4 p.250 top	3	12-10-10	**Optional** p.259 middle	1-2	15 per set
Optional p.250 bottom	1-2	12 (10)	**9** p.291 top	2-3	15 to 20 per set
5 p.279 bottom	2-3	12-10 (10)	**Optional** p.290 top	1-2	10 per set each leg
6 p.204 top	3	12-10-10	**Optional** p.289 middle	1-2	10 per set each leg

GETTING STRONGER ©1986 Bill Pearl & Shelter Publications, Inc.

Tennis In-Season Program

This is designed to maintain the strength levels acquired during the off- and/or pre-season.

Days per week: 2, with 1-2 days rest between workouts and 2 days rest before matches.

exercises		sets	reps	exercises		sets	reps
1 p.197 bottom		1	20 to 40 each side	**5** p.202 top		2	12-10
2 p.191 top		1	15 to 30	**Optional** p.306 middle		1-2	12 (10)
3 p.248 bottom		2	12-10	**6** p.297 bottom		2	12 to 15 per set each leg
Optional p.251 bottom		1-2	12 (10)	**Optional** p.289 middle		1	10 each leg
4 p.275 bottom		2	12-10	**Optional** p.263 top		1	Floor to top

Additional exercises:

1. Dumbbells may be substituted
2. Machines may be substituted
3. Bent-over barbell twist
4. Nautilus shoulder flys
5. Hand grippers or tennis balls
6. Bent-over low pulley rear deltoid raise
7. Nautilus pull-overs
8. Medicine ball work—rotational
9. Stroke work with surgical tubing
10. Stroke work with light dumbbells

Exercise options:

1. Circuit training and par course training
2. Weighted racquets
3. Stairs and stadiums for agility, footwork or cardio-vascular endurance
4. Plyometrics: depth jumping
5. Short sprints and agility runs
6. Running the lines on tennis courts—up, back, across
7. Overload on-court workouts
8. Aerobics dance classes
9. Isokinetic training

Problem areas:

1. Stretch year-round for maximum flexibility.
2. Make sure you do enough torso work: abdominals, obliques or erector spinal (lower back). □

TRACK AND FIELD

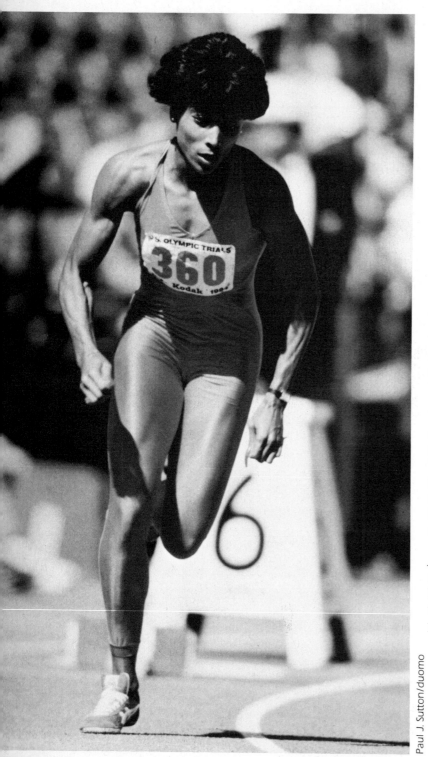

Paul J. Sutton/duomo

By Sam Adams, Head Coach, University of California at Santa Barbara; Coach, U.S. Olympic Decathletes, 1984.

Strength and explosiveness in track and field are more important than in just about any other sport. For this reason, a well-designed weight training program is especially important for track and field athletes. In track and field, each event has its own special demands, and must have its own strength development program to meet these demands. I also feel that strength development has a direct relationship to endurance development.

Tailor your weight training program to your event. Throwers need significant leg and trunk strength. Sprinters and jumpers need significant leg strength. Middle distance and distance runners need upper body development and flexibility. All track and field athletes should include a comprehensive stretching program, based on static stretching or PNF concepts (see p. 67), in their program.

At U.C. Santa Barbara, we use a 10-exercise circuit weight training program for general conditioning and toning. This prepares the athlete for the more intensive off-season and in-season weight training programs where the focus will be more closely tailored to the specific demands of each event.

Aims: Generally, to strengthen all major muscle groups and develop muscle balance; specifically, to strengthen those muscle groups used in the athlete's particular event.

Track & Field Circuit Weight Training Program For All Athletes

This is a balanced program aimed at developing power, muscular endurance, cardiovascular endurance and flexibility. Whatever your event, follow this program for four weeks before starting your off-season program.

Use approximately 60% on all lifts. Start with any of the exercises shown and stay in the sequence shown. If possible, work in groups of three; when all have completed the exercise, move immediately to the next station and begin.

Try to complete the circuit three times in one hour or less.

Days per week: 3, with 1 day rest between workouts.

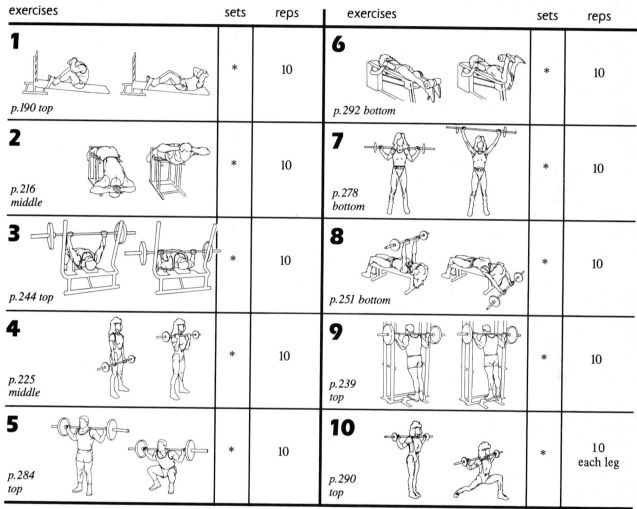

exercises	sets	reps	exercises	sets	reps
1 p.190 top	*	10	**6** p.292 bottom	*	10
2 p.216 middle	*	10	**7** p.278 bottom	*	10
3 p.244 top	*	10	**8** p.251 bottom	*	10
4 p.225 middle	*	10	**9** p.239 top	*	10
5 p.284 top	*	10	**10** p.290 top	*	10 each leg

*Do one set of Exercise 1, then one set of Exercise 2, etc., until all 10 are completed. Do this three times.

Note: Although free weights are shown here, this program (except for lunges) can also be done on a Universal-type multi-station machine.

Track & Field - Sprinters, Jumpers, Hurdlers Off-Season Program

Begin this after 4 weeks of "Circuit Weight Training Program" on previous page. Follow this program until season begins.

Days per week: 3, with 1-2 days rest between workouts and at least 2 before meets.

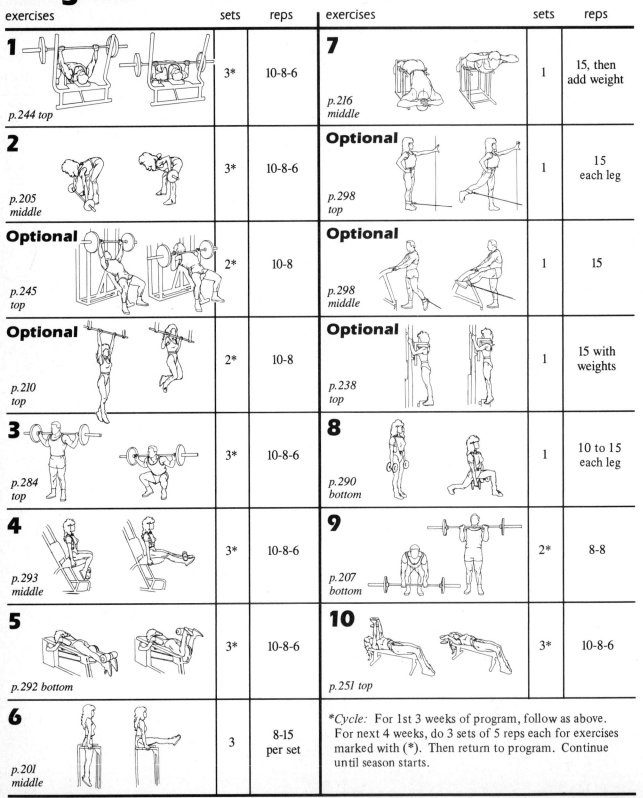

exercises	sets	reps	exercises	sets	reps
1 p.244 top	3*	10-8-6	**7** p.216 middle	1	15, then add weight
2 p.205 middle	3*	10-8-6	**Optional** p.298 top	1	15 each leg
Optional p.245 top	2*	10-8	**Optional** p.298 middle	1	15
Optional p.210 top	2*	10-8	**Optional** p.238 top	1	15 with weights
3 p.284 top	3*	10-8-6	**8** p.290 bottom	1	10 to 15 each leg
4 p.293 middle	3*	10-8-6	**9** p.207 bottom	2*	8-8
5 p.292 bottom	3*	10-8-6	**10** p.251 top	3*	10-8-6
6 p.201 middle	3	8-15 per set			

Cycle: For 1st 3 weeks of program, follow as above. For next 4 weeks, do 3 sets of 5 reps each for exercises marked with (*). Then return to program. Continue until season starts.

Track & Field - Sprinters, Jumpers, Hurdlers In-Season Program

To maintain strength gains of off-season program, sets and reps are here cut back to maintenance level. Increase weight and reduce reps for more strength. Circuit training can be continued if desired.

Days per week: 2 with 1-2 days rest between workouts and at least 2 before meets.

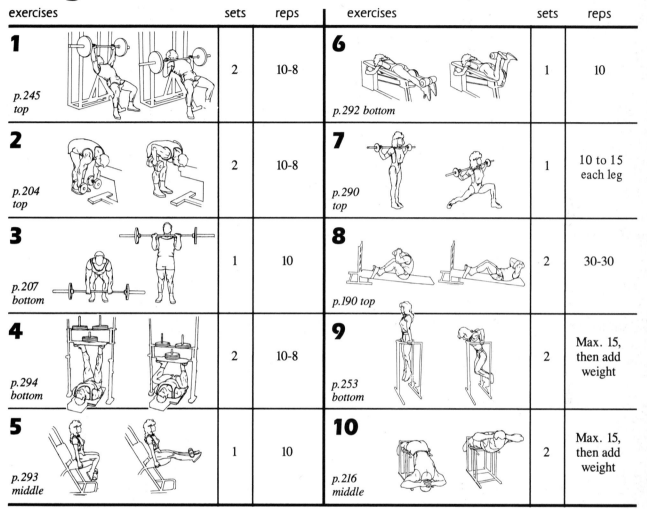

exercises	sets	reps	exercises	sets	reps
1 p.245 top	2	10-8	**6** p.292 bottom	1	10
2 p.204 top	2	10-8	**7** p.290 top	1	10 to 15 each leg
3 p.207 bottom	1	10	**8** p.190 top	2	30-30
4 p.294 bottom	2	10-8	**9** p.253 bottom	2	Max. 15, then add weight
5 p.293 middle	1	10	**10** p.216 middle	2	Max. 15, then add weight

Additional exercises:

1. Dumbbells may be substituted
2. Machines may be substituted
3. Step ups with weight
4. Good mornings
5. Rotary torso work
6. Clean and jerk
7. Dumbbell flys
8. Close grip bench press
9. Chest shoulder press

Problem Areas:

1. Stretch year-round for maximum flexibility.
2. Conditioning: Do some type of running workouts year-round.
3. Joints: Pay attention to ankle and knee stress, let joints adapt gradually to work load. □

Exercise Options:

1. Plyometrics: bounding, box and depth jumping
2. Medicine ball exercises
3. Ask your coach

Track & Field Vaulters, Decathletes, Heptathletes Off-Season Program

Vaulters and competitors in multi-sport events need both upper and lower body strength. Begin this program after 4 weeks of the "Track & Field Circuit Weight Training Program."

Days per week: 3, with 1 day rest between workouts.

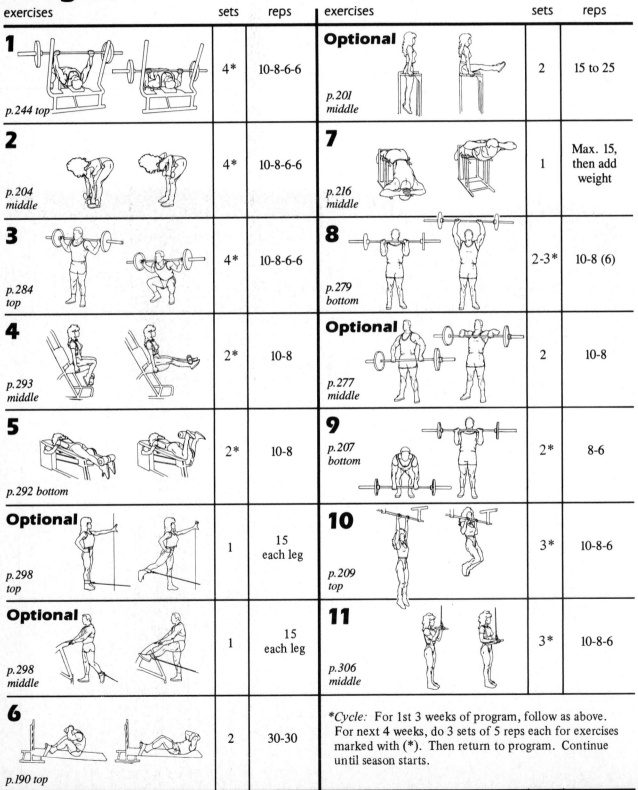

exercises		sets	reps	exercises		sets	reps
1 p.244 top		4*	10-8-6-6	**Optional** p.201 middle		2	15 to 25
2 p.204 middle		4*	10-8-6-6	**7** p.216 middle		1	Max. 15, then add weight
3 p.284 top		4*	10-8-6-6	**8** p.279 bottom		2-3*	10-8 (6)
4 p.293 middle		2*	10-8	**Optional** p.277 middle		2	10-8
5 p.292 bottom		2*	10-8	**9** p.207 bottom		2*	8-6
Optional p.298 top		1	15 each leg	**10** p.209 top		3*	10-8-6
Optional p.298 middle		1	15 each leg	**11** p.306 middle		3*	10-8-6
6 p.190 top		2	30-30				

Cycle: For 1st 3 weeks of program, follow as above. For next 4 weeks, do 3 sets of 5 reps each for exercises marked with (*). Then return to program. Continue until season starts.

Track & Field Vaulters, Decathletes, Heptathletes In-Season Program

Aim here is to maintain strength levels from off-season program. Exercises, sets and reps are cut back to a maintenance level. For greater strength, increase weights and reduce reps to 8-6(6). Circuit training is an option for additional in-season work.

Days per week: 2, with 1-2 days rest between workouts and at least 2 before meets.

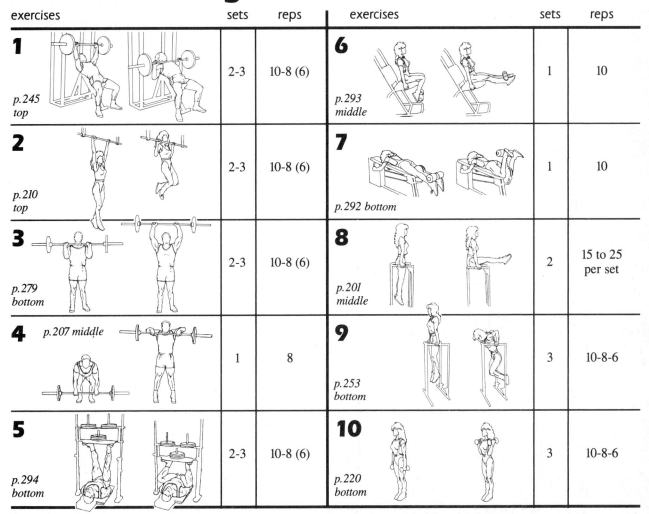

exercises		sets	reps	exercises		sets	reps
1 p.245 top		2-3	10-8 (6)	**6** p.293 middle		1	10
2 p.210 top		2-3	10-8 (6)	**7** p.292 bottom		1	10
3 p.279 bottom		2-3	10-8 (6)	**8** p.201 middle		2	15 to 25 per set
4 p.207 middle		1	8	**9** p.253 bottom		3	10-8-6
5 p.294 bottom		2-3	10-8 (6)	**10** p.220 bottom		3	10-8-6

Additional Exercises:

1. Dumbbells may be substituted
2. Machines may be substituted
3. Step ups with weight
4. Lunges with weight
5. Good mornings
6. Rotary torso work
7. Close-grip bench press
8. Dumbbell flys
9. Inverted pull-ups

Exercise Options:

1. Hang from chin bar. Raise body to upside-down vertical position. Tuck on way up. Keep arms straight.
2. Circuit training on the field with pole vault skills

3. Plyometrics, both upper and lower body
4. Medicine ball exercises
5. Pole vault skill practice year-round—running with pole, planting

Problem Areas:

1. Stretch year-round.
2. Cardiovascular conditioning. Run year-round (distance, interval, speedwork).
3. Joint stress and soreness from repeated pole plants (shoulders)
4. Endurance for long competitions, long waiting period between jumps. □

Track & Field Throwers Off-Season Program

This program emphasizes strength, power lifts and rotational work. In addition, you should do wrist and finger exercises as shown in the "Forearms" section. For three major lifts—the bench press, squat and power clean, follow a year-round cycle of changing sets and reps, as shown at lower right. With squats, exercise no. 5, alternate between holding barbell in back, as shown and in front as in Flat-Footed Barbell Front Squat (p. 287 middle).

Days per week: 3, with 1 day rest between workouts.

exercises		sets	reps	exercises		sets	reps
1 p.244 top		*	*	**9** p.213 top		1	10 to 20 ea. side
2 p.204 middle		4	10-8-6-4	**Optional** p.279 bottom		3	8-6-6
3 p.245 top		2-3	8-6 (6)	**Optional** p.277 bottom		3	10-10-8
4 p.210 top		2-3	8-6 (6)	**10** p.207 middle		*	*
5 p.284 top		*	*	**11** p.220 bottom		3	10-8-6
6 p.293 middle		2	10-8	**12** p.306 middle		3	10-8-6
7 p.292 bottom		2	10-8	Cycle: for Exercises marked (*) above			
				Sept., Oct., Nov.		4-5	8 to 10 per set
				Dec. (power phase)		6	8-6-5-3-3-1
8 p.190 top		2	30-30	Jan., Feb.		5	5 to 8 per set
				March, April, May, June: Follow In-Season Program			
				July, Aug.		3-6	10-8-6 (5) (3) (3)

Track & Field Throwers In-Season Program

This program is designed to maintain the strength levels gained during the off-season program. For three major lifts—power pulls, squats and bench press—follow a cycle from March through June as shown at bottom. The dates shown here can be modified to correspond to your actual season.

Days per week: 2, with 1-2 days rest between workouts and at least 2 days before meets.

exercises	sets	reps	exercises	sets	reps
1 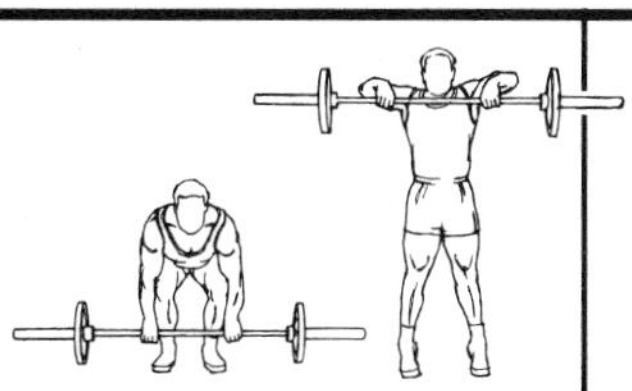 p.207 middle	*	*	**6** 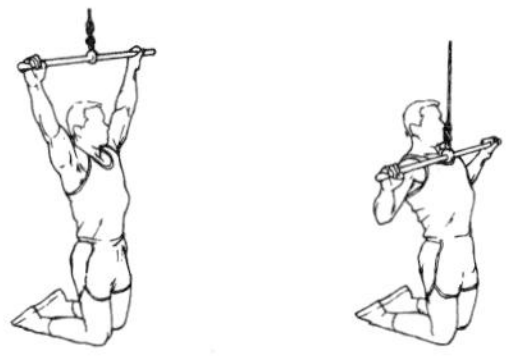 p.202 middle	3-4	10-8-6 (6)
2 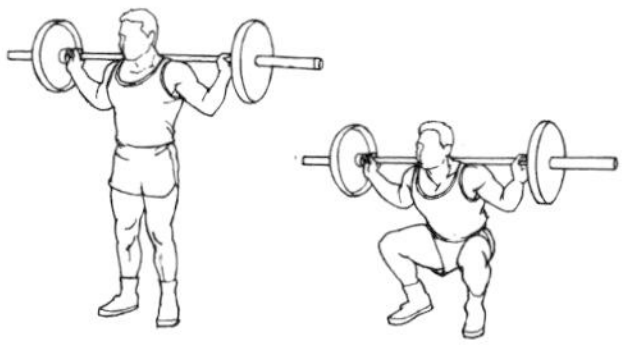 p.284 top	*	*	**7** 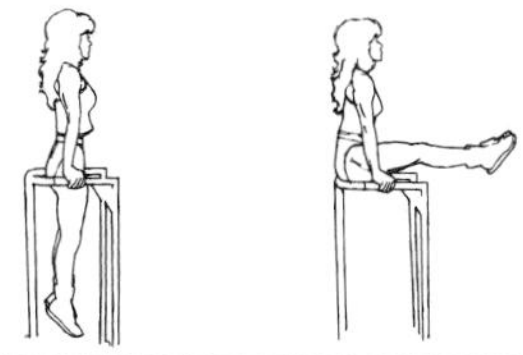 p.201 middle	2	10 to 20 per set
3 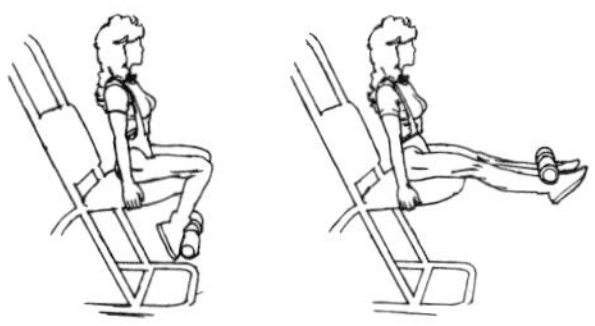 p.293 middle	1-2	10 (8)	**8** 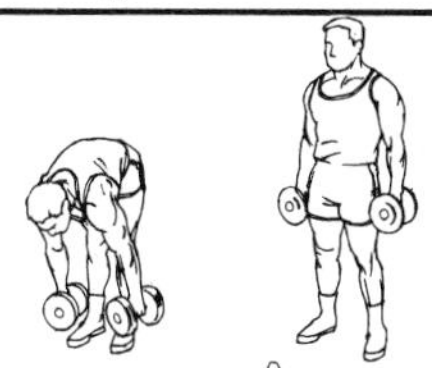 p.206 bottom	1-2	10 (10)
4 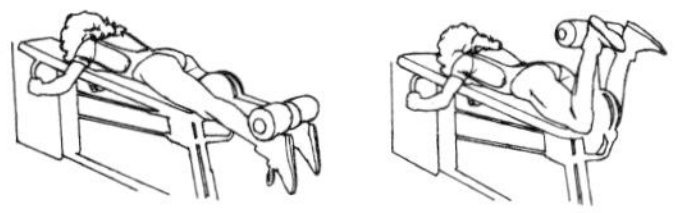 p.292 bottom	1-2	10 (8)	**9** 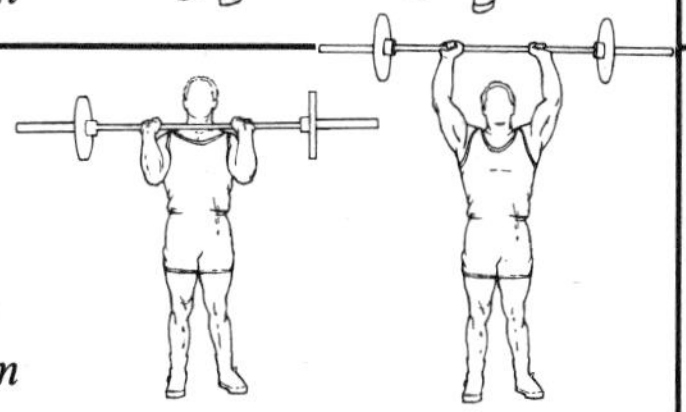 p.279 bottom	1-3	10 (8) (6)
5 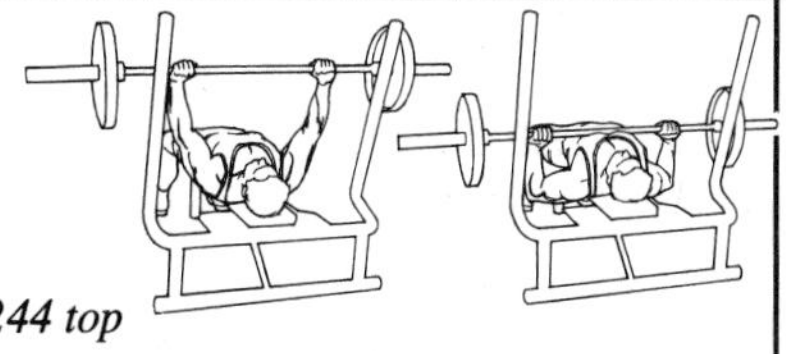 p.244 top	*	*	**10** 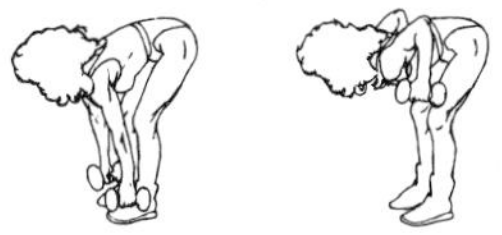 p.204 middle	1-3	10 (8) (6)

*Cycle:

March — 2-3 times per week, 6 sets of 10-8-6-5-3-3
April — 2-3 times per week, 3-5 sets of 5-3(3)-3(1)
May, June — 2 times per week, 3-4 sets of 5-3-3(1)

See next page for additional exercises, exercise options and problem areas for throwers.

Additional Exercises:

1. Dumbbells may be substituted
2. Machines may be substituted
3. Dumbbell and barbell wrist curls; wrist-roller wrist curl
4. Clean and jerk
5. Good mornings
6. Rotary torso work
7. Step ups with weight
8. Lunges with weight
9. Leg press
10. Close-grip bench press
11. Dumbbell or cable chest flys
12. Squeezing exercises: grippers, rubber balls
13. Fingertip push-ups
14. Toe raises

Exercise Options:

1. Circuit weight training program
2. Plyometrics, both upper and lower body
3. Medicine ball exercises
4. Skill movements: practice throwing movement skills year-round
5. Light implements for throwing
6. Split routines for upper and lower body on weight workout days
7. Bar rotations, hip turns, dumbbell turns, trunk twisters, footwork

Problem Areas:

1. Stretch year-round.
2. Some type of running workouts year-round.
3. Implements: throw light when doing 10's, heavy when 8's or 5's (winter)
   March-April: light implements for speed
   April-June: less throw per practice (adjust per individual)
   Sept-March: High volume throws (90-100 per practice)
4. Fingers, wrists & forearms: make sure they are strong and flexible.□

Budd Symes

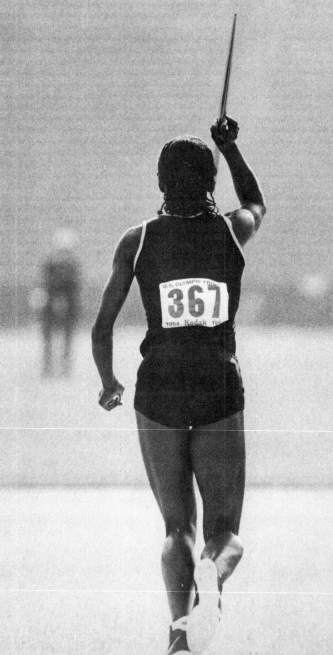

TRIATHLON

By Gary T. Moran, Ph.D., Human Anatomy and Kinesiology; M.S., Exercise Physiology; Runner and Triathlete.

A triathlete is subjected to an enormous amount of stress in training, and thus it's important to develop sufficient strength in order to prevent injuries. Muscular balance and flexibility are necessary to assure smooth, fluid, coordinated movements. This program will enable the tri-athlete to increase muscular strength, balance opposing muscle groups and help prevent injuries.

The triathlon strength training program is based on the following needs:
- *Bike:* arm and leg strength (endurance comes from on-bike training)
- *Swim:* upper body strength and stamina
- *Run:* total body strength

Work hardest on the event in which you are weakest. By the same token, concentrate your weight training on your weakest body part. For example:
- Shoulder and arm work for swimming and to prevent fatigue on bike
- Quad strength to prevent knee pain from cycling
- Lat work for added power in free-style arm pull
- Hip exercises for stamina and proper biomechanics in running.

Aims: To build muscular endurance, increase strength, balance major muscle groups and prevent injuries.

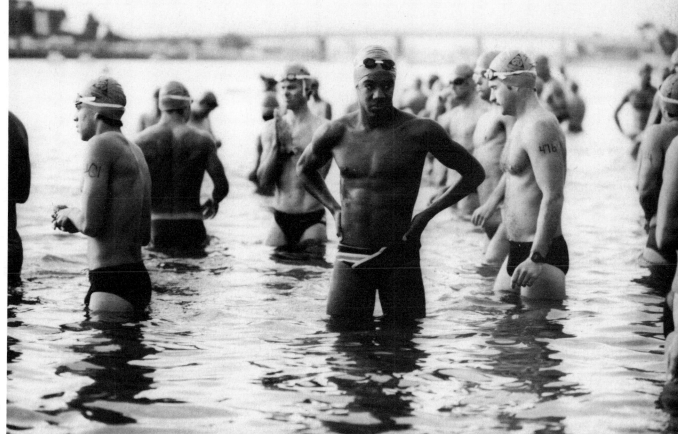

Budd Symes

Triathlon Off-Season Program

This program is designed to build strength and stamina and to prevent injuries.

Days per week: You can do either a regular routine or a split routine:
(a) *Regular routine:* 3 days per week, with 1 day rest between workouts
(b) *Split routine:* M-W-F, exercises 1-3; T-Th-Sat, exercises 4-7
   Caution: Don't overtrain. For example, don't do an upper body weight workout on your heavy swim day. Don't do a lower body weight workout on your heavy cycling or running day.

Supersets: Do the first set of exercise 1(a), then immediately do the first set of exercise 1(b). Rest 1-2 minutes, then go on to second set of 1(a), 1(b).

exercises		sets	reps	exercises		sets	reps
1 (a) *p.244 top*		3	10-10-8	**3** *p.190 top*		1-2	25 to 50 per set
(b) *p.202 bottom*		3	12-10-10 each arm	**4** *p.284 top*		3	12-10-10
Optional (a) *p.278 bottom*		3	12-10-10	**Optional** (a) *p.297 bottom*		2	10-10 each leg
Optional (b) *p.202 middle*		3	12-10-10	**Optional** (b) *p.289 middle*		1-2	10 to 15 per set each leg
Optional (a) *p.277 middle*		2	10-10	**5** (a) *p.293 middle*		3	12-10-8
Optional (b) *p.253 bottom*		2	10-10	(b) *p.292 bottom*		3	12-10-8
2 (a) *p.251 top*		3	12-10-10	**6** *p.213 top*		1	20 to 30 each side
(b) *p.219 middle*		3	12-10-8 each arm	**7** *p.194 middle*		1-2	15 to 25 per set

Triathlon In-Season Program

This program is designed to maintain the strength gains achieved during the off-season to maximize performance and prevent injuries.

Days per week: You can do either a regular routine or a split routine:
(a) *Regular routine:* 3 days per week, with 1 day rest between workouts
(b) *Split routine:* M-W-F, exercises 1-3; T-Th-Sat, exercises 4-7
  Caution: Don't overtrain. For example, don't do an upper body weight workout on your heavy swim day. Don't do a lower body weight workout on your heavy cycling or running day.

exercises	sets	reps	exercises	sets	reps
1 (a) p.248 bottom	2	10-10	**4** p.296 bottom	2	10-10
(b) p.214 top	2	10-10	**Optional** p.297 bottom	1	10 each leg
Optional (a) p.277 middle	1-2	10 (10)	**5** (a) p.293 middle	2	10-10
Optional (b) p.253 bottom	1-2	10 (10)	(b) p.292 bottom	2	10-10
2 (a) p.307 bottom	2	10-8	**Optional** (a) p.298 bottom	1	10 each leg
(b) p.218 middle	2	10-8	(b) p.299 top	1	10 each leg
3 p.190 middle	2	20 to 50	**6** p.298 middle	1	10 each side
Optional p.216 middle	1	15-25	**7** p.196 top	1-2	15 to 25 per set

Additional exercises:

1. Dumbbells may be substituted
2. Machines may be substituted
3. Lunges with weight
4. Seated lat row
5. Chins
6. Stiff-legged barbell deadlift
7. Neck, rotary torso and wrist work
8. Dumbbell flys
9. Straight arm pull-over

Exercise options:

1. Depth jumping
2. Box jumping
3. Running stadium steps
4. Stretching year-round for maximum flexibility
5. Circuit training
6. For swimming: biokinetic and isokinetic machines; pulleys, cables and tubing to simulate stroke with resistance

Problem areas:

1. Bike: wrists from grip, neck and lower back fatigue, shoulder soreness, knees (work medial quads)
2. Swim: shoulder flexibility and strength, knee and hip soreness
3. Run: joint soreness (ankle, knee, hip stress) from excessive pounding □

VOLLEYBALL

Budd Symes

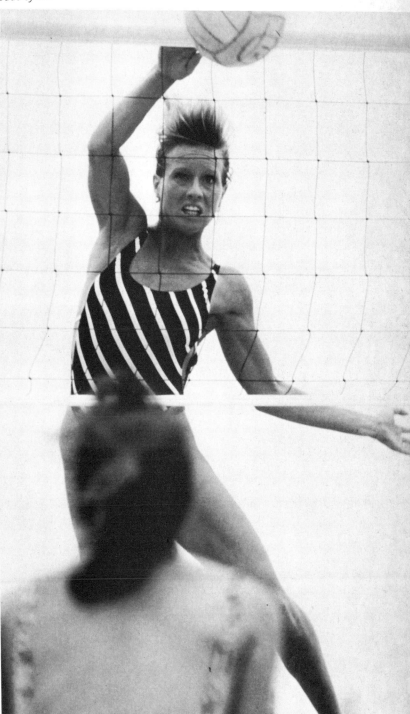

By Doug Beal, Ph.D., U.S.A. National Teams Director; Coach, 1984 Men's Olympic Volleyball team (gold medalists); 5-time U.S. Volleyball Association All-American while playing for U.S. National Team, 1970-1976; All-American and Big Ten Conference Most Valuable Player at Ohio State, 1969.

Our athletes all participate in a weight training program with goals of increasing strength, power and explosiveness. Because of the repetitive jumping required in volleyball, great emphasis is placed on lower body power. But we also work on the abdominals and core muscle stability.

National team volleyball players have a long season. They play year-round. In fact, in preparing for the Olympics, their season lasts for four solid years. Weight training is essential to survive such intensive training. Of course, high school, college and other teams have more typical seasons. All our players take part in:

1. *Jumping training:* Our most significant training. We do approach jumps, jumps with weighted tubes on shoulders, jumps over barriers, against resistance from elastic surgical tubing, etc. We do 300-500 jumps per each 45-minute session.
2. *Weight training:* I prefer free weights, but we also use machines. While we emphasize lower body power and strength, we also do shoulder and arm weight work for injury reduction.
3. *Interval running:* By running short bursts at high speeds, we increase endurance.

Aims: To increase and maintain strength levels, to create muscle balance, and to prevent injuries from intensive training.

Volleyball Off-Season Program

Start this program 1-2 weeks after the season ends.

Days per week: 3, with 1 day rest between workouts.

exercises	sets	reps	exercises	sets	reps
1 p.284 top	4	10-8-8-6	**Optional** p.252 top	1-2	15 to 30 per set on fingertips
2 p.291 top	2	15 to 30 per set	**7** p.222 top	3	10-8-8 each arm
3 p.248 bottom	4	10-8-8-6	**8** p.194 middle	1-2	10 to 25 per set
4 p.214 bottom	4	12-10-10-8	**Optional** p.195 top	1-2	15 to 25 per set
Optional p.202 top	2	10-10	**9** p.192 bottom	1	25 to 50 each side
Optional p.216 middle	1-2	Max. 15 per set, then add weight	**10** p.196 top	1	25 to 50
5 p.277 bottom	3	10-8-8	**Optional** p.198 bottom	1	25 to 50 each leg
6 p.306 middle	3	10-8-8	**Optional** p.201 top	1	10 to 20 each leg

Volleyball In-Season Program

This program is designed to maintain strength levels acquired during the off-season program.

Days per week: 2, with 1-2 days rest between workouts and 2 days rest before games.

exercises	sets	reps	exercises	sets	reps
1 *p.296 bottom*	3	12-12-10	**4** *p.202 top*	3	12-10-8
Optional *p.297 bottom*	2	12-10 each leg	**5** *p.301 top*	3	12-10-8 each arm
2 *p.251 top*	3	12-10-8	**Optional** *p.225 top*	2	15-15
3 *p.207 bottom*	2	10-8	**6** *p.195 top*	1-2	15 to 25 per set
Optional *p.248 bottom*	2	10-8	**Optional** *p.201 bottom*	1-2	10 to 20 per set each leg

Additional exercises:

1. Dumbbells may be substituted
2. Machines may be substituted
3. Chins
4. Seated lat row
5. Dumbbell lat rows
6. Leg extensions
7. Good mornings
8. Barbell shoulder shrug
9. Rotary torso work
10. Lunges with weight

Exercise options:

1. Circuit training in weight room or on-the-court conditioning (agility or footwork)
2. Plyometrics: box or depth jumping, weighted jumps, sponge jumps
3. Conditioning: stairs, stadium, form running, agility drills
4. Conditioning exercises that include all possible court movements

Problem areas:

1. Stretch year-round for maximum flexibility.
2. Watch out for knee pain in relation to work load.

WRESTLING

By Joe Seay, *Head Wrestling Coach, Oklahoma State University and Head Coach, 1985 U.S.A. World Team;* **Jerry Palmieri**, *Head Assistant Strength and Conditioning Coach, Oklahoma State University.*

There are 4 phases in our weight training program, and each phase has its own strength goal:
1. Off-season (mid-March to mid-October) — develop strength and power.
2. Pre-season (mid-October to January) — strength and power is maintained while the wrestlers are active in several tournaments.
3. In-season (January to mid-March)
   a) Lactic Acid (January to mid-February) — we attempt to acclimate the athletes' bodies to the buildup of lactic acid, a fatigue substance, during this busy time in a wrestler's season.
   b) Peaking (mid-February to mid-March) — by emphasizing strenuous muscular endurance through a circuit program, we try to peak the wrestlers for the conference and national championships.

Specifically, wrestlers need hip strength and power since many wrestling moves originate from the hips. Strength is also needed in the muscles responsible for pulling movements: biceps, forearms, mid-back and upper back. Wrestlers from each weight class follow the same strength program, except for the heavy-weights. Heavyweights have no weight limitation, so stay on a strength and power program to continue developing strength and lean body mass until the peaking phases, when they join the circuit program.

Our wrestlers also do intense interval running for endurance and longer slow runs (3-5 miles) for weight control.

Aims: To strengthen all the major muscle groups and to develop muscle balance. Special emphasis is placed on hips, thighs, neck and the pulling muscles.

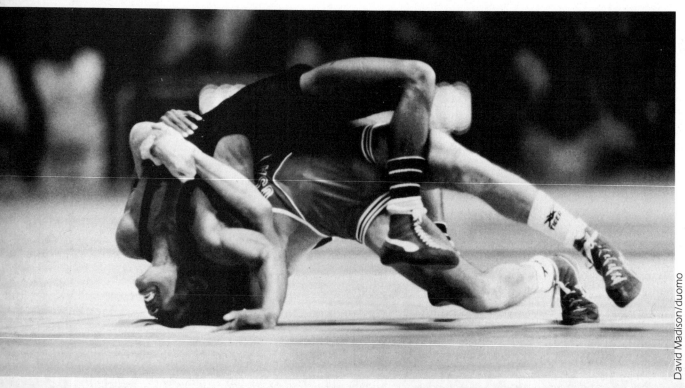

David Madison/duomo

Wrestling Off-Season Program

This program is designed to strengthen all major muscle groups and develop muscle balance.

Days per week: 3, with 1 day rest between workouts.

exercises		sets	reps	exercises		sets	reps
1 p.195 top		1-2	15 to 30 per set	**7** p.212 top		3	15-15-15
Optional p.193 bottom		1	25 to 50 each side	**Optional** p.250 bottom		1-2	12 (10)
2 p.216 middle		1-2	Max. 15 per set, then add weight	**8** p.306 middle		3	10-8-8
3 p.295 bottom		3	12-10-8	**9** p.229 top		3	10-8-8
4 p.253 top		3	10-8-8	**10** p.259 bottom		2	20-20
Optional p.244 top		2	8-8	**11** p.259 middle		2	15-15
5 p.275 bottom		3	10-8-8	**12** p.269 bottom		1-2	5 to 10 per set
6 p.214 bottom		3	12-10-8				

Wrestling Pre-Season Program

This program is designed to maximize strength.

Days per week: 3, with 1 day rest between workouts. (As wrestling and conditioning workouts increase, you may choose to cut back to 2 weight workouts per week.)

exercises	sets	reps	exercises	sets	reps
1 p.194 middle	1-2	15 to 30 per set	**7** p.305 bottom	3	10-8-8
Optional p.192 bottom	1	25 to 50 each side	**8** p.218 middle	3	10-8-8
2 p.201 middle	1-2	15 to 30 per set	**9** p.259 bottom	2	20-20
3 p.244 top	3	10-8-6	**10** p.259 middle	2	15-15
4 p.251 top	3	10-8-8	**11** p.289 bottom	3	10-10-10 each side
5 p.277 middle	3	10-8-6	**12** p.293 middle	3	10-10-10
6 p.214 top	3	12-10-8	**Optional** p.238 top	1-3	15 to 25 per set
Optional p.207 bottom	2	8-8			

GETTING STRONGER ©1986 Bill Pearl & Shelter Publications, Inc.

Wrestling In-Season Program

This program is designed to maintain strength levels achieved during the off- and pre-season programs. Different coaches employ different in-season programs. Some do strictly high-rep high-intensity circuit training, some combine one maintenance weight workout and one circuit workout and some use two maintenance weight workouts and let actual wrestling take care of the lactic acid and endurance-recovery work. The program here is one viable program. Be sure to consult with your coach.

Days per week: 2, with 2 days rest between workouts and at least 2 days rest before competitions.

exercises		sets	reps	exercises		sets	reps
1 p.190 top		1-2	20 to 50 per set	**6** p.204 middle		2	12-12
2 p.201 middle		1-2	15 to 25 per set	**7** p.215 top		3	10 to 15 per set
3 p.191 top		1	25 to 50	**8** p.306 top		3	10 to 15 per set
4 p.245 top		3	12-10-10	**9** p.293 middle		2-3	15-15 (15)
5 p.251 top		3	12-10-10	**10** p.292 bottom		2-3	10-10 (10)

Additional exercises:

1. Machines may be substituted
2. Dumbbells may be substituted
3. Power pulls
4. Dead lift
5. Rotary torso work
6. Chest flys
7. Step-ups with weight
8. Grip strength: rubber ball, hand gripper
9. Seated buddy-system neck resistance
10. Neck assistance on Universal leg extension machine

Exercise options:

1. Circuit training involving wrestling skills on the mat
2. Medicine ball exercises
3. You may alternate heavy-medium days on major lifts: bench, power cleans

Problem areas:

1. Stretch year-round for maximum flexibility.
2. Do neck work at least 3 times a week in off-season every day in practice.
3. A year-round conditioning program can be used:
   - Sprint interval work = 2-3 times a week
   - Distance endurance work = 2-3 times a week □

FINE TUNING

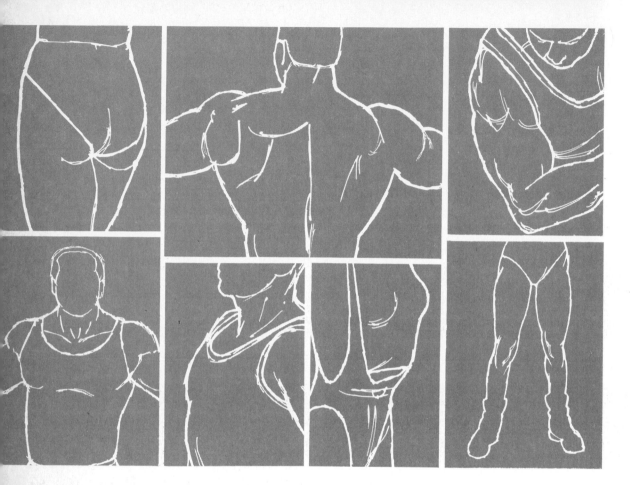

On the following seven pages are specialized programs for individual body parts. All the other programs in the book are overall body workouts focusing on the major muscle groups—for general conditioning, bodybuilding or strength training for sports.

The aim here is not to replace any of the other programs. But in addition to your other training, you can use these supplemental exercises to get very specific about shaping any one major muscle group.

If you are currently using one of the other programs in the book and on a tight time schedule, you may want to cut back on some of the exercises in that program so you can include some of these.

Exercises for:

Muscular Arms. . . . p. 177
Strong Back. . . . . . p. 178
Tight Bottom. . . . . p. 179
Larger Chest. . . . . .p. 180
Shapely Legs. . . . . p. 181
Broad Shoulders. . .p. 182
Flat Stomach. . . . . p. 183

Exercises for Muscular Arms

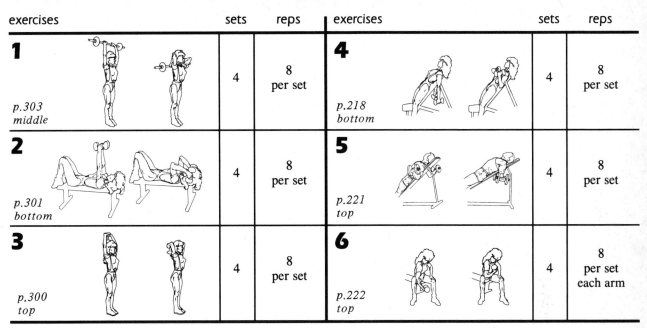

exercises		sets	reps	exercises		sets	reps
1 p.303 middle		4	8 per set	**4** p.218 bottom		4	8 per set
2 p.301 bottom		4	8 per set	**5** p.221 top		4	8 per set
3 p.300 top		4	8 per set	**6** p.222 top		4	8 per set each arm

GETTING STRONGER ©1986 Bill Pearl & Shelter Publications, Inc.

Tips:

- This program of six exercises recommends 3 sets each. Do not increase the sets to 5 or 6 in hopes of faster growth. You can overwork a muscle just as you can fail to work it enough. The sets and reps shown are ideal for these exercises.
- The triceps exercises shown here (and in general) are excellent for replacing the fat that tends to accumulate on the backs of arms with muscle.
- Concentrate while doing the exercises. Think of the muscles being worked and focus your energy and effort there.
- Try to get a complete extension and contraction on each exercise; handle a poundage that allows you to do this.
- Train at a speed that keeps the muscles warm.
- Keep a daily record of poundages for each exercise in order to train progressively.

To train progressively—Suppose you start the **Close Grip Triceps Curl** (number 1) with 50 pounds:

First 3 workouts — Use 50 lbs. for all four sets.
Fourth workout — Use 50 lbs. for 3 sets, 60 lbs. for one set.
Fifth workout — Use 50 lbs. for 1 set, 60 lbs. for 3 sets.
Sixth workout — Use 60 lbs. for all four sets.

Continue to increase the poundage in this gradual manner. This is only an example. Find the right weights for you. Start light and remember to use proper form.

Exercises for a Strong Back

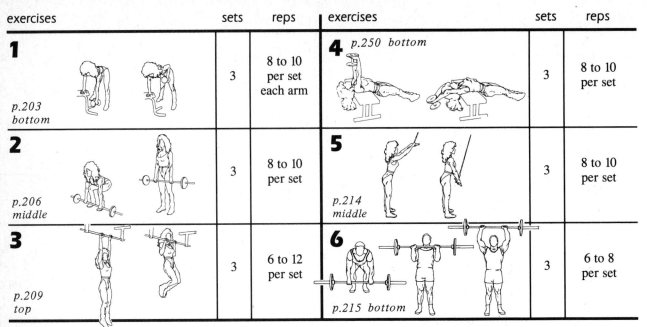

exercises		sets	reps	exercises		sets	reps
1 p.203 bottom		3	8 to 10 per set each arm	**4** p.250 bottom		3	8 to 10 per set
2 p.206 middle		3	8 to 10 per set	**5** p.214 middle		3	8 to 10 per set
3 p.209 top		3	6 to 12 per set	**6** p.215 bottom		3	6 to 8 per set

GETTING STRONGER ©1986 Bill Pearl & Shelter Publications, Inc.

Tips:

- Upper lat development will have a more dramatic effect on the look of the overall physique, but don't neglect the lower lats. See the "Back" section (pp. 202-217) for the different exercises for lower and upper lats.
- Isolation is difficult when working the lats because any lat exercise also works the arms. Beginners generally have stronger arms than lats, so they use them more. The arms, by taking the load, keep getting stronger and the lats suffer accordingly. The best solution is to get some coaching or watch an experienced bodybuilder train; you will see how the lats can be isolated in an exercise, so the arms merely go along for the ride.
- Study yourself when lifting and learn to recognize that particular feeling when the lats are pulling exclusively, with no aid from the arms. Think *lats*. Visualize them working (and stretching).

Exercises for a Tight Bottom

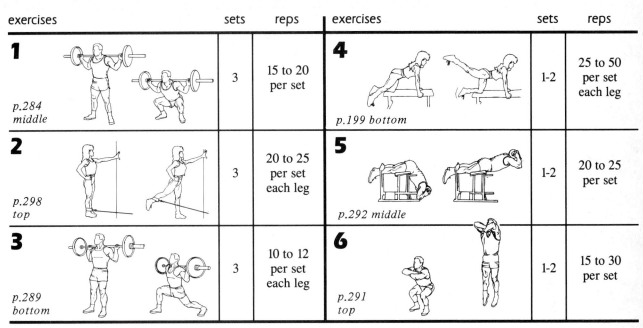

exercises		sets	reps	exercises		sets	reps
1 p.284 middle		3	15 to 20 per set	**4** p.199 bottom		1-2	25 to 50 per set each leg
2 p.298 top		3	20 to 25 per set each leg	**5** p.292 middle		1-2	20 to 25 per set
3 p.289 bottom		3	10 to 12 per set each leg	**6** p.291 top		1-2	15 to 30 per set

GETTING STRONGER ©1986 Bill Pearl & Shelter Publications, Inc.

Tips:

- As with the other major fat depot of the body, the stomach, the bottom requires a 3-phase program for reducing fat and creating firmness.
    1. Good diet: Control your food intake so you do not consume more calories than you burn, and cut back on the amount of fat in your diet.
    2. Regular cardiovascular exercise: Aerobic exercise activates the fat-burning muscles.
    3. Weight training: Regularly following this program will work wonders.
- These exercises are powerful. Start out easy and increase poundages as this area becomes used to the increased workload.
- Go particularly easy on squats and lunges. Overdoing these can make you extremely sore.
- The muscles in this area are exceptionally strong and will respond quickly to the program prescribed here, if followed regularly and sensibly.

Exercises for a Larger Chest

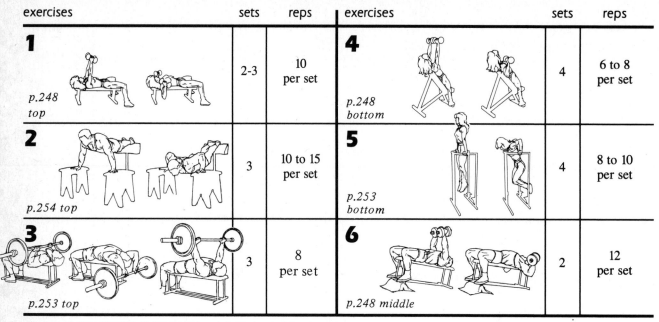

exercises	sets	reps	exercises	sets	reps
1 p.248 top	2-3	10 per set	**4** p.248 bottom	4	6 to 8 per set
2 p.254 top	3	10 to 15 per set	**5** p.253 bottom	4	8 to 10 per set
3 p.253 top	3	8 per set	**6** p.248 middle	2	12 per set

GETTING STRONGER ©1986 Bill Pearl & Shelter Publications, Inc.

Tips:

- Although the bench press is a great asset in increasing power, I believe it is considerably overrated as a chest development exercise. I have found that the best exercises for pectoral development are: bent arm laterals, chest cross-overs, incline presses, decline movements and flies.
- Try to keep the stress on the pectorals, rather than the triceps, front shoulders or back when doing near-maximum poundages for these exercises. *Concentrate* on the pecs, think of them doing the work.
- Practice deep breathing. It gives your system more oxygen to work with, helps in recovery time and increases chest expansion.
- Posture is very important. No matter how hard you work to build your chest, slouching, slumping or rounding your shoulders is counterproductive. Standing erect—head high, back straight, chest up and out—can add 2-4 inches to the size of your chest.

Exercises for Shapely Legs

Thighs		sets	reps	exercises		sets	reps
1 p.284 middle		4	8 to 10 per set	**4** p.293 middle		3	10 to 12 per set
2 p.294 bottom		4	10 to 12 per set	**5** p.292 bottom		4	8 to 10 per set
3 p.287 bottom		4	8 to 10 per set	**6** p.289 bottom		3	10 to 12 per set each leg

Calves		sets	reps			sets	reps
1 p.238 top		6	15 to 20 per set	**3** p.240 top		6	20 to 25 per set
2 p.242 middle		6	15 to 20 per set	**4** p.236 top		2	25 to 50 per set each leg

GETTING STRONGER ©1986 Bill Pearl & Shelter Publications, Inc.

Tips:

- Thigh and calf exercises *can* be done at home, but machines found in most gyms are more efficient than free weights for leg work.
- Thigh work is hard work. It will probably entail more exertion and sweat than any other body part.
- Squats are excellent for the upper thigh. They also bring the buttocks into play. Large buttocks can be helpful in many sports, but to minimize this effect when doing squats:
    - Do not dip your rear end too low
    - Do not bend your back too far forward

- The calf consists of three main areas. Varying the position of your feet during calf exercises can alter the effect:
    - To work the inner calf: Toes pointing out, heels together.
    - To work the main head: Toes pointing straight ahead.
    - To work the outer head: Toes pointing in, heels out.

Exercises for Broad Shoulders

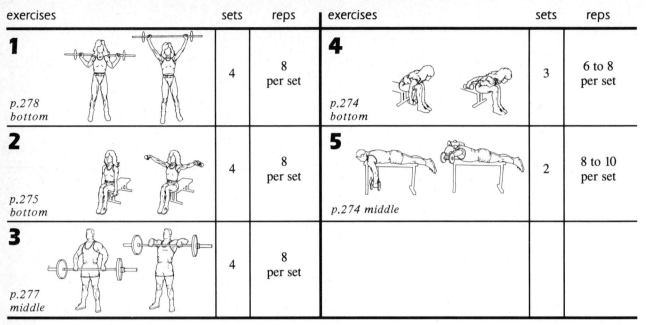

exercises		sets	reps	exercises		sets	reps
1 *p.278 bottom*		4	8 per set	**4** *p.274 bottom*		3	6 to 8 per set
2 *p.275 bottom*		4	8 per set	**5** *p.274 middle*		2	8 to 10 per set
3 *p.277 middle*		4	8 per set				

GETTING STRONGER ©1986 Bill Pearl & Shelter Publications, Inc.

Tips:

- Analyze your development and decide which parts of the deltoids need the most work. You can reduce sets on the stronger or better developed part, and add sets on the weaker part. Try to find a balance.
- If you have a history of shoulder injuries, consult your doctor before starting training. Use light weights and restricted, controlled exercises at first. Do *not* do straight arm pullovers, chins or similar exercises. Recommended shoulder rehabilitation exercises are:
    1. *Close-Grip Military Press:* Keep tension on the muscles at all times. Do not stretch out overhead, but make a complete extension and lock out the elbows.
    2. *Upright Barbell Rowing:* Use a shoulder-width grip and light weights. Extend the barbell to arms' length, keeping tension on the bar and shoulders rigid.
    3. *Presses* in the prone position: Use a close grip and light weights. Keep muscles under tension at all times.

Exercises for a Flat Stomach

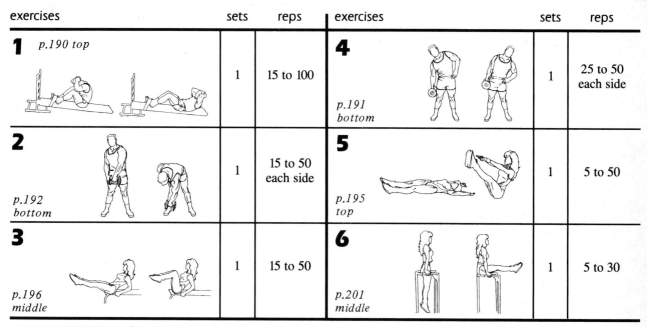

exercises		sets	reps	exercises		sets	reps
1 *p.190 top*		1	15 to 100	**4** *p.191 bottom*		1	25 to 50 each side
2 *p.192 bottom*		1	15 to 50 each side	**5** *p.195 top*		1	5 to 50
3 *p.196 middle*		1	15 to 50	**6** *p.201 middle*		1	5 to 30

Tips:

- There are 3 phases to a complete abdominal program:
  1. Diet: If you are taking in more calories than you are burning, or eating a high-fat diet, the excess will be stored somewhere, and the mid-section is a major fat storage area (nature stores fat where people are the least active).
  2. Aerobic exercise: Cardiovascular exercise develops fat-burning muscles. With regular aerobic exercise, these muscles burn fat not just when you are exercising but hours later—even when you are sitting or sleeping.
  3. Weight training: Follow this program.
- Think in terms of the entire mid-section, not just the upper and lower abdominals. Work the lower back, external obliques, intercostal muscles (muscles between the ribs). All are equally important.
- Pay more attention to the number of reps than to the weight you can handle. Start each new abdominal exercise with a manageable number of reps and add a few more each workout.
- If abdominal muscles are weak, the lower back is liable to injury. Strong abdominal muscles carry the load when you lift heavy objects. Weak abdominal muscles mean the load is transferred to the lower back.□

EXERCISES FOR FREE WEIGHTS

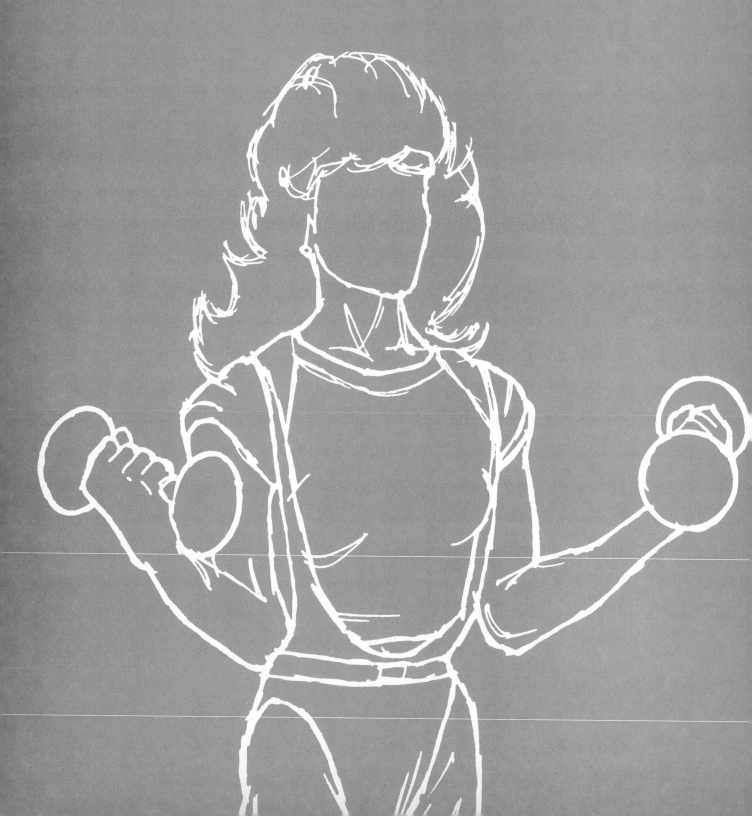

General Information on Exercises for Free Weights

- In the following section are 325 exercises for free weights, grouped according to body parts.
- These are by no means *all* the exercises that can be done with free weights, but they are the ones we consider most important.
- Please read the instructions with each exercise carefully, since body placement, grip, stance and procedure are all important.
- Some of the exercises shown in this "free weights" section are done with machines. These machines are commonly found in almost any gym that has free weights.
- Categorizing the exercises by body part ("Abdominals" or "Biceps," for example) is often arbitrary, since many of the exercises work more than one body part.
- There are two indexes for the exercises: by *drawings,* on pp. 426-442 and by *titles* on pp. 433-432.

Exercises for:

Abdominals pp. 190-201
Back 202-217
Biceps 218-235
Calves 236-243
Chest 244-257
Forearms 258-265
Neck 266-271
Shoulders 272-283
Thighs 284-299
Triceps 300-310

BODY PARTS

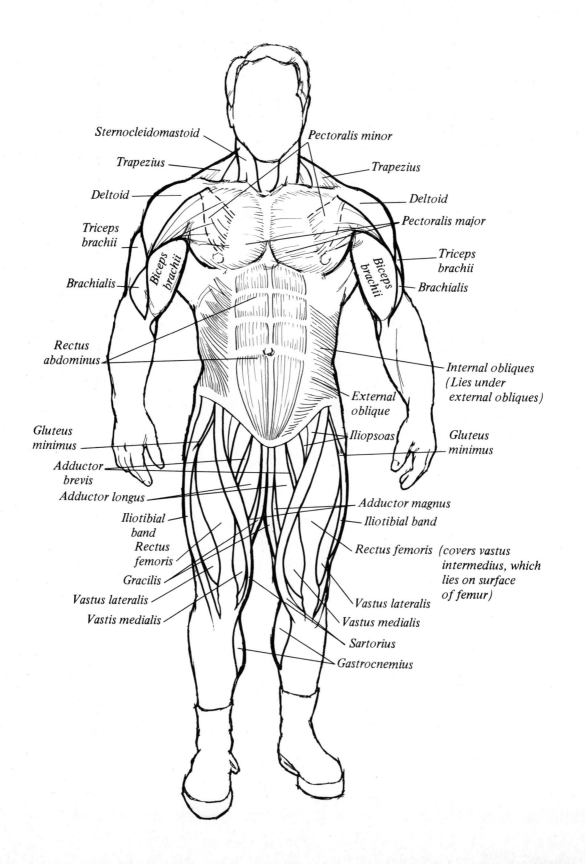

Sternocleidomastoid

Trapezius

Deltoid

Triceps
brachii

Brachialis

*Biceps
brachii*

Rectus
abdominus

Gluteus
minimus

Adductor
brevis

Adductor longus

Iliotibial
band
Rectus
femoris

Gracilis

Vastus lateralis

Vastis medialis

Pectoralis minor

Trapezius

Deltoid

Pectoralis major

*Biceps
brachii*

Triceps
brachii

Brachialis

Internal obliques
(Lies under
external obliques)

External
oblique

Iliopsoas

Gluteus
minimus

Adductor magnus

Iliotibial band

Rectus femoris (covers vastus
intermedius, which
lies on surface
of femur)

Vastus lateralis

Vastus medialis

Sartorius

Gastrocnemius

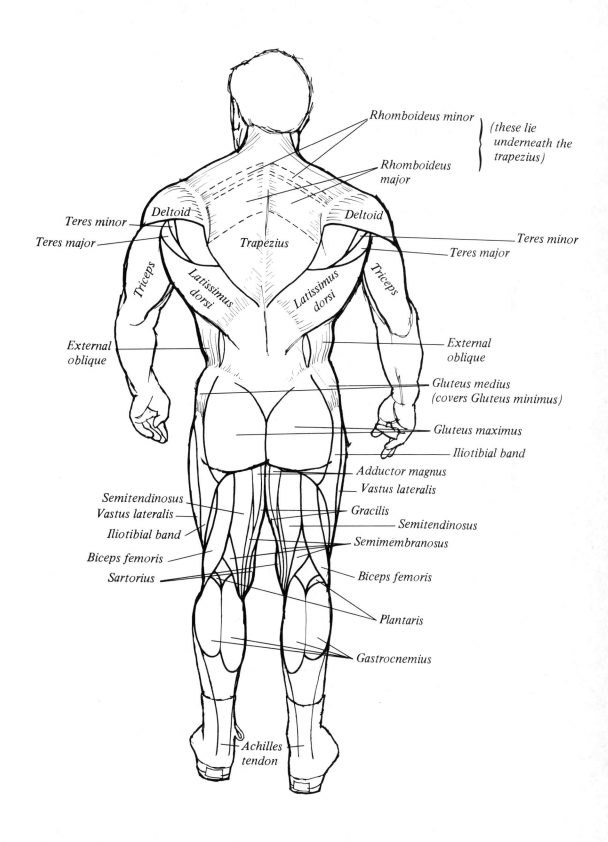

Rhomboideus minor

(these lie
underneath the
trapezius)

Rhomboideus
major

Deltoid

Teres minor

Teres major

Triceps

Deltoid

Teres minor

Teres major

Triceps

Trapezius

Latissimus
dorsi

Latissimus
dorsi

External
oblique

External
oblique

Gluteus medius
(covers Gluteus minimus)

Gluteus maximus

Iliotibial band

Adductor magnus

Vastus lateralis

Semitendinosus

Vastus lateralis

Gracilis

Semitendinosus

Iliotibial band

Semimembranosus

Biceps femoris

Biceps femoris

Sartorius

Plantaris

Gastrocnemius

Achilles
tendon

BODY PARTS

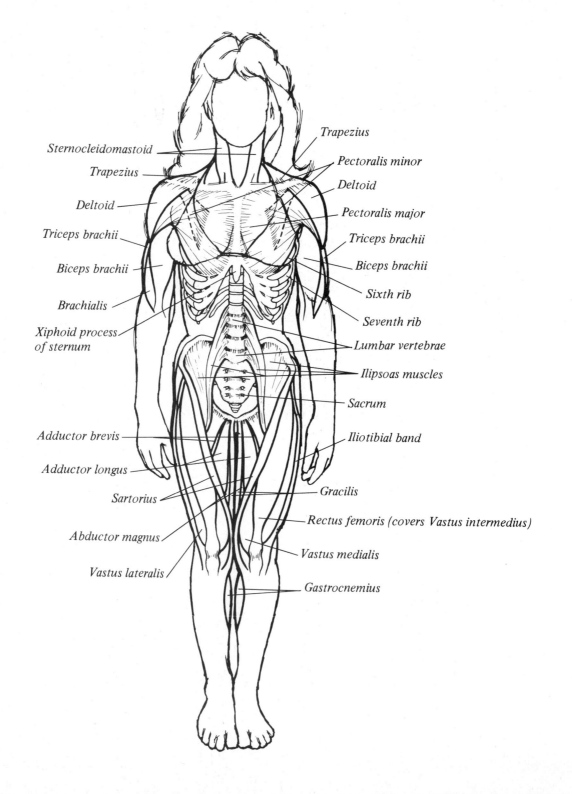

Sternocleidomastoid

Trapezius

Deltoid

Triceps brachii

Biceps brachii

Brachialis

Xiphoid process
of sternum

Adductor brevis

Adductor longus

Sartorius

Abductor magnus

Vastus lateralis

Trapezius

Pectoralis minor

Deltoid

Pectoralis major

Triceps brachii

Biceps brachii

Sixth rib

Seventh rib

Lumbar vertebrae

Ilipsoas muscles

Sacrum

Iliotibial band

Gracilis

Rectus femoris (covers Vastus intermedius)

Vastus medialis

Gastrocnemius

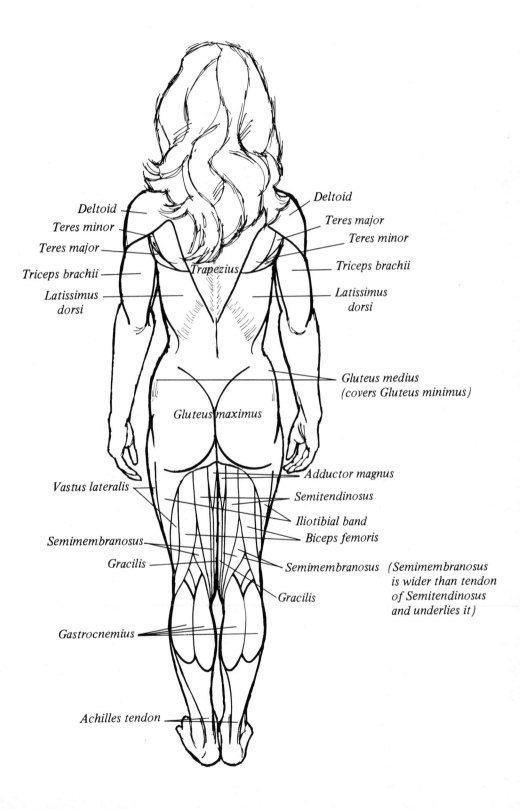

Deltoid

Teres minor

Teres major

Triceps brachii

Latissimus
dorsi

Deltoid

Teres major

Teres minor

Triceps brachii

Latissimus
dorsi

Trapezius

Gluteus medius
(covers Gluteus minimus)

Gluteus maximus

Adductor magnus

Semitendinosus

Iliotibial band

Biceps femoris

Vastus lateralis

Semimembranosus

Gracilis

Semimembranosus

Gracilis

Gastrocnemius

(Semimembranosus
is wider than tendon
of Semitendinosus
and underlies it)

Achilles tendon

ABDOMINALS

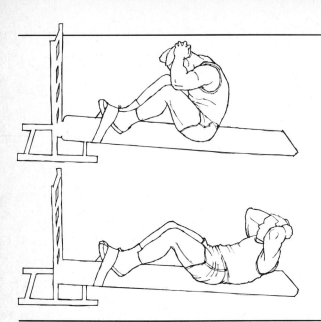

Bent-Knee Sit-Up
Upper Abdominals

- Hook feet under strap of sit-up board.
- Keep knees bent 45°.
- Put hands behind head, chin on chest.
- Lie back until lower back touches.
- Return to starting position.
- Inhale down, exhale up.
- To make harder, adjust bench to higher angle.

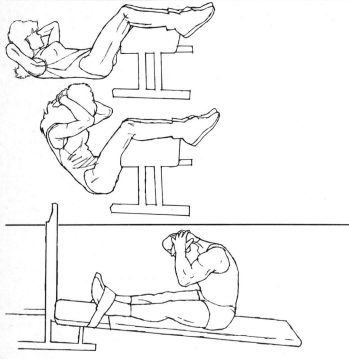

Heel-High Sit-Up
Upper Abdominals

- Lie on floor with lower legs on top of bench.
- Position body so thighs are at a 45° angle.
- With hands behind head, pull up as far as possible.
- Return to starting position.
- Do not swing body up and down but concentrate on abdominal muscles.
- Exhale up, inhale down.
- To make harder, hold light weight on chest.

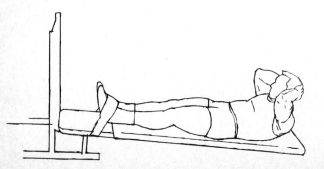

Sit-Up
Abdominals

- Hook feet under strap of sit-up board, knees slightly bent.
- Hand behind head, chin on chest.
- Lie down until lower back touches board. Do not lie completely back, but keep tension on abdominal muscles.
- Return to starting position.
- Inhale down, exhale up.
- Can also be done on floor (hook feet under coach, etc.) or on decline bench.

Note: Straight-legged sit-ups put more pressure on the lower back than bent-knee sit-ups. Bent knees isolate and work the abdominal muscles to a greater degree. We include straight-legged sit-ups since it also works the hip flexors (*ilipsoas* and *rectus femoris*), but it should not be used if you have lower back problems.

Barbell Good Morning
Lower Back and Abdominals

- Stand erect, feet 16" apart.
- Place light barbell on shoulders.
- Keep back straight, head up.
- Bend forward until upper body is parallel to floor.
- Return to starting position.
- Keep knees locked.
- Inhale down, exhale up.

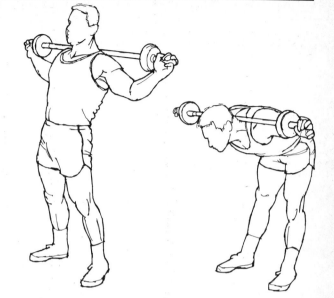

Barbell Side Bend
Obliques

- Stand erect, feet 16" apart.
- Place light barbell on shoulders.
- Keep back straight, head up.
- Bend to right as far as possible, then bend to left as far as possible.
- Bend at waist only, not at hips or knees.
- This exercise can also be done seated.
- Inhale to right, exhale to left.

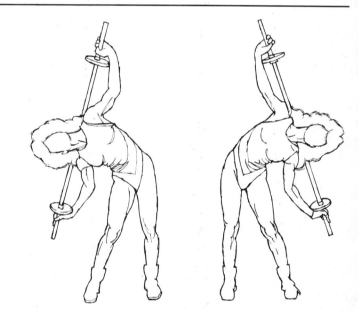

Dumbbell Side Bend
Obliques

- Stand erect, feet 16" apart.
- Hold dumbbell in right hand, palms in.
- Place left hand on waist.
- Keep back straight.
- Bend to right as far as possible, then bend to left as far as possible.
- Change weight to left hand and repeat movement.
- Bend at waist only, not at hips or knees.
- Inhale to right, exhale to left.
- Can be done with free hand on side of head.

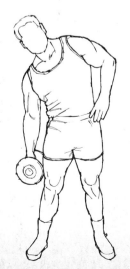
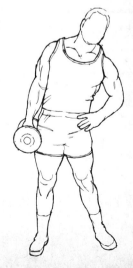

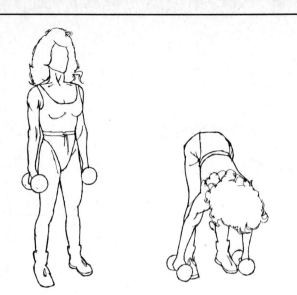

Stiff-Legged Dumbbell Dead Lift
Obliques and Lower Back

- Stand erect, feet 16" apart.
- Hold dumbbells, palms in.
- Keep back straight, head up, hips and knees locked.
- Bend forward until dumbbells touch floor.
- Return to starting position.
- Inhale down, exhale up.

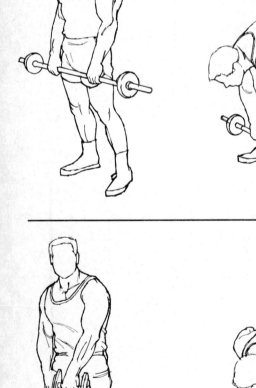

Stiff-Legged Barbell Dead Lift
Obliques and Lower Back

- Place barbell on floor in front of you.
- With feet 16" apart, bend and grasp bar just to outside of legs.
- Keep knees locked, back straight, head up.
- Using only back muscles, stand erect with arms locked.
- Lower weight to floor.
- Inhale up, exhale down.

Bend to Opposite Foot
Obliques and Lower Back

- Stand erect, feet 16" apart.
- Grasp dumbbell with left hand, palm in.
- Place right hand on upper right thigh.
- Bend until dumbbell nearly touches right foot.
- Return to starting position.
- Change dumbbell to right hand and repeat.
- Inhale down, exhale up.

Alternated Twisting Dumbbell Bend to Opposite Foot
Obliques and Lower Back

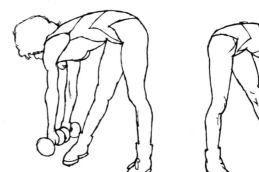

- Stand erect, feet 16" apart.
- Hold dumbbells, palms in.
- Keep back straight, head up, hips and knees locked.
- Inhale and twist torso to right, then bend, holding twist until dumbbells nearly touch right foot.
- Return to starting position and exhale.
- Repeat movement to left side.
- A movement to the right and left equals one rep.

Warm-Up (Dumbbell Swing-Through)
Most Large Muscle Groups

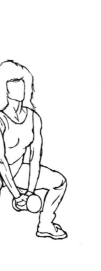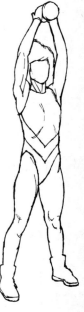

- Hold dumbbell with both hands.
- Stand erect, feet 16" apart.
- With arms straight, squat until upper thighs are parallel to floor.
- Raise up in semicircular motion with dumbbell at arms' length until overhead.
- Lower dumbbell to starting position in same path.
- Swing dumbbell through legs for better stretch.
- Inhale up, exhale down.

Seated Barbell Twist
Obliques

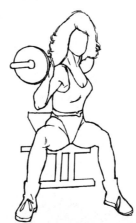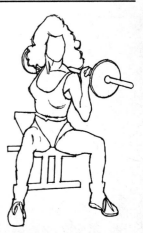

- Place light barbell on shoulders.
- Sit at end of bench, feet firmly on floor.
- Twist torso to right, then to left by twisting at waist only.
- Do not move head from side to side.
- Keep back straight, head up.
- Inhale to right, exhale to left.
- Can also be done standing.
- Can also be done holding dumbbell next to chest.

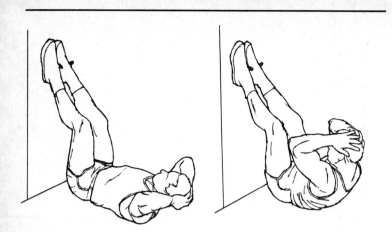

Feet-Against-Wall Sit-Up
Upper Abdominals

- Lie on floor with body close to wall.
- Put feet against wall, knees slightly bent.
- Place hands behind head.
- Pull up as far as possible.
- Return to starting position.
- Inhale up, exhale down.

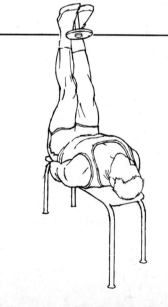

Over-a-Bench Sit-Up
Upper Abdominals

- Sit on bench.
- Put feet under something to support body.
- Keep knees slightly bent.
- Bend back and down until you are just below parallel to floor.
- Return to starting position.
- Inhale down, exhale up.
- To make harder, hold light weight on chest.

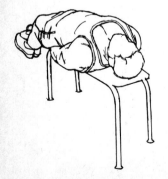

Flat Bench Weighted Leg Raise
Lower Abdominals

- Place light weight between feet.
- Lie on flat bench with legs off the end.
- Place hands under buttocks, palms down.
- Keep legs straight, knees locked.
- Raise legs as high as possible.
- Lower legs until they are about 3" off floor.
- Inhale up, exhale down.
- To make easier, do not use weight.

Jackknife Sit-Up
Upper and Lower Abdominals

- Lie on floor on your back.
- Place arms straight back behind head.
- Bend at waist while raising legs and arms to meet in jackknife position.
- Lower arms and legs to floor.
- Inhale up, exhale down.
- Keep elbows and knees locked.

Incline Leg Pull-In
Lower Abdominals

- Put sit-up board at 25-30° angle.
- Lie with head at top.
- Hold bar.
- Bend knees, pulling upper thighs into midsection.
- Return to starting position.
- Do not let feet touch board once exercise has started.
- Concentrate on lower abdominals.
- Inhale up, exhale down.
- To make harder, hold lightweight dumbbell between feet.
- Can also be done off floor.

Incline Arms-Extended Sit-Up
Upper Abdominals

- Put sit-up board at 25-30° angle.
- Sit with feet at high side under strap.
- Keep knees slightly bent, arms above head, elbows locked.
- Lower torso until lower back touches.
- Raise straight up as far as possible.
- Inhale down, exhale up.
- To make easier, lower angle of bench.

See "Note," bottom page 190.

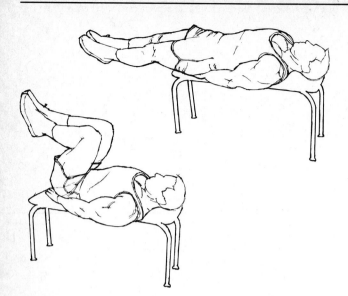

Flat Bench Leg Pull-In
Lower Abdominals

- Lie on flat bench with legs off end.
- Place hands under buttocks, palms down, legs out straight.
- Bend knees, pulling upper thighs into midsection.
- Return to starting position.
- Concentrate on lower abdominals.
- Inhale up, exhale down.
- To make harder, hold lightweight dumbbell between feet.

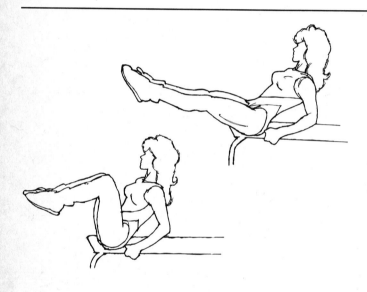

Seated Flat Bench Leg Pull-In
Lower Abdominals

- Sit on flat bench.
- Place hands behind buttocks and grasp sides of bench.
- Extend legs straight out.
- Bend knees, pulling upper thighs into midsection.
- Return to starting position.
- Keep lower legs parallel to floor when extended.
- Concentrate on abdominals.
- Inhale up, exhale down.
- To make harder, hold light dumbbell between feet.

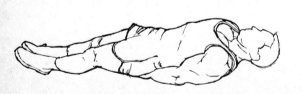
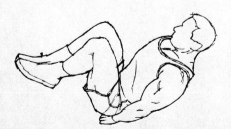

Leg Pull-In
Lower Abdominals

- Lie on floor with hands under buttocks, palms down, legs extended.
- Bend knees, pulling upper thighs into midsection.
- Return to starting position.
- Concentrate on lower abdominals.
- Inhale up, exhale down.
- To make harder, hold light dumbbell between feet.

Extension Machine Leg Pull-In
Hip Flexors and Lower Abdominals

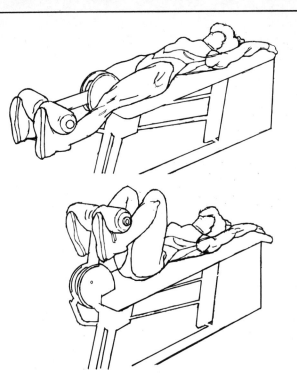

- Lie on back on leg extension machine.
- Grasp either back of board or bar behind head for support.
- Place feet behind pads used for leg biceps curls.
- Pull knees up as far as possible.
- Pause, then lower pads to starting position.
- Keep tension on abdominals.
- Inhale up, exhale down.
- Can also be done by hooking feet to straps of low wall pulley.

Seated Flat Bench Leg Tuck
Lower Abdominals

- Sit on flat bench.
- Place hands behind buttocks and hold sides of bench.
- Sit back slightly and raise feet about 6" off floor.
- Bend knees, bringing torso slightly forward until upper thighs and chest touch.
- Return to starting position.
- Keep tension on abdominals.
- Inhale up, exhale down.

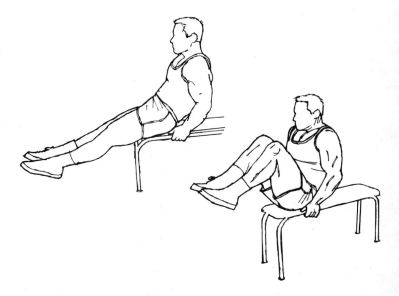

Hip Roll
Obliques

- Lie on your back.
- Hold an object behind your head for support or place hands under buttocks, palms down.
- Bend knees, feet firmly on floor.
- Lower legs to right side until upper thigh touches floor.
- Return to starting position, then repeat to left side.
- Do all bending at waist.
- Do not let shoulders come off floor.
- Inhale to right, exhale to left.

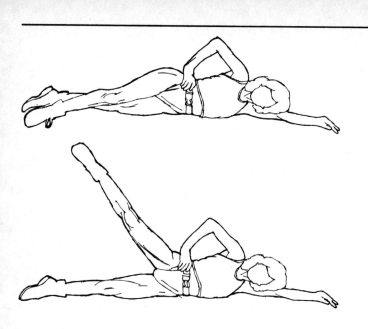

Lying Side Leg Raise
Hips

- Lie on left side.
- Tilt body slightly forward.
- Raise right leg as far as possible.
- Keep leg straight, do not bend at waist.
- Return leg to starting position.
- Lie on right side and repeat with left leg.
- Inhale up, exhale down.
- Can also be done on standing incline bench.

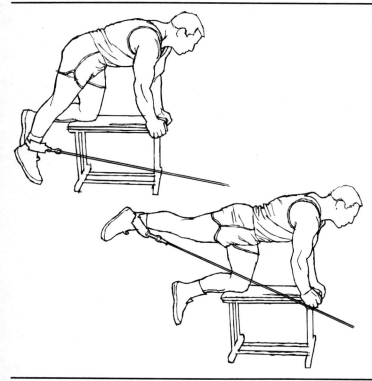

Kneeling Low-Pulley Back-Kick
Lower Back and Hips

- Place ankle strap on right ankle and have bench far enough from pulley so right leg can support weight stack while it hangs straight down.
- Kneel with left knee on flat bench.
- Grasp outer side of bench with arms locked.
- Raise leg straight back as far as you can.
- Do not bend knee.
- Return leg to starting position.
- Place strap on left ankle and repeat with left leg.
- Inhale up, exhale down.

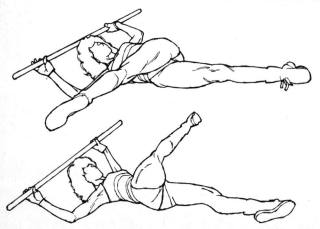

Lying Leg Crossover
Hips and Obliques

- Lie on back.
- Hold an object behind head with a wider-than-shoulder grip.
- Keep shoulders on floor.
- Swing right leg over left leg, as far to the side as possible until it is nearly as high as your head.
- Keep leg close to floor.
- Return to starting position, then repeat movement with left leg.
- Keep knees locked, legs as straight as possible.
- Inhale as you swing leg, exhale as you lower it.

Incline Back-Kick
Hips

- Lie face down on incline bench.
- Raise right leg straight back.
- Return leg to starting position.
- Keep leg as straight as possible.
- Repeat with left leg.
- Inhale up, exhale down.
- Can also be done lying on floor.

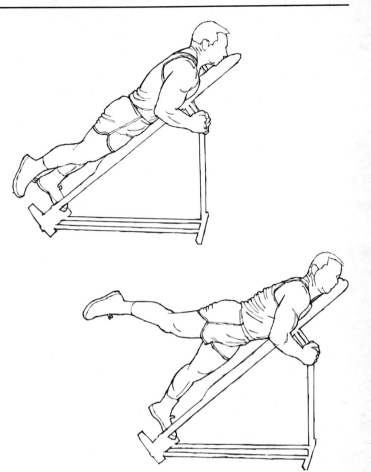

Kneeling Back-Kick
Lower Back and Hips

- Kneel with left knee on flat bench.
- Hold outer sides of bench, arms locked.
- Let right leg hang down.
- Raise right leg straight back as far as possible.
- Do not bend leg at knee.
- Return leg to starting position.
- Repeat with left leg.
- Inhale up, exhale down.

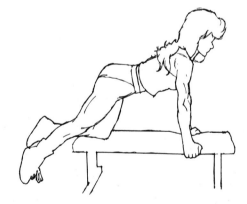

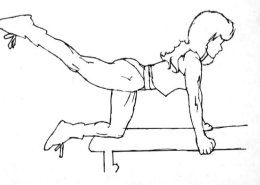

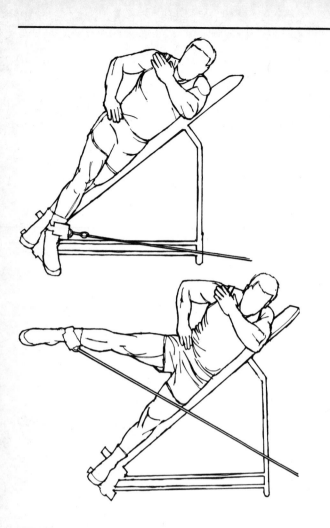

Incline Low-Pulley Side Leg Raise
Hips and Obliques

- Lie on left side on incline bench.
- Tilt body slightly forward.
- Put ankle strap on right ankle.
- Have bench far enough from pulley so leg supports the weight stack while right leg hangs to side of bench.
- Raise leg as far as possible.
- Keep leg straight, do not bend at waist.
- Return leg to starting position.
- Lie on right side and repeat with left leg.
- Inhale up, exhale down.

Incline Side Leg Circle
Hips

- Lie on right side on incline bench with torso tilted slightly forward.
- Raise left leg up and move in a circle.
- The top of the circle should be nearly parallel to body.
- Keep leg straight, do not bend at waist.
- Return leg to starting position.
- Lie on left side and repeat with right leg.
- Inhale up, exhale down.

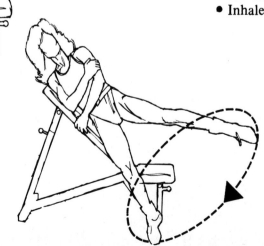

Alternated Low-Pulley Leg Pull-In
Lower Abdominals

- Lie on back in front of wall pulley, feet towards machine.
- Strap both ankles to lower pulley cables.
- Lie far enough from machine to raise weight stacks when legs are straight.
- Place hands under buttocks, palms down.
- Bend right knee, pulling right thigh up as far as possible.
- When lowering right leg to starting position, start raising left leg.
- As one leg goes up the other comes down— like cycling.
- Inhale on right, exhale on left.

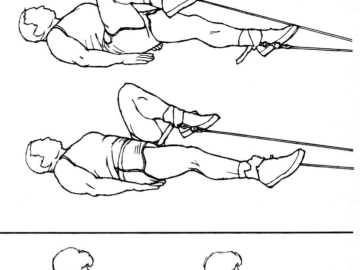

Dip Stand Leg Raise
Lower Abdominals

- Get on dip stand facing out.
- Arms straight, legs locked.
- Raise legs until parallel to floor.
- Keep knees straight.
- Return to starting position.
- Inhale up, exhale down.
- To make harder, hold light weight between feet.

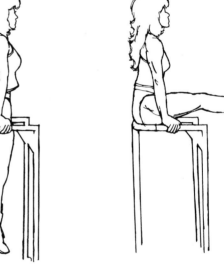

Alternated Dip Stand Leg Raise
Lower Abdominals

- Get on dip stand facing out.
- Arms straight, legs locked.
- Raise right leg up until parallel to floor.
- As you lower right leg, start raising left leg.
- Inhale on right, exhale on left. □

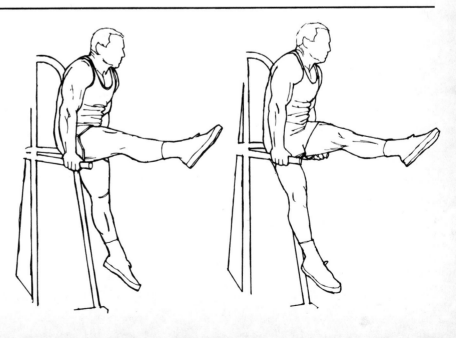

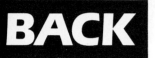
BACK

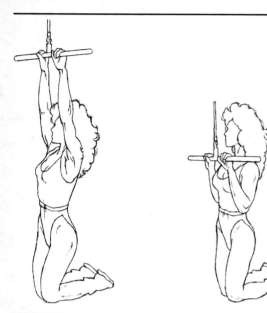

Close-Grip Front Lat Pull-Down
Lower Lats

- Hold lat bar with hands about 8" apart.
- Kneel down far enough to support weights with arms extended overhead.
- Pull bar straight down until even with upper chest.
- Return to starting position.
- Inhale down, exhale up.
- Can also be done with medium grip.

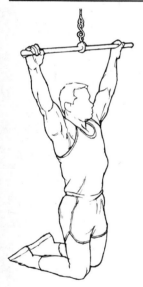
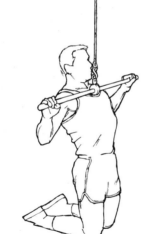

Wide-Grip Front Lat Pull-Down
Upper Lats

- Hold lat bar with hands about 36" apart.
- Kneel down far enough to support weights with arms extended overhead.
- Pull bar straight down until even with upper chest.
- Return to starting position.
- Inhale down, exhale up.

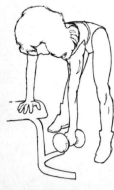
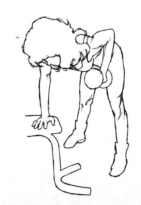

Hand-on-Bench One-Arm Dumbbell Rowing
Upper and Lower Lats

- Place dumbbell on floor in front of bench.
- Put left leg back, knee locked.
- Bend right knee slightly.
- Bend over and hold dumbbell with left hand, palm in, about 6" off floor.
- Put right hand on bench, elbow locked.
- Pull dumbbell straight up to side of chest keeping arm close to side.
- Return to starting position using same path.
- Inhale up, exhale down.
- Reverse position and repeat movement on right side.

Wide-Grip Rear Lat Pull-Down
Upper Lats

- Hold lat bar with hands about 36" apart.
- Kneel down far enough to support weights with arms extended overhead.
- Pull bar straight down until it touches back of neck just above shoulders.
- Return to starting position.
- Inhale down, exhale up.
- Can also be done with medium grip.

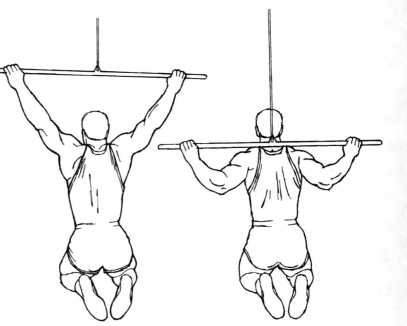

Medium-Grip Front-to-Rear Lat Pull-Down
Lats

- Hold lat bar with hands about 24" apart.
- Kneel down far enough to support weights with arms extended overhead.
- Pull bar straight down until even with upper chest.
- Return to starting position.
- Pull bar straight down until it touches back of neck just above shoulders.
- Return to starting position.
- Inhale down, exhale up.

Bent-Over Dumbbell Rowing
Lats

- Place dumbbell on floor in front of a waist-high object.
- Rest right forearm and forehead on object.
- Put left foot back about 36", leg straight.
- Bend right knee slightly.
- Hold dumbbell with left hand.
- Pull straight up to side of chest.
- Lower to starting position.
- Inhale up, exhale down.
- Reverse position and repeat movement on right side.

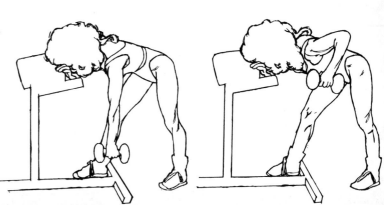

Bent-Over Head-Supported Two-Arm Dumbbell Rowing
Upper Back and Lats

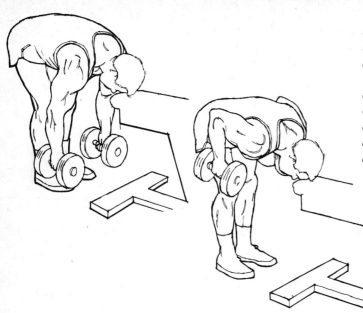

- Put feet close together.
- Place dumbbell outside of each foot.
- Bend forward and rest forehead on comfortable waist-high bench.
- Keep knees slightly bent.
- Pull dumbbells straight up to sides of chest.
- Lower to starting position.
- Inhale up, exhale down.
- Do not let dumbbells touch floor during exercise.

Bent-Over Two-Arm Dumbbell Rowing
Upper Back and Lats

- Put feet close together.
- Place dumbbell outside of each foot.
- Bend forward and grasp dumbbells.
- Keep knees slightly bent, torso parallel to floor.
- Pull dumbbells straight up to sides of chest.
- Inhale up, exhale down.
- Do not let dumbbells touch floor during exercise.
- Keep head up, back straight.

Standard Bent-Over One-Arm Long Bar Rowing
Upper Back and Lats

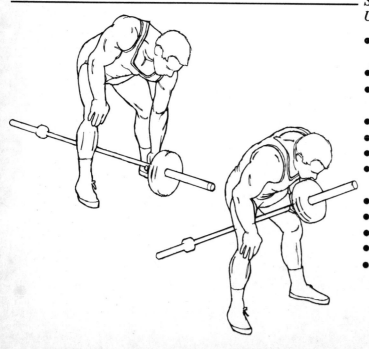

- Place empty barbell bar in a corner or against something.
- Put weights on other end of bar.
- Straddle bar and bend forward until torso is parallel to floor.
- Keep knees slightly bent.
- Grasp bar just behind plates with left hand.
- Place right hand on right knee.
- Pull bar straight up, elbow in, until plates touch chest.
- Lower bar to starting position.
- Inhale up, exhale down.
- Do not let plates touch floor during exercise.
- Keep back straight.
- Reverse position and repeat with right arm.

Standard Bent-Over Two-Arm Long Bar Rowing
Upper Back and Lower Lats

- Place empty barbell bar in a corner or against something.
- Put weights on other end of bar.
- Straddle bar and bend forward until torso is parallel to floor.
- Keep knees slightly bent.
- Hold bar just behind plates with both hands.
- Pull bar straight up, elbows in, until plates touch chest.
- Lower bar to starting position.
- Inhale up, exhale down.
- Do not let plates touch floor during exercise.
- Keep back straight.

Bent-Over Wide-Grip Barbell Rowing
Upper Back and Lats

- Place barbell on floor in front of you.
- Keep feet 18" apart.
- Bend over and hold bar with hands about 6-8" wider than shoulders.
- Keep legs slightly bent, torso parallel to floor.
- Pull bar straight up to lower part of chest.
- Lower to starting position.
- Inhale up, exhale down.
- Do not let bar touch floor during exercise.
- Keep head up, back straight.
- Can also be done with close or wide grip.

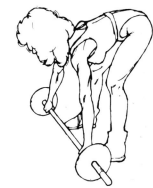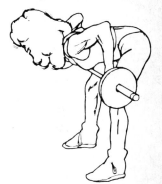

Bent-Over Head-Supported Wide-Grip Barbell Rowing
Upper Back and Upper Lats

- Place barbell on floor in front of you.
- Keep feet 18" apart.
- Place forehead on comfortable waist-high bench.
- Bend down and hold bar as wide as is comfortable.
- Keep legs slightly bent and torso parallel to floor.
- Pull bar straight up to chest.
- Lower to starting position.
- Inhale up, exhale down.
- Do not let bar touch floor during exercise.
- Keep back straight.
- Can also be done with close or medium grip.

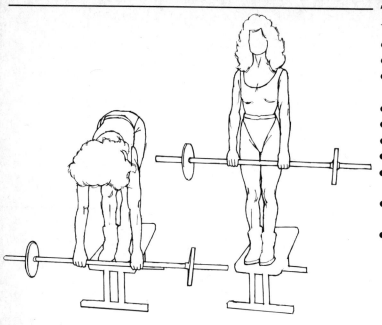

Stiff-Legged Barbell Dead Lift off Bench
Lower Back and Leg Biceps

- Place barbell on end of bench.
- Stand on bench.
- Bend at waist, head up, back straight, knees locked.
- Hold bar with hands about 16" apart.
- Straighten up, holding bar at arms' length.
- Lower back to bench.
- Inhale up, exhale down.
- Use muscles of the lower back for most of the pulling.
- If flexible enough, step closer to end of bench to allow bar to go below bench top.
- Can also be done with dumbbells.

Barbell Dead Lift
Buttocks, Thighs, Lower Back

- Place barbell on floor in front of you.
- Keep feet 16" apart.
- Bend down and hold bar just outside of knees.
- Keep knees bent, back straight, head up.
- Using thighs and back, stand erect, arms locked.
- Inhale up, exhale down.
- Can also be done with dumbbells.

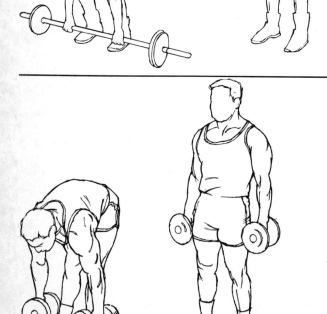

Stiff-Legged Dumbbell Dead Lift
Buttocks, Thighs, Lower Back

- Stand with feet about 8" apart.
- Place dumbbell outside of each foot.
- Reach down and grasp dumbbells.
- Keep legs straight, back straight, head up.
- Straighten up, elbows locked.
- Lower dumbbells to floor with legs straight.
- Inhale up, exhale down.
- Can also be done with barbell.

Wide-Grip High Pull
Legs and Back

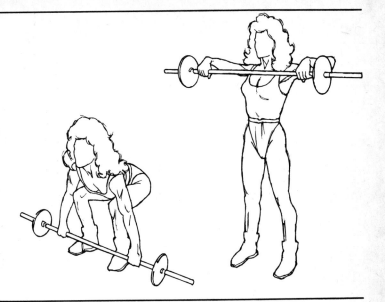

- Place barbell on floor in front of you.
- Keep feet about 16" apart.
- Step close to bar until shins are nearly touching it.
- Hold bar with hands 36" apart.
- Bend knees until upper thighs are nearly parallel to floor.
- Keep head up, back straight and at 45° angle.
- Stand erect, pulling straight up to shoulder level.
- For better pulling power, continue pull by throwing head back and raising high on toes at top position.
- Lower bar to arms' length, then to floor.
- Inhale up, exhale down.

Medium-Grip High Pull
Legs and Back

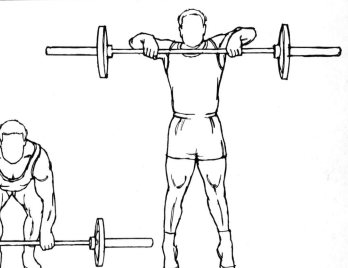

- Place barbell on floor in front of you.
- Keep feet about 16" apart.
- Step close to bar until shins are nearly touching it.
- Hold bar with hands 24" apart.
- Bend knees until upper thighs are nearly parallel to floor.
- Keep head up, back straight and at 45° angle.
- Stand erect pulling bar straight up to shoulder level.
- For better pulling power, continue pull by throwing head back and raising high on toes at top position.
- Lower bar to arms' length, then to floor.
- Inhale up, exhale down.
- Can also be done with dumbbells.

Barbell Power Clean
Legs and Back

- Place barbell on floor in front of you.
- Keep feet about 16" apart.
- Step close to bar until shins are nearly touching it.
- Hold bar with hands 24" apart.
- Bend legs until upper thighs are nearly parallel to floor.
- Keep head up, back straight and at 45° angle.
- Stand erect, pull bar to shoulders.
- Flip bar over and back until it rests on upper chest.
- Lower bar to floor.
- Inhale up, exhale down.
- Can also be done with dumbbells.

Barbell Push Press
Legs, Back, Shoulders

- Hold barbell with hands 36" apart.
- Either clean bar to top of upper chest or take bar off rack and place on upper chest.
- Squat down about 12", back straight, elbows slightly forward, head up.
- With power from legs and back, push bar overhead to arms' length for short period, then lower back to top of upper chest.
- Inhale up, exhale down.

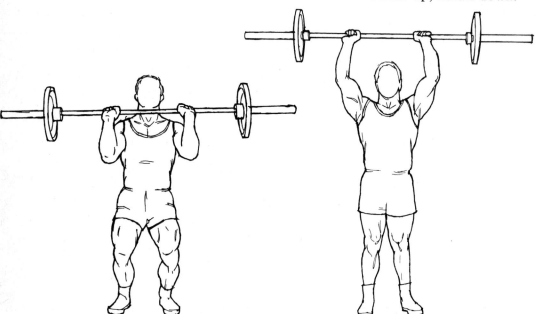

Dumbbell Push Press
Legs, Back, Shoulders

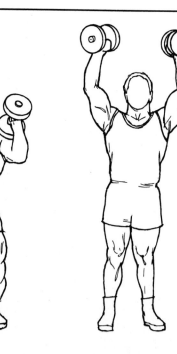

- Clean two dumbbells to height of shoulders, palms in.
- Squat down about 12", back straight, elbows slightly forward, head up.
- With power from legs and back, push dumbbells overhead to arms' length by straightening out legs quickly.
- Hold dumbbells at arms' length for short period, then back to shoulder height.
- Inhale up, exhale down.

Close-Grip Front Chin
Lower Lats

- Use chinning bar about 6" higher off floor than you can reach with arms extended overhead.
- Hold bar with hands 6" to 8" apart.
- Pull up, trying to touch chin to bar.
- Return to starting position.
- Try to keep back slightly hyperextended.
- Do not swing back and forth.
- Inhale up, exhale down.

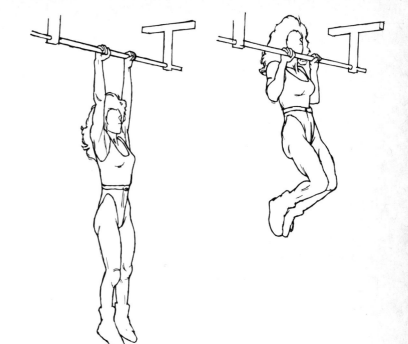

Close-Grip V-Bar Chin
Lower Lats

- Place V-bar attachment on chinning bar.
- Hold handles with both hands.
- Pull up, trying to touch chin to bar.
- Return to starting position.
- Try to keep back slightly hyperextended.
- Do not swing back and forth.
- Inhale up, exhale down.

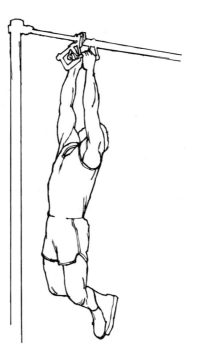
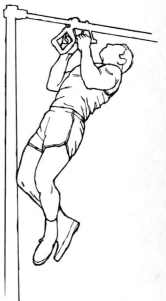

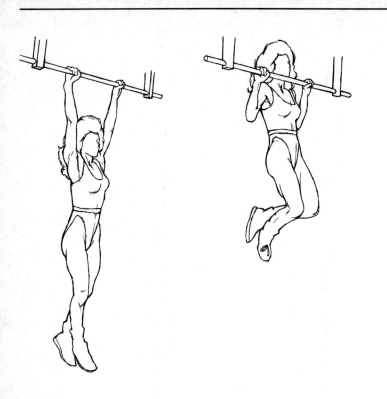

Medium-Grip Front Chin
Lats

- Use chinning bar about 6" higher off floor than you can reach with arms extended overhead.
- Hold bar with hands 18" to 20" apart.
- Pull up, trying to touch chin to bar.
- Return to starting position.
- Try to keep back slightly hyperextended.
- Do not swing back and forth.
- Inhale up, exhale down.

Wide-Grip Rear Chin
Upper Lats

- Use chinning bar about 6" higher off floor than you can reach with arms extended overhead.
- Hold bar with hands 32" to 34" apart.
- Pull up, trying to touch back of neck to bar.
- Return to starting position.
- Do not swing back and forth.
- Inhale up, exhale down.

Medium-Grip Rear Chin
Upper Lats

- Use chinning bar about 6" higher off floor than you can reach with arms extended overhead.
- Hold bar with hands 18" to 20" apart.
- Pull up, trying to touch back of neck to bar.
- Return to starting position.
- Do not swing back and forth.
- Inhale up, exhale down.

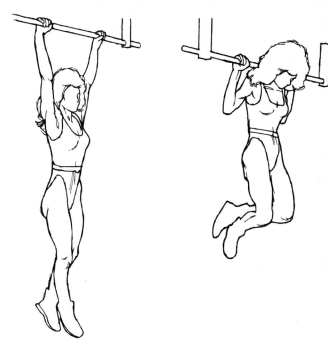

Reverse Close-Grip Front Chin
Lower Lats

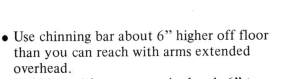

- Use chinning bar about 6" higher off floor than you can reach with arms extended overhead.
- Hold bar with a reverse grip, hands 6" to 8" apart.
- Pull up, trying to touch chin to bar.
- Return to starting position.
- Do not swing back and forth.
- Inhale up, exhale down.

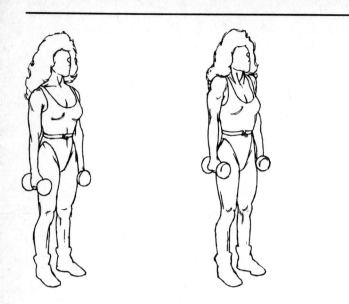

Dumbbell Shoulder Shrug
Trapezius

- Keep feet about 16" apart.
- Hold dumbbells.
- Stand erect, dumbbells hanging at arms' length.
- Droop shoulders down as much as possible.
- Raise shoulders up and rotate in a circular motion from front to rear.
- Inhale at beginning, exhale at end of repetition.

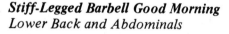

Barbell Shoulder Shrug
Trapezius

- Hold barbell, palms down, with hands 16" apart.
- Keep feet about 16" apart.
- Stand erect, bar hanging at arms' length.
- Droop shoulders down as much as possible.
- Raise shoulders up and rotate in a circular motion from front to rear.
- Inhale at beginning, exhale at end of repetition.

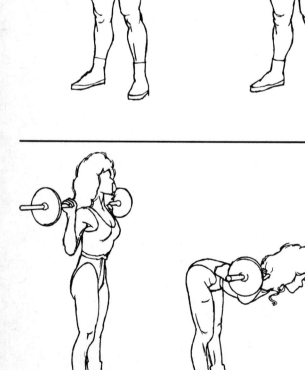

Stiff-Legged Barbell Good Morning
Lower Back and Abdominals

- Place barbell on shoulders.
- Keep head up, back straight.
- Bend at waist, legs locked, until upper body is parallel to floor.
- Return to starting position.
- Inhale down, exhale up.
- Can also be done with knees slightly bent.

Twisting Hyperextension
Lower Back

- Extend upper body over end of high bench.
- Lock legs under support.
- End of bench should be at hips.
- Bend down at waist so upper body is vertical to floor.
- Place hands behind head.
- Raise torso up and to the right until slightly past parallel.
- Return to starting position.
- Do prescribed number of reps to the right, then repeat to the left side.
- Inhale up, exhale down.
- Can also be done with weight behind neck to increase resistance.

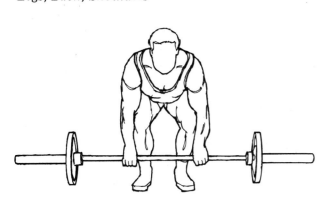

Barbell Power Clean and Press
Legs, Back, Shoulders

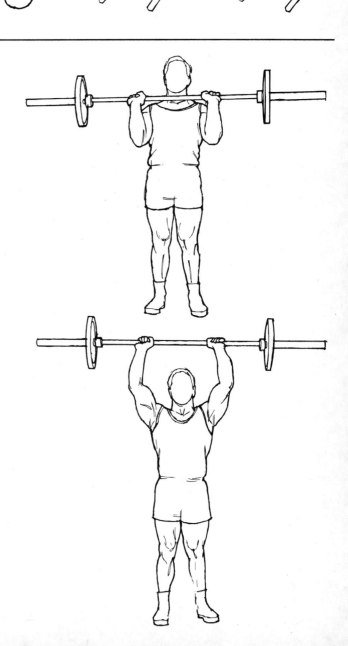

- Place barbell in front of you.
- Keep feet about 16" apart.
- Step close to bar until shins are nearly touching it.
- Hold bar with hands 24" apart.
- Bend knees until thighs are nearly parallel to floor.
- Inhale while pulling bar straight up as you stand erect.
- Lift bar as high as shoulders.
- Flip bar over and back until it rests on upper chest and then exhale.
- Inhale again and press barbell directly overhead to arms' length.
- Pause at top before exhaling.
- Lower bar back to upper chest and down to floor to complete repetition.
- Can also be done with dumbbells.

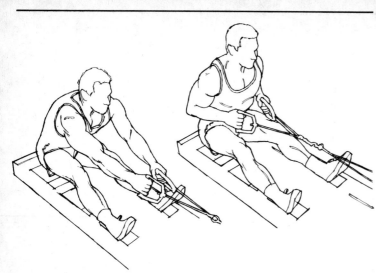

Seated Two-Arm Low Lat Pull-In
Lower Lats and Upper Back

- Sit on floor in front of low pulley.
- Place feet against object for support.
- Hold low pulley handles.
- Bend forward throughout the exercise, do not go back and forth at waist.
- Pull handles directly to sides of chest just below pectorals.
- Return weight stacks to starting position.
- Inhale at beginning, exhale at end of repetition.
- Can also be done one arm at a time.

Straight-Arm Close-Grip Lat Pulldown
Lats

- Hold lat bar with hands 8" apart.
- Step back from machine until arms support weights while extended in front, even with top of head.
- Pull bar straight down, in semicircular motion with arms locked, until it touches top of thighs.
- Return to starting position using same path.
- Inhale down, exhale up.

Seated Two-Arm High Lat Pull-In
Upper Lats and Upper Back

- Sit on floor in front of high pulley.
- Place feet against object for support.
- Hold high pulley handles.
- Bend forward throughout exercise, do not go back and forth at waist.
- Pull handles directly to sides of chest in line with pectorals.
- Return weight stacks to starting position.
- Inhale at beginning, exhale at end of repetition.
- Can also be done one arm at a time.

Universal Machine Shoulder Shrug
Trapezius

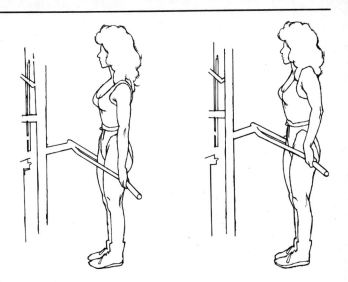

- Stand between handles of Universal bench press station.
- Hold handles close to inside ends.
- Stand erect and raise weight stack with arms locked at sides.
- Droop both shoulders down to front.
- Raise shoulders and rotate in circular motion from front to back.
- Inhale at beginning, exhale at end of repetition.

Barbell Power Clean and Jerk
Legs, Back, Shoulders

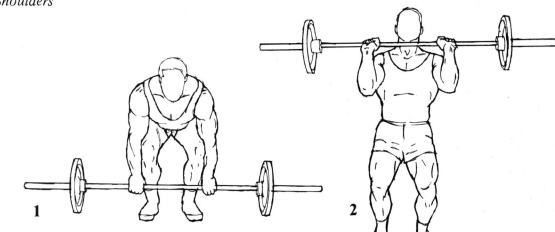

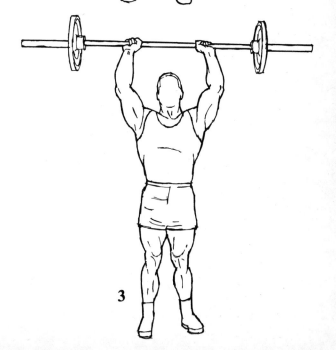

- Place barbell in front of you.
- Keep feet about 16" apart.
- Step close to bar until shins are nearly touching it.
- Hold bar with hands 24" apart.
- Bend knees until upper thighs are nearly parallel to floor.
- Keep arms straight, head up.
- Your back should be at 45° angle.
- Inhale while pulling bar straight up as you stand erect.
- Lift bar as high as shoulders.
- Flip bar over and back until it rests on upper chest, then exhale.
- Inhale again and squat 12" keeping back straight, elbows forward.
- Use power from legs and back to thrust bar overhead to arms' length.
- Pause at top before exhaling.
- Lower bar back to upper chest and down to floor to complete repetition.

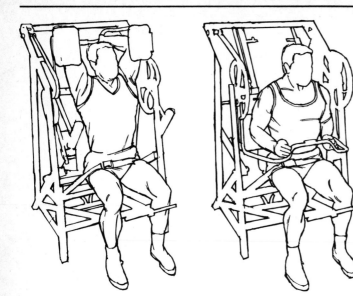

Pullover on Nautilus Machine
Lats, Triceps

- Sit on seat of Nautilus-type pullover machine.
- Strap into machine if required.
- Place elbows on pads behind head.
- Either hold left wrist with right hand or place hands on bar provided farther behind head.
- Keep all pressure on elbows.
- Pull with back muscles until forearms are at sides.
- Return to starting position.
- Inhale at beginning, exhale at end of repetition.

Hyperextension
Lower Back

- Extend upper body over end of high bench.
- Lock legs under support.
- End of bench should be at hips.
- Bend down at waist so upper body is vertical to floor.
- Place hands behind head.
- Raise torso straight up until slightly past parallel.
- Return to starting position.
- Inhale up, exhale down.
- Can also be done with weight behind neck to increase resistance.

Standing Bent-Over Wide-Grip Bar Lat Pull-In on High Pulley
Upper Lats

- Hold bar, palms down, hands 36" apart.
- Stand far enough back to raise weight stack, arms extended.
- Bend at waist, knees slightly bent, head up, back straight, feet 24" apart.
- Pull bar straight in to lower pectorals.
- Return to starting position.
- Inhale in, exhale out.

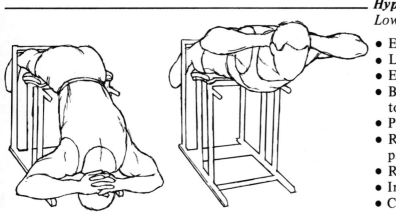

Lying High-Bench Wide-Grip Barbell Lat Pull-Up _____
Upper Lats

- Lie holding barbell at arms' length, palms down, hands 36" apart.
- Pull bar straight up to underside of bench.
- Return to starting position.
- Inhale up, exhale down.☐

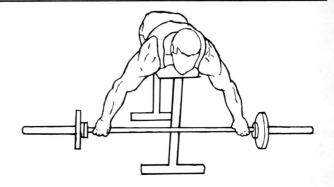

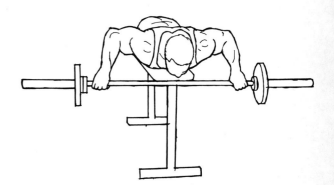

BICEPS

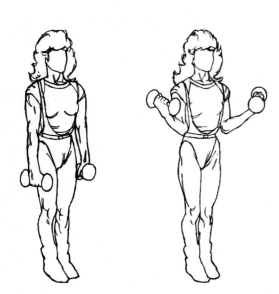

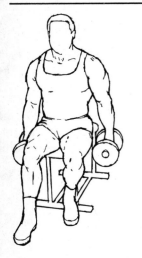

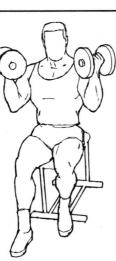

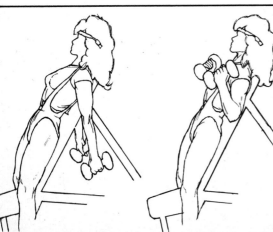

Standing Inner-Biceps Curl
Inner Biceps

- Hold dumbbells.
- Stand erect, feet 16" apart.
- Keep back straight, head up, hips and legs locked.
- Start with dumbbells at arms' length, palms in, at sides of upper thighs.
- Curl dumbbells out and up, rotating wrists to turn palms up.
- Keep forearms in line with outer deltoids.
- Lower dumbbells back to starting position using same path.
- Inhale up, exhale down.
- Can also be done seated or on incline bench.

Note: On all 6 dumbbell curl exercises on these two pages, you start with palms *in,* then rotate wrists as you raise arms.

Seated Dumbbell Curl
Biceps and Arms

- Hold dumbbells.
- Sit at end of bench, feet firmly on floor.
- Keep back straight, head up.
- Start with dumbbells at arms' length, palms in.
- Begin curl with palms in until past thighs, then turn palms up for remainder of curl to shoulder height.
- Keep palms up while lowering until past thighs, then turn palms in.
- Keep upper arms close to sides.
- Concentrate on biceps while raising and lowering weights.
- Inhale up, exhale down.

Incline Dumbbell Curl
Biceps and Arms

- Hold dumbbells.
- Lie back on incline bench.
- Start with dumbbells at arms' length, palms in.
- Begin curl with palms in until past upper thighs, then turn palms up for remainder of curl to shoulder height.
- Keep palms up while lowering until past upper thighs, then turn palms in.
- Keep upper arms close to sides.
- Inhale up, exhale down.

Standing Alternated Dumbbell Curl
Biceps

- Hold dumbbells.
- Stand erect, feet 16" apart.
- Keep back straight, head up, hips and legs locked.
- Start with dumbbells at arms' length, palms in.
- Curl dumbbell in right hand with palm in until past thigh, then palm up for remainder of curl to shoulder height.
- Keep palm up while lowering until past thigh, then turn palm in.
- Keep upper arm close to side.
- Do a repetition with right arm, then curl left arm.
- Inhale up, exhale down.
- Can also be done seated on flat bench or seated incline bench.

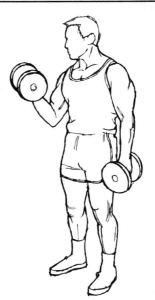
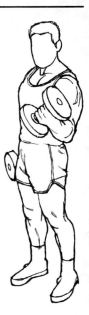

Incline Alternated Dumbbell Curl
Biceps

- Hold dumbbells.
- Lie back on incline bench.
- Start with dumbbells at arms' length, palms in.
- Curl dumbbell in right hand with palm in until past thigh, then turn palm up for remainder of curl to shoulder height.
- Keep palm up while lowering until past thigh, then turn palm in.
- Keep upper arms close to sides.
- Do a repetition with right arm, then curl left arm.
- Inhale up, exhale down.

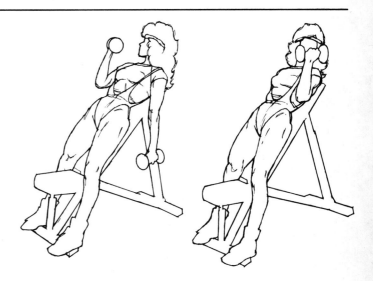

Seated Alternated Dumbbell Curl
Biceps

- Hold dumbbells.
- Sit at end of bench, feet firmly on floor.
- Keep back straight, head up.
- Start with dumbbells at arms' length, palms in.
- Curl dumbbell in right hand with palm in until past thigh, then turn palm up for remainder of curl to shoulder height.
- Keep palm up while lowering until past thigh, then turn palm in.
- Keep upper arm close to side.
- Do a repetition with right arm, then curl left arm.
- Inhale up, exhale down.

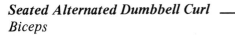
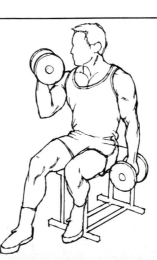
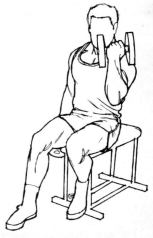

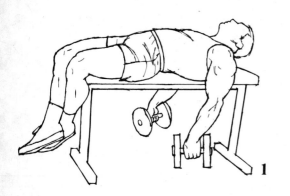

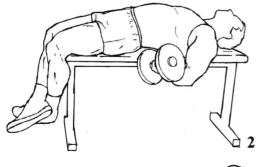

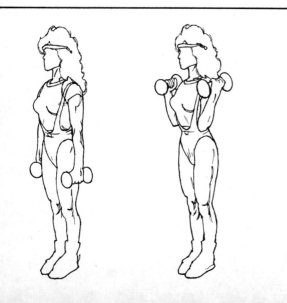

Lying-Supine 4x4x4 Dumbbell Curl
Biceps

- Hold dumbbells.
- Lie on your back on a flat bench.
- Start with dumbbells at arms' length, palms in.
- Begin curl, turning palms up.
- Do 4 complete repetitions from floor to shoulder.
- At the end of the fourth rep, keep the dumbbell at the top position (fig. 3).
- Do 4 partial reps, lowering the weight from your shoulders to where your lower arms are parallel to floor (fig. 2).
- At the end of the fourth rep, lower dumbbells to arms' length (fig. 1).
- Do 4 partial reps from arms' length to where your lower arms are parallel to floor (fig. 2).
- 12 reps completes one set.
- Inhale up, exhale down.

Standing Dumbbell Curl
Biceps

- Hold dumbbells.
- Stand erect, feet 16" apart.
- Keep back straight, head up, hips and legs locked.
- Start with dumbbells at arms' length, palms in.
- Begin curl with palms in until past thighs, then turn palms up for remainder of curl to shoulder height.
- Keep palms up while lowering until past thighs, then turn palms in.
- Keep upper arms close to sides.
- Concentrate on biceps while raising and lowering weights.
- Inhale up, exhale down.

Incline Inner-Biceps Curl
Inner Biceps

- Hold dumbbells.
- Lie back on incline bench.
- Start with dumbbells at arms' length, palms in.
- Curl dumbbells out and up, keeping forearms in line with outer deltoids.
- Lower dumbbells to starting position, using same path.
- Inhale up, exhale down.

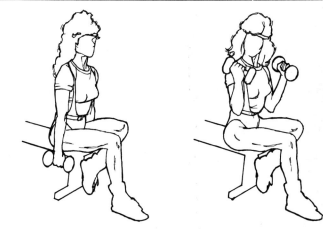

Seated Inner-Biceps Curl
Inner Biceps

- Hold dumbbells.
- Sit at end of bench, feet firmly on floor.
- Keep back straight, head up.
- Start with dumbbells at arms' length, palms in.
- Curl dumbbells out and up, turning palms out as you lift, keeping forearms in line with outer deltoids.
- Lower dumbbells to starting position using same path.
- Inhale up, exhale down.
- Can also be done standing.

Kneeling Isolated Dumbbell Curl
Biceps

- Hold dumbbell in right hand, palm up.
- Kneel on left knee.
- Right leg should be bent at about 45°.
- Hold dumbbell in front of you at arm's length.
- Place left hand on left hip.
- Curl dumbbell up in semicircular motion to shoulder height.
- *Do not* let upper arm rest against upper thigh at all.
- Upper arm should remain vertical to floor.
- Lower dumbbell to starting position using same path.
- Inhale up, exhale down.
- Reverse position and repeat movement with left arm.

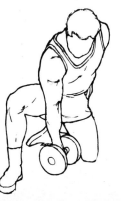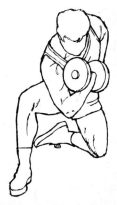

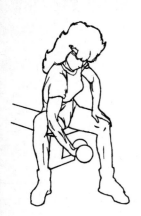
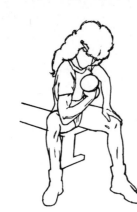

Seated Concentrated Dumbbell Curl
Biceps

- Hold dumbbell in right hand, palm up.
- Sit at end of bench, feet firmly on floor about 24" apart.
- Hold dumbbell in front of you at arm's length.
- Bend slightly forward and place left hand on left knee.
- Rest upper right arm against inner right thigh about 4" above knee.
- Curl dumbbell up in semicircular motion to shoulder height.
- Keep upper arm against inner thigh at all times.
- Lower dumbbell to starting position using same path.
- Inhale up, exhale down.
- Reverse position and repeat movement with left arm.

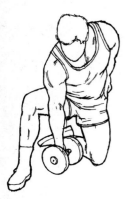
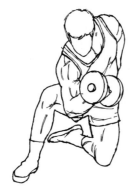

Kneeling Concentrated Dumbbell Curl
Biceps

- Hold dumbbell in right hand, palm up.
- Kneel on left knee.
- Right leg should be bent at about 45°.
- Place right upper arm against inner right thigh.
- Place left hand on left hip.
- Curl dumbbell up in semicircular motion to shoulder height.
- Keep upper arm against inner thigh at all times.
- Lower dumbbell to starting position using same path.
- Inhale up, exhale down.
- Reverse position and repeat movement with left arm.

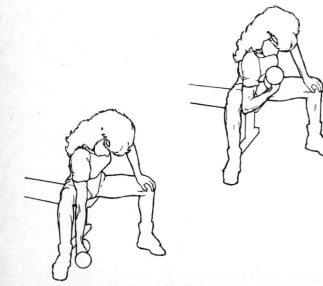

Seated Isolated Dumbbell Curl
Biceps

- Hold dumbbell in right hand, palm up.
- Sit at end of bench, feet firmly on floor about 24" apart.
- Hold dumbbell in front of you at arm's length.
- Bend slightly forward and place left hand on left knee.
- Curl dumbbell up in semicircular motion to shoulder height.
- *Do not* let upper arm rest against inner thigh at all.
- Upper arm should remain vertical to floor.
- Lower dumbbell to starting position using same path.
- Inhale up, exhale down.
- Reverse body position and repeat movement with left arm.

Lying-Supine Dumbbell Curl
Biceps

- Hold dumbbells.
- Lie on back on flat bench, head up, legs to side of bench.
- Start with dumbbells at arms' length, palms in.
- As you begin curl, turn palms up.
- Turn palms in at end of each rep.
- Keep upper arms close to sides.
- Inhale up, exhale down.

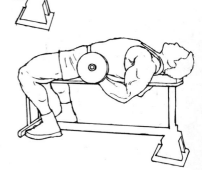

Standing Scott Bench One-Arm Dumbbell Curl
Lower Biceps

- Hold dumbbell in right hand, palm up.
- Stand at Scott bench, arm resting on slanted pad.
- Curl dumbbell up in semicircular motion until forearm touches biceps.
- Keep upper arm drawn in.
- Return to starting position using same path.
- Reverse position and do with left arm.
- Inhale up, exhale down.
- Can also be done with 2 dumbbells.

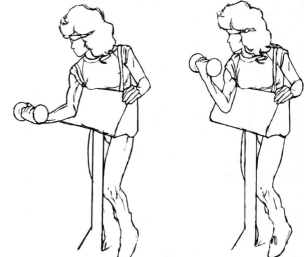

Seated Scott Bench Two-Arm Dumbbell Curl
Lower Biceps

- Hold dumbbells, palms up.
- Sit on Scott bench, arms resting on slanted pad.
- Curl dumbbells up in semicircular motion until forearms touch biceps.
- Keep upper arms drawn in.
- Return to starting position using same path.
- Inhale up, exhale down.
- Can also be done with barbell or easy-curl barbell.

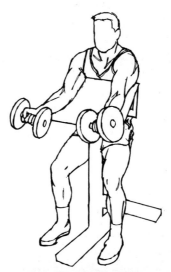
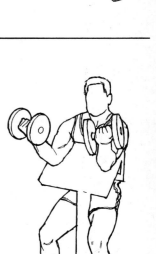

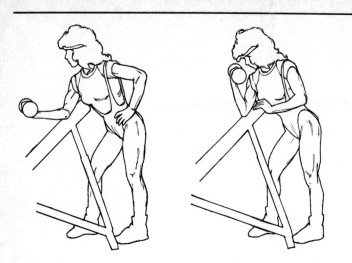

Standing One-Arm Dumbbell Curl Over Incline Bench
Biceps

- Stand behind incline bench.
- Hold dumbbell in right hand, palm up with arm on bench.
- Curl dumbbell up in semicircular motion until forearm touches biceps.
- Return to starting position using same path.
- Inhale up, exhale down.
- Reverse position and repeat movement with left arm.

Standing Close-Grip Barbell Curl Against Wall
Outer Biceps

- Hold barbell with both hands, palms up, 12" apart.
- Stand, back resting against wall, legs slightly out in front, knees locked.
- Start with bar at arms' length against upper thighs.
- Curl bar up in semicircular motion until forearms touch biceps.
- Keep upper arms close to sides.
- Lower to starting position using same path.
- Keep upper body against wall at all times.
- Inhale up, exhale down.
- Can also be done with medium or wide grip.

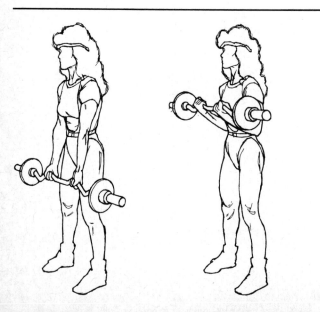

Standing Close-Grip Easy-Curl-Bar Curl Against Wall
Outer Biceps

- Hold easy-curl bar with both hands on first curves of bar, palms up.
- Stand with back resting against wall, legs slightly spread, knees locked.
- Hold bar at arms' length against upper thighs.
- Curl bar up in semicircular motion until forearms touch biceps.
- Keep upper arms against sides.
- Keep back against wall.
- Return to starting position using same path.
- Inhale up, exhale down.

Standing Close-Grip Barbell Curl
Outer Biceps

- Hold barbell with both hands, palms up, 12" apart.
- Stand erect, back straight, head up, feet 16" apart.
- Start with bar at arms' length against upper thighs.
- Curl bar up in semicircular motion until forearms touch biceps.
- Keep upper arms close to sides.
- Lower to starting position using same path.
- Do not swing back and forth to help lift bar.
- Inhale up, exhale down.

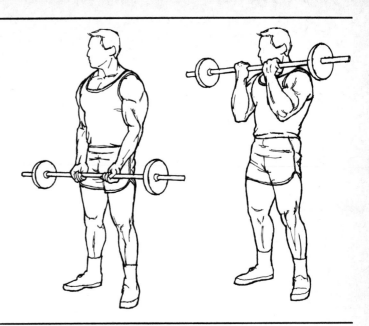

Standing Medium-Grip Barbell Curl
Biceps

- Hold barbell with both hands, palms up, 18" apart.
- Stand erect, back straight, head up, feet 16" apart.
- Start with bar at arms' length against upper thighs.
- Curl bar up in semicircular motion until forearms touch biceps.
- Keep upper arms close to sides.
- Lower to starting position using same path.
- Do not swing back and forth to help lift bar.
- Inhale up, exhale down.
- Can also be done with wide grip.

Flat Preacher Bench One-Arm-Dumbbell Curl
Biceps

- Lie face forward on flat preacher bench.
- Hold dumbbell in right hand, palm up.
- Support upper right arm against pad.
- Curl dumbbell up in semicircular motion until forearm touches biceps.
- Keep upper arm against pad at all times.
- Lower to starting position using same path.
- Reverse position and do with left arm.
- Inhale up, exhale down.
- Can also be done with wide grip.

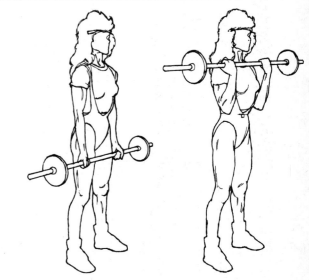

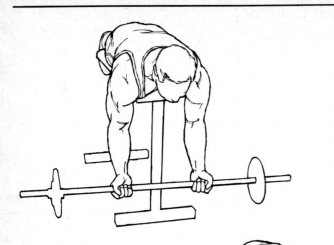

Lying High Bench Medium-Grip Barbell Curl
Lower Biceps

- Lie face forward on tall flat bench.
- Have upper body down to upper pectorals over end of bench.
- Hold barbell with both hands, palms up, 16" apart.
- Start with bar at arms' length.
- Curl bar up in semicircular motion until forearms touch biceps.
- Keep upper arms vertical to floor.
- Return to starting position using same path.
- Inhale up, exhale down.

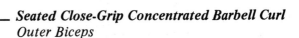

Seated Close-Grip Concentrated Barbell Curl
Outer Biceps

- Place barbell on floor near end of bench.
- Sit at end of bench, feet about 24" apart.
- Bend forward at waist.
- Hold bar with both hands, palms up, 6" apart.
- Rest elbows against inner thighs about 4" up from knees.
- Curl bar up in semicircular motion until forearms touch biceps.
- Lower bar to starting position using same path.
- Inhale up, exhale down.

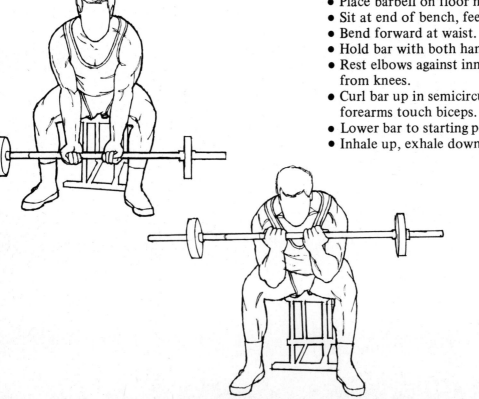

Lying High Bench Close-Grip Barbell Curl
Outer and Lower Biceps

- Lie face forward on tall flat bench.
- Have upper body down to upper pectorals over end of bench.
- Hold barbell with both hands, palms up, 12" apart.
- Start with bar at arms' length.
- Curl bar up in semicircular motion until forearms touch biceps.
- Keep upper arms vertical to floor.
- Return to starting position using same path.
- Inhale up, exhale down.

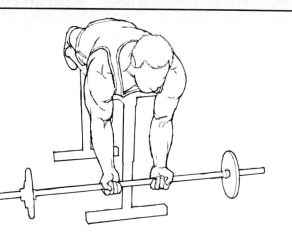

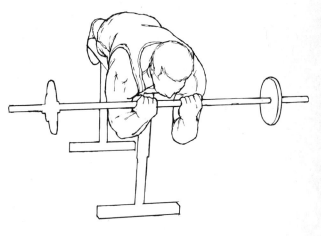

Flat Preacher Bench Close-Grip Barbell Curl
Outer Biceps

- Lie face forward on flat preacher bench.
- Have upper body down to upper pectorals over end of bench.
- Hold barbell with both hands, palms up, 12" apart.
- Start with bar at arms' length.
- Keep upper arms against pad.
- Curl bar up in semicircular motion until forearms touch biceps.
- Try to keep upper arms from moving outward as you curl.
- Return to starting position using same path.
- Inhale up, exhale down.

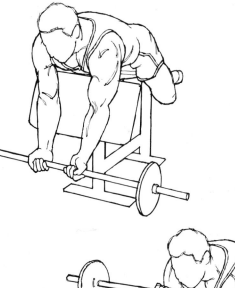

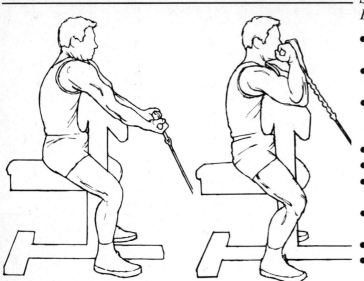

Seated Scott Bench Bar Curl on Low Pulley
Biceps

- Attach short bar to low pulley cables of wall pulley.
- Place Scott bench in front of pulley, facing machine.
- Have bench far enough away from machine to allow arms to support weight with bar at arms' length.
- Hold bar with both hands, palms up.
- Sit on bench with upper arms resting on pad.
- Curl bar up in semicircular motion until forearms touch biceps.
- Try to keep upper arms from moving outward as you curl.
- Return to starting position using same path.
- Inhale up, exhale down.

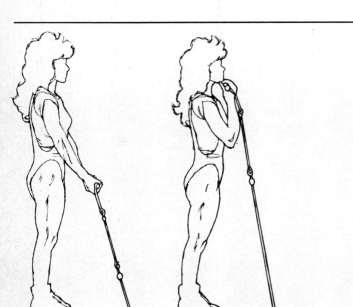

Standing Bar Curl on Universal Machine
Biceps

- Stand facing low pulley station of Universal machine.
- Hold short bar attached to low cable, palms up.
- Stand back from pulley to allow arms to support weight with arms extended.
- Curl bar up in semicircular motion until forearms touch biceps.
- Keep upper arms close to sides.
- Return to starting position using same path.
- Inhale up, exhale down.

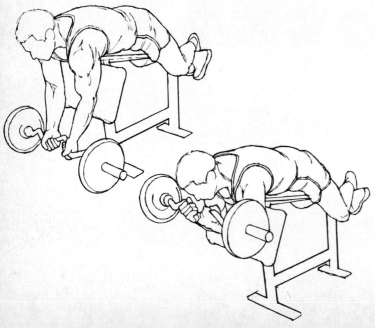

Flat Preacher Bench Close-Grip Easy-Curl-Bar Curl
Outer Biceps

- Hold easy-curl bar with both hands on first curves of bar, palms up.
- Lie face forward on preacher bench.
- Support upper arms against pad.
- Curl bar up in semicircular motion until forearms touch biceps.
- Try to keep upper arms from moving outward as you curl.
- Return to starting position using same path.
- Inhale up, exhale down.

Standing Medium-Grip Easy-Curl-Bar Curl
Biceps

- Hold easy-curl bar with both hands on second curve of bar, palms up.
- Stand erect, back straight, head up, feet 16" apart.
- Hold bar at arms' length against upper thighs.
- Curl bar up in semicircular motion until forearms touch biceps.
- Keep upper arms against sides.
- Return to starting position using same path.
- Inhale up, exhale down.

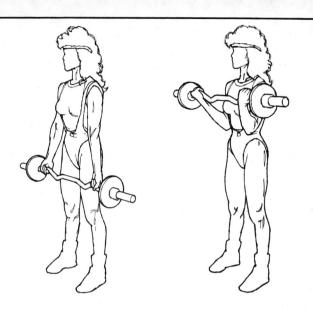

Flat Preacher Bench Medium-Grip Barbell Curl
Biceps

- Lie face forward on flat preacher bench.
- Have upper body down to upper pectorals over end of bench.
- Hold barbell with both hands, palms up, 16" apart.
- Start with bar at arms' length.
- Keep upper arms against pad.
- Curl bar up in semicircular motion until forearms touch biceps.
- Try to keep upper arms from moving outward as you curl.
- Return to starting position using same path.
- Inhale up, exhale down.

Seated Close-Grip Easy-Curl-Bar Concentrated Curl
Outer and Lower Biceps

- Hold easy-curl bar with both hands on first curves of bar, palms up.
- Sit at end of flat bench.
- Bend forward at waist, back straight, head up, feet firmly on floor 16" apart.
- Place upper arms against side of upper thighs.
- Hang arms straight down.
- Curl bar up in semicircular motion until forearms touch biceps.
- Return to starting position using same path.
- Inhale up, exhale down.

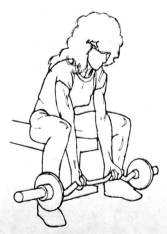
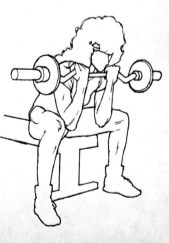

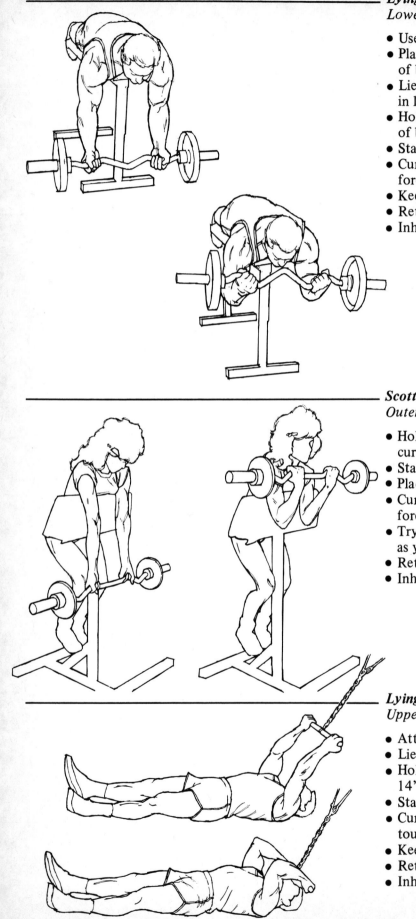

Lying High Bench Medium-Grip Easy-Curl-Bar Curl
Lower Biceps

- Use a bench that is about 30" high.
- Place easy-curl bar on floor at one end of bench.
- Lie face down on bench with end of bench in line with shoulders.
- Hold bar with both hands on second curve of bar, palms up.
- Start with bar at arms' length.
- Curl bar up in semicircular motion until forearms touch biceps.
- Keep upper arms vertical to floor.
- Return to starting position using same path.
- Inhale up, exhale down.

Scott Bench Close-Grip Easy-Curl-Bar Curl
Outer Biceps

- Hold easy-curl bar with both hands on first curves of bar, palms up.
- Stand at (or sit on) Scott curling bench.
- Place upper arms against pad.
- Curl bar up in semicircular motion until forearms touch biceps.
- Try to keep upper arms from moving outward as you curl.
- Return to starting position using same path.
- Inhale up, exhale down.

Lying Floor Head-Forward High-Pulley Bar Curl
Upper Biceps

- Attach short bar to top pulley cable.
- Lie on floor with head toward machine.
- Hold bar with both hands, reverse grip, 14" apart.
- Start with arms extended.
- Curl bar down in semicircular motion until it touches chin.
- Keep upper arms vertical at all times.
- Return to starting position using same path.
- Inhale down, exhale up.

Squatting Close-Grip Easy-Curl-Bar Concentrated Curl
Outer and Lower Biceps

- Hold easy-curl bar with both hands on first curves of bar, palms up.
- Squat until upper thighs are nearly parallel to floor.
- Keep back straight, head up.
- Place upper arms against inner thighs.
- Hang arms straight down.
- Curl bar up in semicircular motion until forearms touch biceps.
- Keep upper arms against inner thighs at all times.
- Return to starting position using same path.
- Inhale up, exhale down.

Flat Preacher Bench Medium-Grip Easy-Curl-Bar Curl
Biceps

- Hold easy-curl bar with both hands on second curves of bar, palms up.
- Lie face forward on preacher bench.
- Support upper arms against pad.
- Curl bar up in semicircular motion until forearms touch biceps.
- Try to keep upper arms from moving outward as you curl.
- Return to starting position using same path.
- Inhale up, exhale down.

Lying One-Arm Biceps Curl on High Pulley
Biceps

- Hold pulley handle with right hand.
- Lie on your back in front of pulley with head toward machine.
- Lie far enough from machine to allow arm to support weight stack while vertical to floor.
- Curl handle down in semicircular motion to chin.
- Keep upper arm vertical at all times.
- Return to starting position using same path.
- Inhale down, exhale up.
- Reverse position and repeat movement with left arm.

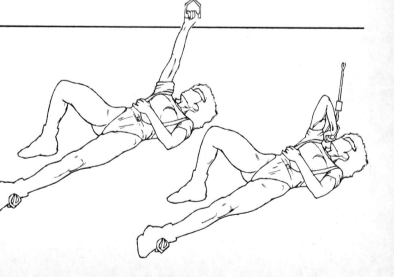

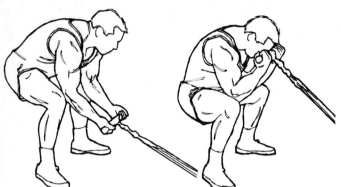

Squatting Concentrated Bar Curl on Low Pulley
Outer Biceps

- Attach short bar to low pulley cable.
- Stand facing machine.
- Hold bar with both hands, palms up, 6" apart.
- Stand far enough from machine to allow arms to support weight.
- Squat until upper thighs are parallel to floor.
- Rest elbows against inner thighs about 4" from knees.
- Curl bar up in semicircular motion until forearms touch biceps.
- Return to starting position using same path.
- Inhale up, exhale down.

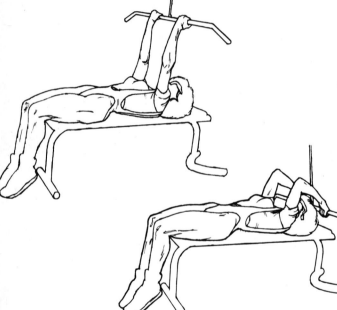

Lying Flat Bench Close-Grip Bar Curl on Lat Machine
Outer Upper Biceps

- Place flat bench below bar of lat machine.
- Position bench about 6" behind bar.
- Hold bar with both hands, reverse grip, 8" apart.
- Lie on your back with head over end.
- Extend arms straight above shoulders.
- Curl bar down in semicircular motion until it touches chin.
- Keep upper arms vertical at all times.
- Return to starting position using same path.
- Inhale down, exhale up.

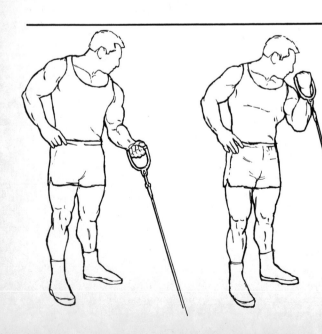

Standing One-Arm Curl on Low Pulley
Biceps

- Hold left pulley cable with left hand.
- Stand far enough from machine so weight stack is supported with arm at side, palm facing thigh.
- Curl handle, turning palm up when hand clears thigh.
- Curl until biceps and forearm touch.
- Keep upper arm in close to side.
- Return to starting position, turning palm in when nearing thigh.
- Inhale up, exhale down.
- Repeat with right arm.
- Can also be done with both arms together or alternating arms.

Lying-Supine Close-Grip Bar Curl on High Pulley
Outer Biceps

- Place flat bench in front of high pulley.
- Hold bar with both hands, palms down, 8" apart.
- Lie on your back with head over end of bench.
- Extend arms straight above shoulders.
- Curl bar down in semicircular motion until it touches chin.
- Keep upper arms vertical at all times.
- Return to starting position using same path.
- Inhale down, exhale up.

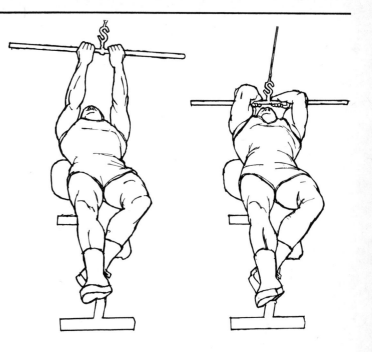

Lying Bar Curl on Universal Machine
Biceps

- Stand facing low pulley station of Universal machine.
- Hold short bar attached to low cable, palms up.
- Lie on your back with feet facing machine.
- Position body far enough from machine to allow arms to support weight at arms' length.
- Rest arms against upper thighs.
- Curl bar up in semicircular motion until forearms touch biceps.
- Keep upper arms close to sides at all times.
- Return to starting position using same path.
- Inhale up, exhale down.

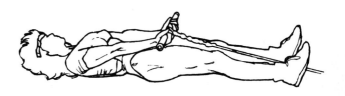

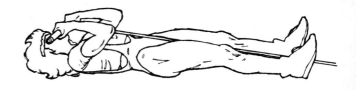

Seated Medium-Grip Curl on Biceps Machine
Biceps

- Sit on seat of biceps curling machine.
- Hold bar at second curves, palms up.
- If machine has straight bar, keep hands 16" apart.
- Place upper arms against pad.
- Curl bar up in semicircular motion until forearms touch biceps.
- Try to keep upper arms from moving outward.
- Return to starting position using same path.
- Inhale up, exhale down.

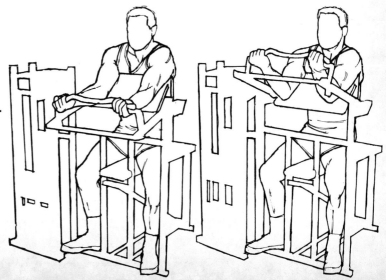

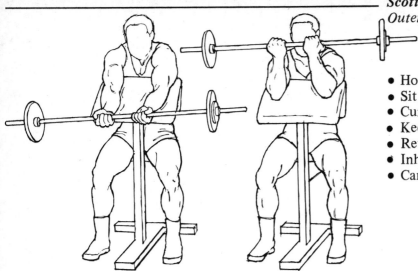

Scott Bench Close-Grip Barbell Curl
Outer Biceps

- Hold barbell, palms up, 12" apart.
- Sit on bench, upper arms against pad.
- Curl bar until forearms and biceps touch.
- Keep upper arms in close.
- Return to starting position.
- Inhale up, exhale down.
- Can also be done with medium or wide grip.

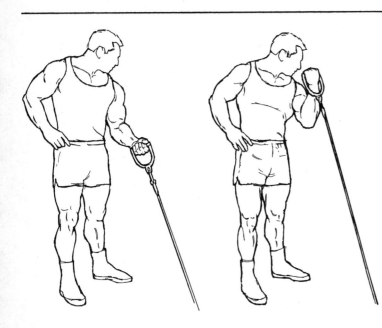

Standing One-Arm Curl on Low Pulley
Biceps

- Hold left pulley cable with left hand.
- Stand far enough from machine so weight stack is supported with arm at side, palm facing thigh.
- Curl handle, turning palm up when hand clears thigh.
- Curl until biceps and forearm touch.
- Keep upper arm close to side.
- Return to starting position, turning palm in when nearing thigh.
- Inhale up, exhale down.
- Repeat with right arm.
- Can also be done with both arms together or alternating arms.

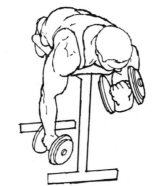

Lying High Bench Alternated Dumbbell Curl
Lower Biceps

- Place two dumbbells on floor.
- Lie face down, end of bench in line with shoulders.
- Grasp dumbbells, palms up.
- Curl right hand dumbbell in semicircular motion until it is directly under chin.
- Curl by bending elbow only, keep upper arm vertical to floor at all times.
- Return to starting position.
- Curl left hand dumbbell in same manner.
- Continue curling back and forth.
- A curl to the right and to the left equals one rep.
- Inhale up, exhale down.

Standing Bar Curl on Universal Machine
Biceps

- Hold short bar attached to lower pulley, palms up.
- Stand far enough back to raise weight stack, bar resting on upper thighs.
- Curl bar until biceps and forearms touch.
- Return to starting position.
- Inhale up, exhale down. ☐

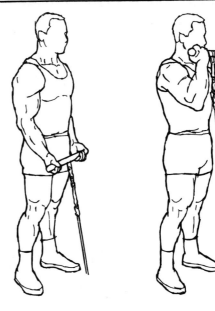

CALVES

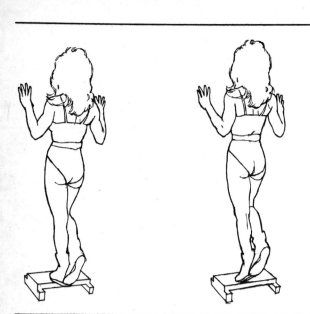

Standing Freehand One-Legged Toe Raise on 2x4
Main Calf Muscles

- Place 2x4 or raised object on floor about 24" away from wall.
- Stand erect, balls of feet on board.
- Keep back straight, head up, legs locked.
- Balance yourself by placing hands against wall.
- Put right foot against left heel.
- Do not let hips move backward or forward.
- Raise up on toes as high as possible.
- Hold position momentarily, then return to starting position.
- Inhale up, exhale down.
- Reverse position and repeat movement with right leg.

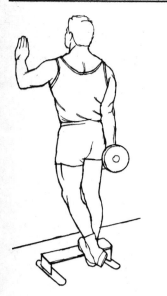

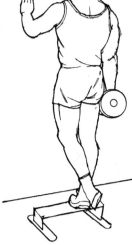

Standing Dumbbell One-Legged Toe Raise
Main Calf Muscles

- Hold dumbbell in right hand, hanging down at side, palm in.
- Step up with ball of right foot on raised object, about 24" away from wall.
- Place left hand against wall.
- Keep back straight, head up, leg locked.
- Put left foot against right heel.
- Do not let hips move backward or forward.
- Raise up on toes as high as possible.
- Hold position momentarily, then return to starting position.
- Inhale up, exhale down.
- Reverse position and repeat movement with left leg.

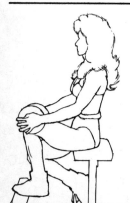

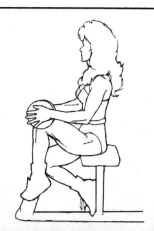

Seated Dumbbell One-Legged Toe Raise
Main Calf Muscles

- Place raised object on floor about 12" away from end of bench.
- Sit at end of bench.
- Rest dumbbell on left upper thigh about 3" above knee.
- Place ball of left foot on object.
- Raise up on toes as high as possible.
- Hold position momentarily, then return to starting position.
- Inhale up, exhale down.
- Reverse position and repeat movement with right leg.

Standing One-Legged Calf Stretch Against Wall
Main Calf Muscles

- Stand facing wall about 40" back.
- Lean forward with outstretched arms, hands against wall.
- Keep back straight, head up, legs locked.
- Put right foot against left heel.
- Do not let hips move backward or forward.
- Raise up on toes as high as possible.
- Hold position momentarily, then return to starting position.
- Inhale up, exhale down.
- Reverse position and repeat movement with right leg.

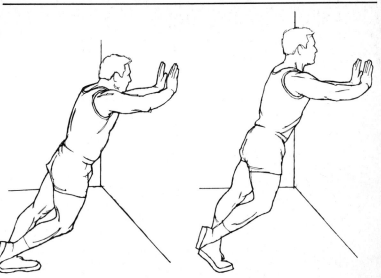

Standing Calf Stretch Against Wall
Main Calf Muscles

- Stand facing wall about 40" back.
- Lean forward with outstretched arms, hands against wall.
- Keep back straight, head up, legs locked.
- Do not let hips move backward or forward.
- Raise up on toes as high as possible.
- Hold position momentarily, then return to starting position.
- Inhale up, exhale down.

Seated Barbell Toe Raise
Main Calf Muscles

- Place raised object on floor about 12" away from end of bench.
- Sit at end of bench.
- Hold barbell on upper thighs about 3" above knees.
- Place balls of feet on object.
- Raise up on toes as high as possible.
- Hold position momentarily, then return to starting position.
- Inhale up, exhale down.

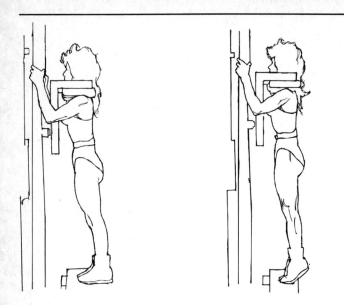

Standing Toe Raise on Wall Calf Machine
Main Calf Muscles

- Position shoulders under bars of wall calf machine.
- Stand erect with balls of feet on foot pad.
- Keep back straight, head up, legs locked.
- Do not let hips move backward or forward.
- Raise up on toes as high as possible.
- Hold position momentarily, then return to starting position.
- Inhale up, exhale down.

Standing One-Legged Toe Raise on Wall Calf Machine
Main Calf Muscles

- Position shoulders under bars of wall calf machine.
- Stand erect and place ball of left foot on foot pad.
- Put right foot against left heel.
- Keep back straight, head up, leg locked.
- Raise up on toes as high as possible.
- Hold position momentarily, then return to starting position.
- Inhale up, exhale down.
- Reverse position and repeat movement with right leg.

Seated Toe Raise on Nautilus-type Machine
Main Calf Muscles

- Sit on seat of machine.
- Place hands under buttocks and hold end of bench.
- Place balls of feet on foot pad.
- Keep legs straight, knees locked.
- Press forward with toes.
- Hold momentarily, then return to starting position.
- Inhale forward, exhale back.
- Toes out, heels in, works inner calves.
- Feet straight works main calf muscles.
- Toes in, heels out, works outer calves.

Standing Toe Raise on Power Rack
Main Calf Muscles

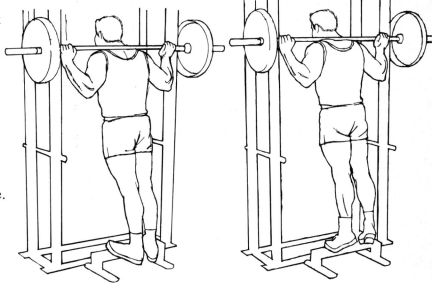

- Place barbell on pegs of power rack just below shoulder height.
- Position raised object on floor directly under bar.
- Place bar on upper back with bar against power rack.
- Stand erect with balls of feet on object.
- Keep back straight, head up, legs locked.
- Do not let hips move backward or forward.
- Raise up on toes as high as possible.
- Hold position momentarily, then return to starting position.
- Inhale up, exhale down.

Seated Negative-Resistance Toe Raise on Universal Leg Press Machine
Main Calf Muscles

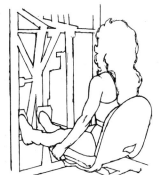
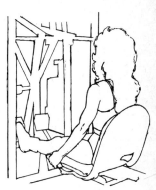

- Sit on chair of machine.
- Hold sides of seat.
- Place balls of feet on lower pads.
- Press weight stack out until legs are straight, knees locked.
- Keep legs in this position at all times.
- Hold this position for short period, then shift all weight to left leg, pressing forward.
- Hold for short period, then shift all weight to right leg, pressing forward.
- Shift back and forth from left to right leg for prescribed number of reps.
- Inhale out, exhale back.

Lying Face Down One-Legged Toe Raise on Wall Leg Press Machine
Main Calf Muscles

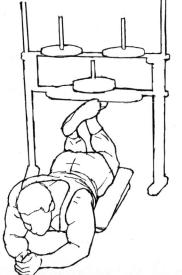
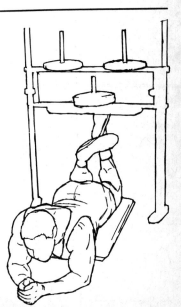

- Lie face down on support pad under machine.
- Position yourself so lower legs are vertical to floor when bent at knees.
- Place balls of feet on foot pad.
- Press toes upward and have training partner release safety stop.
- Now, shift weight on to left leg and place right foot against left heel.
- Lower left toes as far as possible.
- Hold momentarily, then return to starting position.
- Inhale up, exhale down.
- Reverse position and repeat movement with right leg.
- Toes out, heel in, works inner calf.
- Foot straight works main calf muscle.
- Toes in, heel out, works outer calf.

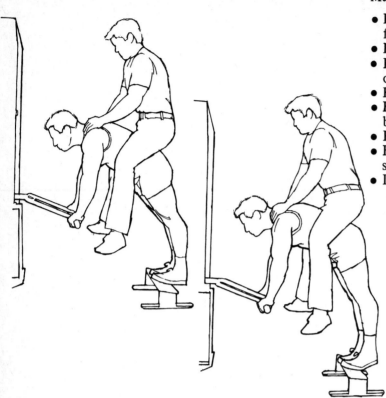

Donkey Toe Raise
Main Calf Muscles

- Place raised object on floor about 36" away from a waist-high object.
- Place balls of feet on raised object, legs locked.
- Bend forward and support upper body with outstretched arms.
- Keep legs straight.
- Have training partner sit on lower back with bulk of his weight on your hips.
- Raise up on toes as high as possible.
- Hold position momentarily, then return to starting position.
- Inhale up, exhale down.

Donkey One-Legged Toe Raise
Main Calf Muscles

- Place raised object on floor about 36" away from a waist-high object.
- Place ball of left foot on board, leg locked.
- Bend forward and support upper body with outstretched arms.
- Put right foot against left heel.
- Keep leg straight.
- Have training partner sit on lower back with bulk of his weight on your hips.
- Raise up on toes as high as possible.
- Hold position momentarily, then return to starting position.
- Inhale up, exhale down.
- Reverse position and repeat movement with right leg.

Standing Toe Raise on Ram Thrust Machine
Main Calf Muscles

- Face machine.
- Position shoulders unders bars of machine, grasp bars on each side of sled, arms straight.
- Do not let hips move backward or forward.
- Raise up on toes as high as possible.
- Hold momentarily, then return to starting position.
- Inhale up, exhale down.

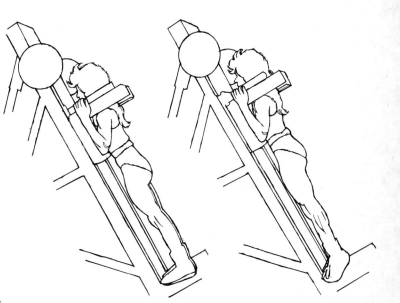

Standing One-Legged Toe Raise on Power Rack
Main Calf Muscles

- Place barbell on pegs of power rack just below shoulder height.
- Position raised object on floor directly under bar.
- Place bar on upper back with bar against power rack.
- Stand erect with ball of left foot on object.
- Keep back straight, head up, leg locked.
- Put right foot against left heel.
- Raise up on toes as high as possible.
- Hold position momentarily, then return to starting position.
- Inhale up, exhale down.
- Reverse position and repeat movement with right leg.

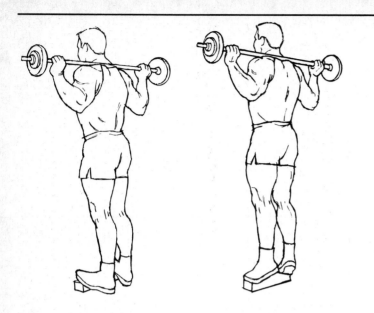

Standing Barbell Toe Raise
Main Calf Muscles

- Place barbell on back of shoulders.
- Put toes on raised object, heels on floor.
- Slowly push up on toes.
- Slowly lower heels to floor.
- Inhale up, exhale down.
- Toes out, heels in, works inner calves.
- Feet straight works main calf muscles.
- Toes in, heels out, works outer calves.

Toe Raise on Seated Calf Machine
Main Calf Muscles

- Sit on seat of machine.
- Place upper thighs under leg pad just above knees.
- Raise up on toes and release safety stop.
- Lower heels to lowest possible comfortable position.
- Raise up on toes as high as possible.
- Hold momentarily, then return to starting position.
- Inhale up, exhale down.

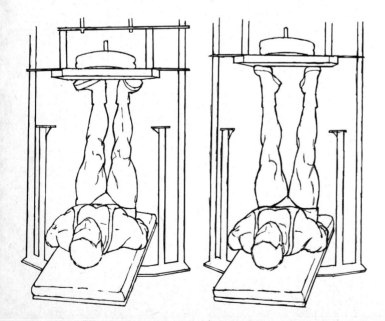

Lying Supine Toe Raise on Wall Leg Press Machine
Main Calf Muscles

- Lie on floor pad under machine, hips directly under foot pad.
- Place balls of feet on foot pad.
- Press weight rack up until legs are straight, knees locked.
- Release safety stops, then place hands under buttocks, palms down.
- Press up with toes, raising rack as high as possible.
- Hold, then return to starting position.
- Inhale up, exhale down.
- Toes out, heels in, works inner calves.
- Feet straight works main calf muscles.
- Toes in, heels out, works outer calves.
- Can also be done one leg at a time.

Seated Lower Pad Toe Raise on Universal Leg Press Machine _____
Main Calf Muscles

- Sit holding side of seat.
- Place balls of feet on lower pads.
- Press until legs are straight, knees locked.
- Keep legs straight at all times.
- Press feet forward as far as possible.
- Hold, then return feet back as far as possible.
- Inhale forward, exhale back.
- Toes out, heels in, works inner calves.
- Feet straight works main calf muscles.
- Toes in, heels out, works outer calves.
- Can also use upper toe pads.

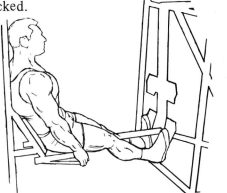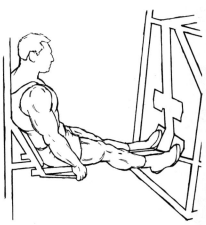

Standing One-Legged Toe Raise on Ram Thrust Machine _____
Main Calf Muscles

- Face into machine.
- Position shoulders under extended portion of machine, grasp bars on each side of sled, arms straight.
- Keep back straight, head up, legs locked.
- Put left foot against right heel.
- Raise up on toes as high as possible.
- Hold momentarily, then return to starting position.
- Inhale up, exhale down.
- Reverse position and repeat movement with left leg. □

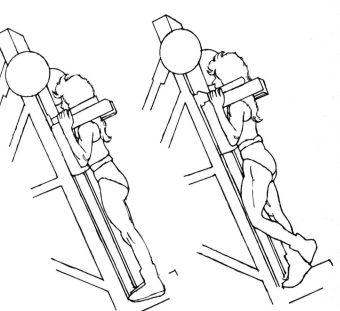

CHEST
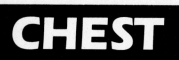

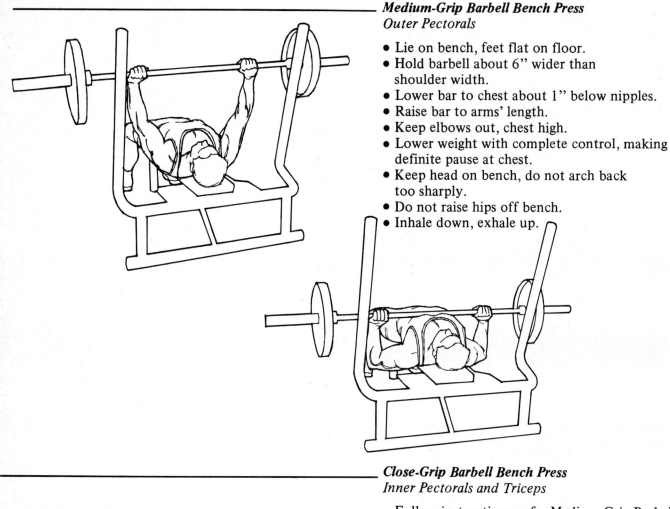

Medium-Grip Barbell Bench Press
Outer Pectorals

- Lie on bench, feet flat on floor.
- Hold barbell about 6" wider than shoulder width.
- Lower bar to chest about 1" below nipples.
- Raise bar to arms' length.
- Keep elbows out, chest high.
- Lower weight with complete control, making definite pause at chest.
- Keep head on bench, do not arch back too sharply.
- Do not raise hips off bench.
- Inhale down, exhale up.

Close-Grip Barbell Bench Press
Inner Pectorals and Triceps

- Follow instructions as for Medium-Grip Barbell Bench Press above, except use a hand grip 12-14" wide.

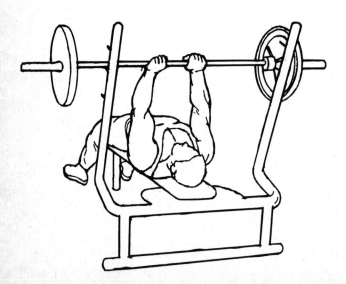
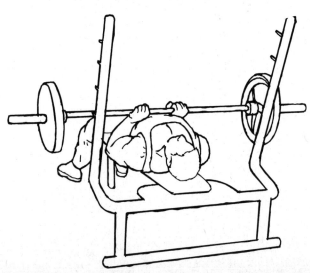

Medium-Grip Incline Barbell Bench Press
Upper Pectorals

- Lie on incline bench, feet flat on floor.
- Hold barbell about 6" wider than shoulder width.
- Lower bar to chest about 3" above nipples.
- Raise bar to arms' length.
- Keep elbows out, chest high.
- Lower weight with complete control, making definite pause at chest.
- Keep head on bench, do not arch back too sharply.
- Do not raise hips off bench.
- Inhale down, exhale up.
- Can also be done with close or wide grip.

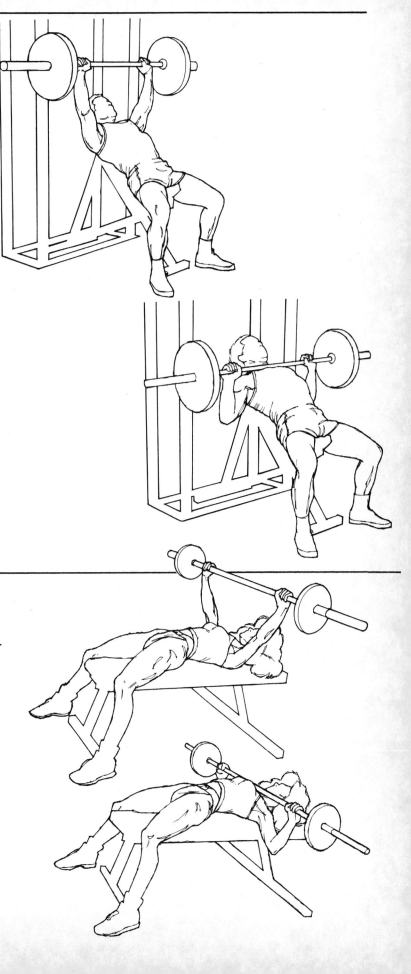

Wide-Grip Barbell Bench Press
Outer Pectorals

- Lie on bench, feet flat on floor.
- Use collar-to-collar grip.
- Lower barbell to chest about 1" below nipples.
- Raise bar to arms' length.
- Keep elbows out, chest high.
- Lower weight with complete control, making definite pause at chest.
- Keep head on bench, do not arch back too sharply.
- Do not raise hips off bench.
- Inhale down, exhale up.

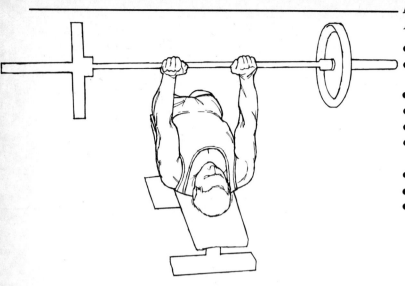

Medium-Grip Decline Barbell Bench Press
Lower Pectorals

- Lie on decline bench.
- Hold barbell about 6" wider than shoulder width.
- Lower bar to chest about 3" below nipples.
- Raise bar to arms' length.
- Keep elbows out, chest high.
- Lower weight with complete control, making definite pause at chest.
- Keep head on bench, chest held high.
- Inhale down, exhale up.
- Can also be done with close grip.

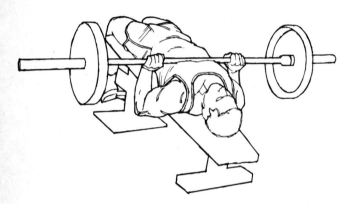

Decline Barbell Bench Press to Neck
Outer and Lower Pectorals

- Lie on decline bench.
- Hold barbell about 10" wider than shoulder width.
- Lower bar to highest part of chest just below neck.
- Raise bar to arms' length.
- Keep elbows back almost in line with ears.
- Lower weight with complete control, making definite pause at chest.
- Keep head on bench and hold chest high.
- Inhale down, exhale up.
- Can also be done with wide grip.

Wide-Grip Incline Barbell Bench Press _____
Outer and Upper Pectorals

- Lie on incline bench, feet flat on floor.
- Use collar-to-collar grip.
- Lower barbell to chest about 3" above nipples.
- Raise bar to arms' length.
- Keep elbows back almost in line with ears.
- Lower weight with complete control, making definite pause at chest.
- Keep head on bench, do not arch back too sharply.
- Do not raise hips off bench.
- Inhale down, exhale up.

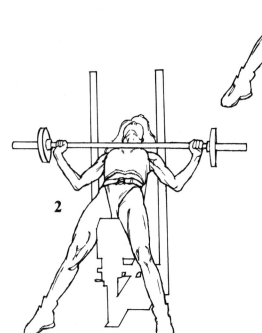

Wide-Grip Decline Barbell Bench Press _____
Outer and Lower Pectorals

- Lie on decline bench.
- Use collar-to-collar grip.
- Lower barbell to chest about 3" below nipples.
- Raise bar to arms' length.
- Keep elbows out, chest high.
- Lower weight with complete control, making definite pause at chest.
- Keep head on bench, chest held high.
- Inhale down, exhale up.

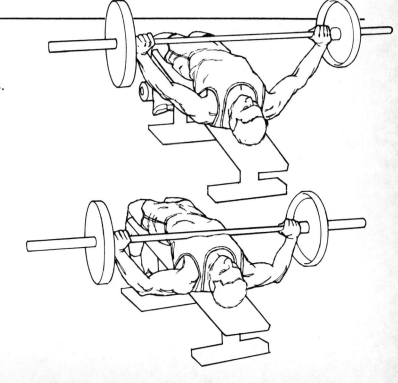

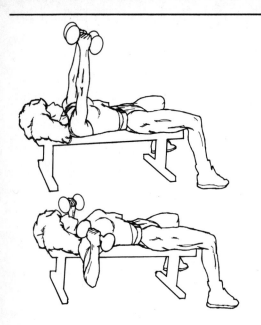

Bent-Arm Lateral
Outer Pectorals

- Lie on bench, feet flat on floor.
- Hold dumbbells together at arms' length above shoulders, palms facing each other.
- Slowly lower dumbbells so they are even with chest and 10" from each side.
- Elbows in line with ears.
- Forearms slightly out of vertical position.
- Return to starting position using same path.
- Inhale down, exhale up.

Decline Dumbbell Fly
Lower Pectorals

- Lie on decline bench.
- Hold dumbbells together at arms' length above shoulders, palms facing each other.
- Keep arms as straight as possible.
- Lower dumbbells out to each side of chest in semicircular motion.
- Weights should be even with sides of chest but back slightly, in line with ears.
- Return to starting position using same path.
- Inhale down, exhale up.
- Breathe heavily, hold chest high, keep head on bench, concentrate on pectorals.

Incline Lateral
Upper Pectorals

- Lie on incline bench.
- Hold dumbbells together at arms' length above shoulders, palms forward.
- Slowly lower dumbbells to chest until 10" from each side of chest.
- Elbows in line with ears.
- Forearms slightly out of vertical position.
- Return to starting position using same path.
- Inhale down, exhale up.

Incline Dumbbell Press
Upper Pectorals

- Lie on incline bench.
- Hold dumbbell in each hand above shoulders, palms facing each other.
- Lower dumbbells straight down to sides of chest, arms close to sides.
- Push back to starting position using same path.
- Arms must be in close at all times.
- Inhale down, exhale up.

Incline Dumbbell Fly
Upper Pectorals

- Lie on incline bench.
- Hold dumbbells together at arms' length, palms facing each other.
- Keep arms as straight as possible.
- Lower dumbbells out to each side of chest in semicircular motion.
- Weights should be even with sides of chest but back slightly, in line with ears.
- Return to starting position using same path.
- Inhale down, exhale up.
- Breathe heavily, hold chest high, keep head on bench, concentrate on pectorals.

Bent-Arm Dumbbell Pullover
Pectorals and Rib Cage

- Lie on bench, head over end, feet flat on floor.
- Hold dumbbell in each hand at sides of chest in line with nipples.
- Keep elbows in at all times.
- Lower weights just past ears in a semicircular motion towards floor.
- Lower dumbbells to floor or as low as possible without pain.
- Pull dumbbells back to sides of chest using same path.
- Inhale down, exhale up.
- Breathe heavily, keep elbows in, hold chest high.

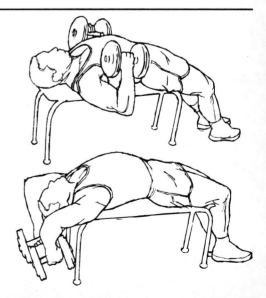

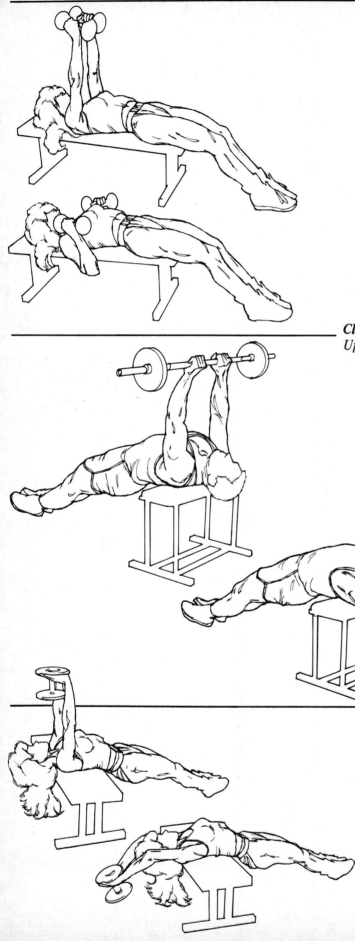

Flat Dumbbell Press
Pectorals

- Lie on bench, feet flat on floor.
- Hold dumbbells at arms' length, palms facing each other.
- Lower dumbbells straight down to sides of chest, arms close to sides.
- Push back to starting position using same path.
- Arms must be in close at all times.
- Inhale down, exhale up.

Close-Grip Straight-Arm Barbell Pullover Across Bench
Upper Pectorals and Rib Cage

- Lie across bench, upper back supporting torso.
- Have head off bench hanging down.
- Keep body and legs nearly straight, drop hips to raise rib cage.
- Hold barbell at arms' length, hands 10" apart.
- Lower weight in semicircular motion behind head as far as possible without pain.
- Return to starting position, keeping elbows locked.
- Inhale down, exhale up.
- Breathe heavily, keep head down, do not raise hips.

Straight-Arm Dumbbell Pullover Across Bench
Pectorals and Rib Cage

- Lie across bench, upper back supporting torso.
- Have head off bench, hanging down.
- Keep body and legs nearly straight, drop hips to raise rib cage.
- Hold dumbbell, hands flat against inside plate, at arms' length above chest.
- Lower dumbbell in semicircular motion behind head as far as possible without pain.
- Return to starting position, elbows locked.
- Inhale down, exhale up.
- Breathe heavily, keep head down, do not raise hips.

Straight-Arm Dumbbell Pullover
Pectorals and Rib Cage

- Lie on bench, head at end, feet flat on floor.
- Start with hands flat against inside plate of dumbbell at arms' length above chest.
- Lower dumbbell in semicircular motion behind head as far as possible without pain.
- Return dumbbell to starting position, elbows locked.
- Inhale down, exhale up.
- Breathe heavily, keep head down, chest high, hips on bench.
- Can also be done with barbell.

Bent-Arm Barbell Pullover
Upper Pectorals, Rib Cage, Triceps

- Lie on bench, head over end, feet flat on floor.
- Rest barbell on chest in line with nipples.
- Hold bar with hands 14" apart.
- Keep elbows in at all times.
- Lower bar off bench, keeping it as close to head as possible.
- Lower bar to floor or as low as comfortable.
- Pull bar back to chest using same path.
- Inhale down, exhale up.
- Breathe heavily, keep head down, do not raise hips.

Medium-Grip Straight-Arm Barbell Pullover
Pectorals and Rib Cage

- Lie on bench, head at end, feet flat on floor.
- Hold barbell above shoulders, hands 24" apart.
- Lower bar in semicircular motion over head as far as possible without pain.
- Return bar to starting position, elbows locked.
- Inhale down, exhale up.
- Breathe heavily, keep head down, chest high, hips on bench.

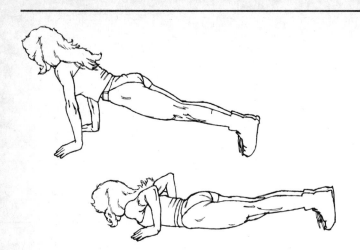

Medium-Grip Push-Ups on Floor
Pectorals and Triceps

- Kneel on floor, hands 24" apart.
- Place legs straight behind, back straight, head up.
- Keeping body rigid, lower yourself until chest touches floor.
- Pause at bottom, then press to starting position.
- Inhale down, exhale up.
- Keep elbows in.

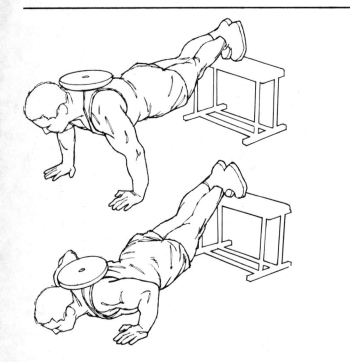

Weighted Medium-Grip Push-Ups, Feet on Bench
Pectorals and Triceps

- Kneel on floor in front of flat bench, hands 24" apart.
- Place feet on bench, knees locked, back straight, head up.
- Have training partner place barbell plate high on upper back.
- Keeping body rigid, lower yourself until nose touches floor.
- Pause at bottom, then press to starting position.
- Inhale down, exhale up.

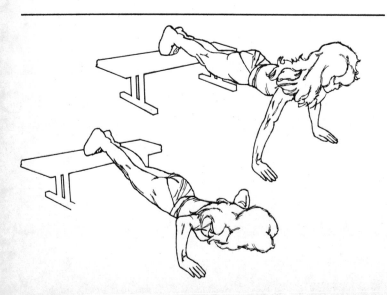

Medium-Grip Push-Ups, Feet on Bench
Pectorals and Triceps

- Kneel on floor in front of flat bench, hands 24" apart.
- Place feet on bench, knees locked, back straight, head up.
- Keeping body rigid, lower yourself until nose touches floor.
- Pause at bottom, then press to starting position.
- Inhale down, exhale up.

Bent-Arm Barbell Pullover and Press
Pectorals, Rib Cage, Triceps

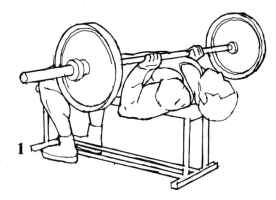
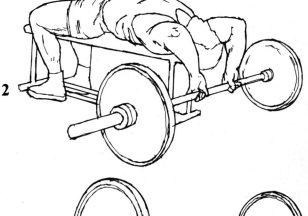
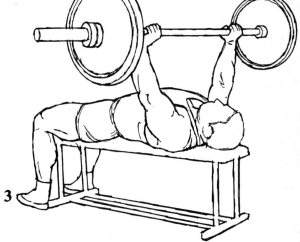
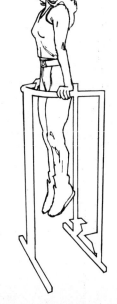

- Lie on bench, head over end, feet flat on floor.
- Rest barbell on chest in line with nipples.
- Hold bar, hands 14" apart.
- Keep elbows in at all times.
- Lower bar off bench, keeping it as close to head as possible.
- Lower bar to floor or as low as comfortable.
- Pull bar back to chest using same path.
- Press bar to arm's length above chest.
- Lower weight to chest.
- Both movements equal one repetition.
- Inhale to start, exhale to end repetition.
- Breathe heavily, hold rib cage high.
- Can also be done with dumbbells.

Dips
Pectorals and Triceps

- Hold yourself erect on bars.
- Keep elbows into sides, lower body by bending shoulders and elbows.
- Continue down as far as you can.
- Pause, then press back to arms' length.
- Do not let body swing back and forth.
- Inhale down, exhale up.

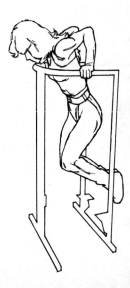

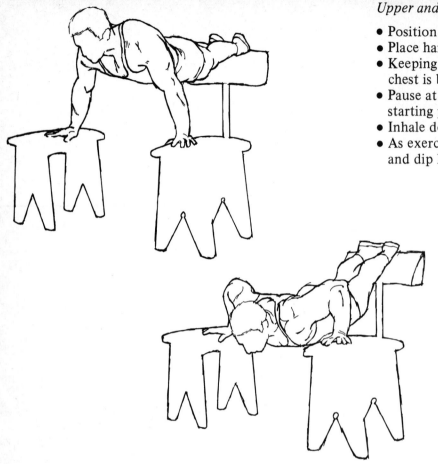

Medium-Grip Push-Ups Between Stools
Upper and Outer Pectorals

- Position stools and foot rest as shown.
- Place hands about 24" apart on stools.
- Keeping body rigid, lower yourself until chest is between stools.
- Pause at bottom, then press to starting position.
- Inhale down, exhale up.
- As exercise gets easier, separate stools and dip lower.

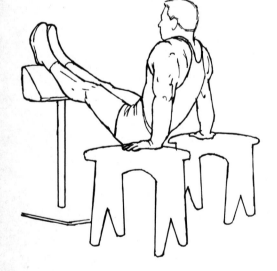

Feet-Elevated Dip Between Stools
Lower Pectorals and Triceps

- Place two stools, or chairs, about 4' in front of waist-high object.
- Position stools slightly wider than shoulder width.
- Place yourself as shown.
- Lower yourself by unlocking elbows until upper arms are nearly parallel to floor.
- Keep legs straight, head up.
- Inhale down, exhale up.

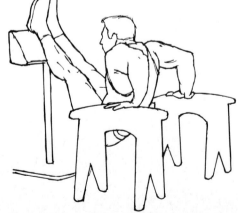

Inner-Pec Press on Inner-Pec Machine
Upper and Inner Pectorals

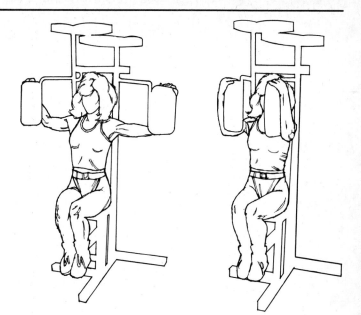

- Position yourself comfortably on machine.
- Keep upper arms high, in line with shoulders.
- Keep forearms vertical, firm against pads, and contract pectorals.
- Inhale as you squeeze, exhale as arms go back.

Low-Pulley Chest Lateral
Upper and Inner Pectorals

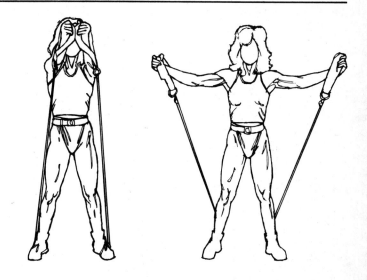

- Face away from machine, hold low pulley handles.
- Step away from machine far enough to raise weight stacks.
- Spread feet about 24" apart.
- Lean forward, bring arms to front, elbows locked, hands in line with nipples.
- Let arms back in semicircular motion, palms facing.
- Bend arms at elbows as you draw arms back until hands are in line with sides.
- Hands should be about 12" away on each side of chest.
- Press hands forward to starting position.
- Inhale back, exhale forward.

Lying Low-Pulley One-Arm Chest Lateral
Pectorals

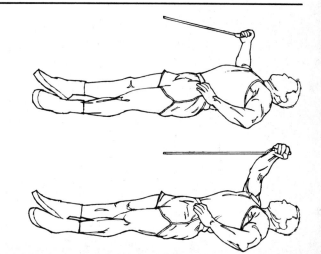

- Lie with body sideways to low wall pulley.
- Hold handle of low pulley in right hand.
- Get far enough away from machine to support weight stack while arm is straight.
- Arm in line with shoulder.
- Raise low pulley cable up in semicircular motion until arm is vertical over chest.
- Lower cable to starting position.
- Reverse position and repeat with left arm.
- Inhale up, exhale down.

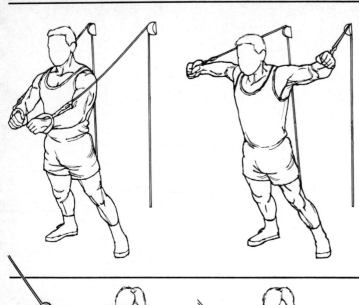

High-Pulley Chest Lateral
Upper and Inner Pectorals

- Face away from machine, hold upper pulley handles.
- Step away from machine far enough to raise weight stacks, feet about 24" apart.
- Lean forward, bring arms to front, elbows locked, hands in line with nipples.
- Let arms back in semicircular motion, palms facing.
- Keep upper arms in line with shoulders.
- Press cables forward to starting position.
- Inhale back, exhale forward.

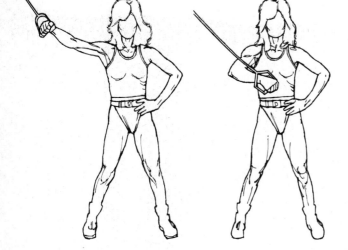

Pec Cross-Over on High Pulley
Lower and Inner Pectorals

- Hold upper pulley handle.
- Stand sideways to pulley.
- Step away from pulley, arm totally extended, with tension on cable.
- Keep arm straight while pulling across chest.
- Do not let hand drop lower than height of shoulders.
- Thumb should face up.
- Concentrate on inner pectorals while pulling.
- Inhale as you begin pull, exhale as you let cable back to starting position.
- Reverse position and repeat with left arm.

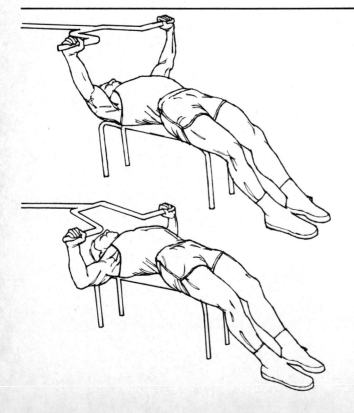

Bench Press on Universal Machine
Pectorals

- Lie on bench, feet flat on floor.
- Bar should be in line with nipples.
- Hold bar with hands about 3" from outside of chest.
- Press bar to arms' length.
- Return to starting position.
- Keep head on bench, hips on bench, rib cage high.
- Inhale up, exhale down.
- Can also be done on seated incline bench.

Incline Compound
Upper Pectorals
(This is a 2-motion exercise,
so study the drawings.)

- Lie on incline bench with dumbbells at arms'
  length overhead.
- With palms out, lower dumbbells in a
  semicircular motion.
- Keep elbows back, in line with ears as
  you lower.
- When dumbbells are even with chest and 10"
  from each side of chest, press back to starting
  position, keeping elbows in line with ears.
- You have completed one-half of the exercise.
- At top position, turn handles so palms
  are facing.
- Lower dumbbells straight down to sides of
  chest, elbows in close to sides.
- Return to starting position.
- Both complete movements equal one rep.
- Inhale at the top and exhale at the top of
  each movement.
- Can also be done on flat or decline bench.

Dips with Weight
Pectorals and Triceps

- Use machine as shown or hang dumbbell from
  waist with webbed belt or piece of rope.
- Hold yourself erect on bars.
- Lower body by bending arms, elbows in close.
- Lower until forearms and biceps touch.
- Pause, then press back to arms' length,
  elbows locked.
- Do not swing body back and forth.
- Inhale down, exhale up. □

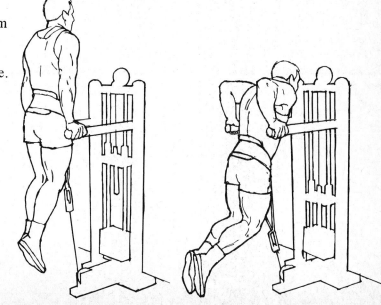

FOREARMS

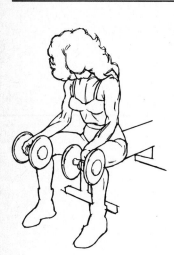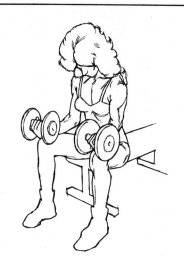

Seated Two-Dumbbell Palms-Up Wrist Curl
Inside Forearms

- Hold dumbbells, sit at end of bench, feet on floor about 20" apart.
- Lean forward, place forearms on upper thighs, palms ups.
- Place back of wrists over knees.
- Lower dumbbells as far as possible, keeping tight grip.
- Curl dumbbells up as high as possible.
- Do not let forearms raise up.
- Inhale up, exhale down.

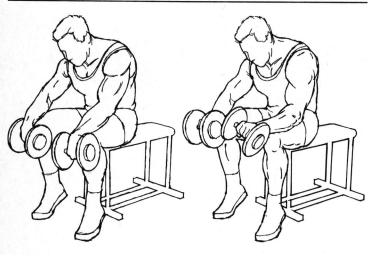

Seated Two-Dumbbell Palms-Down Wrist Curl
Outside Forearms

- Hold dumbbells, sit at end of bench, feet on floor about 20" apart.
- Lean forward, forearms on upper thighs, palms down.
- Place wrists over knees.
- Lower dumbbells as far as possible, keeping tight grip.
- Curl dumbbells as high as possible.
- Do not let forearms raise up.
- Inhale up, exhale down.

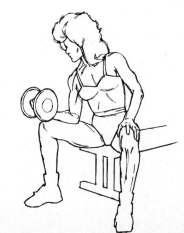

Seated One-Arm Dumbbell Palms-Up Wrist Curl
Inside Forearms

- Hold dumbbell in right hand, sit at end of bench, feet on floor about 20" apart.
- Lean forward, place right forearm on upper right thigh, palm up.
- Place back of wrist on knee.
- Lower dumbbell as far as possible, keeping tight grip.
- Curl dumbbell as high as possible.
- Do not let forearm raise up.
- Inhale up, exhale down.
- Reverse position and repeat with left arm.

Seated One-Arm Dumbbell Palm-Down Wrist Curl
Outside Forearms

- Hold dumbbell in right hand, sit at end of bench, feet on floor about 20" apart.
- Lean forward, place right forearm on upper right thigh, palm down.
- Place wrist over knee.
- Lower dumbbell as far as possible, keeping tight grip.
- Curl dumbbell as high as possible.
- Do not let forearm raise up.
- Inhale up, exhale down.
- Reverse position and repeat with left arm.

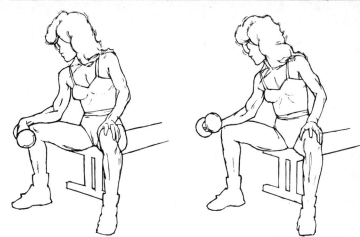

Seated Palms-Down Barbell Wrist Curl
Inside Forearms

- Hold barbell with both hands, palms down, hands 16" apart.
- Sit at end of bench, feet on floor about 20" apart.
- Lean forward, place forearms on upper thighs.
- Place wrists over knees.
- Lower bar as far as possible, keeping tight grip.
- Curl bar as high as possible.
- Do not let forearms raise up.
- Inhale up, exhale down.

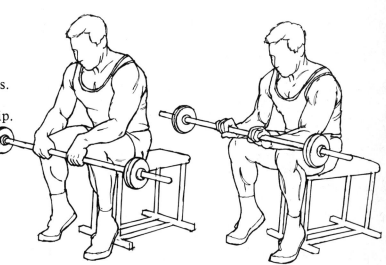

Seated Palms-Up Barbell Wrist Curl
Outside Forearms

- Hold barbell with both hands, palms up, hands 16" apart.
- Sit at end of bench, feet on floor about 20" apart.
- Lean forward, place forearms on upper thighs.
- Place backs of wrists over knees.
- Lower bar as far as possible, keeping tight grip.
- Curl bar as high as possible.
- Do not let forearms raise up.
- Inhale up, exhale down.

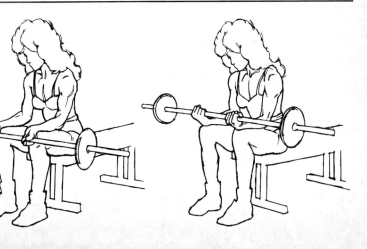

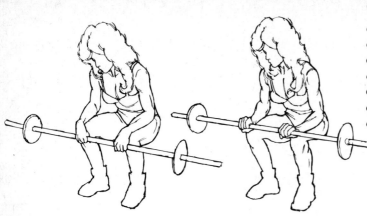

Squatting Palms-Down Barbell Wrist Curl
Outside Forearms

- Hold barbell, palms down, hands 10" apart.
- Squat until upper thighs are parallel to floor.
- Place wrists over knees.
- Lower bar as far as possible, keeping tight grip.
- Curl bar as high as possible.
- Do not let forearms raise up.
- Inhale up, exhale down.

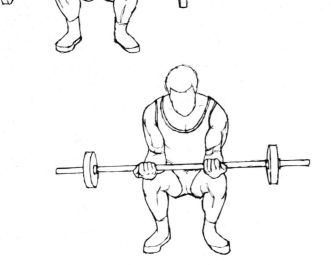

Squatting Palms-Up Barbell Wrist Curl
Inside Forearms

- Hold barbell, palms up, hands 16" apart.
- Squat until upper thighs are parallel to floor.
- Place forearms on upper thighs.
- Place back of wrists over knees.
- Lower bar as far as possible, keeping tight grip.
- Curl bar as high as possible.
- Do not let forearms raise up.
- Inhale up, exhale down.

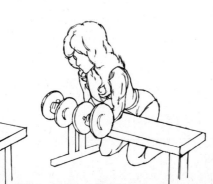

Palms-Up Two-Dumbbells Over-a-Bench Wrist Curl
Inside Forearms

- Place two dumbbells beside flat bench, kneel on opposite side of bench.
- Hold dumbbells, palms up.
- Place forearms flat on bench, back of wrists on edge of bench.
- Lower dumbbells as far as possible, keeping tight grip.
- Curl dumbbells up as high as possible.
- Do not let forearms raise up.
- Inhale up, exhale down.

Palms-Down Two-Dumbbells Over-a-Bench Wrist Curl
Outside Forearms

- Place two dumbbells beside flat bench, kneel on opposite side of bench.
- Hold dumbbells, palms down.
- Place forearms flat on bench, wrists on edge of bench.
- Lower dumbbells as far as possible, keeping tight grip.
- Curl dumbbells as high as possible.
- Do not let forearms raise up.
- Inhale up, exhale down.

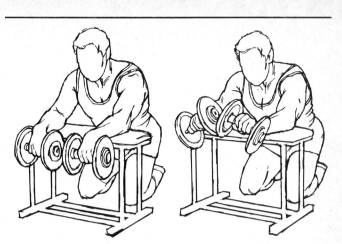

Palms-Up Barbell Over-a-Bench Wrist Curl
Inside Forearms

- Place barbell beside flat bench, kneel on opposite side of bench.
- Hold bar, palms up, hands 16" apart.
- Place forearms flat on bench, backs of wrists on edge of bench.
- Lower bar as far as possible, keeping tight grip.
- Curl bar as high as possible.
- Do not let forearms raise up.
- Inhale up, exhale down.

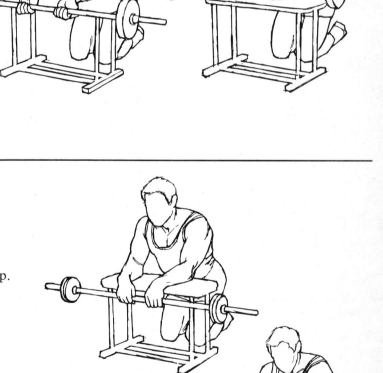

Palms-Down Barbell Over-a-Bench Wrist Curl
Outside Forearms

- Place barbell beside flat bench, kneel on opposite side of bench.
- Hold barbell, palms down, hands 16" apart.
- Place forearms flat on bench, wrists on edge of bench.
- Lower bar as far as possible, keeping tight grip.
- Curl bar as high as possible.
- Do not let forearms raise up.
- Inhale up, exhale down.

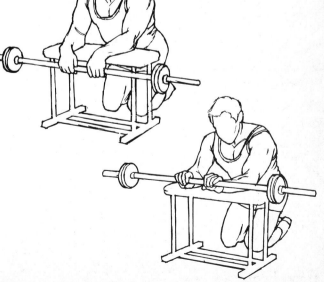

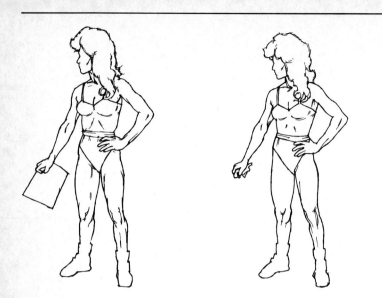

Newspaper Hand and Forearm Exercise
Hand and Forearm Muscles

- Can be done standing, seated or lying.
- Hold sheet of newspaper.
- Start at one corner and gather it into palm of hand.
- Continue gathering, squeeze paper into tight ball.

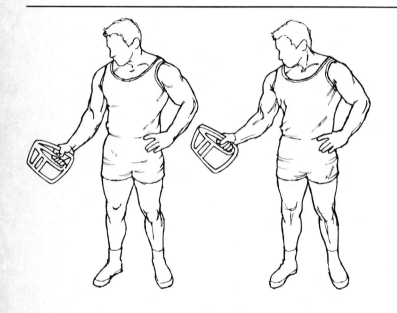

Hand-Gripper Forearm Exercise
Hand and Forearm Muscles

- Can be done standing, seated or lying.
- Grasp gripper handle and tighten as much as possible.
- Continue squeezing until grip or forearms give out, then change hands.
- Do same number of reps with each hand.
- Not all grippers close completely.

Rubber Ball Hand Squeeze
Hand and Forearm Muscles

- Can be done standing, seated or lying.
- Grasp tennis ball in palm and tighten grip as much as possible.
- Release tension, then tighten again.
- Do same number of reps with each hand.

Standing Arms-Extended Wrist-Roller Wrist Curl
Outside Forearms

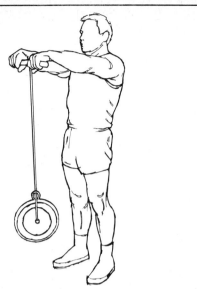
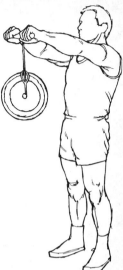

- Place light weight on end of rope of wrist roller.
- Stand erect, back straight, head up.
- Hold wrist roller with both hands, palms down.
- Extend arms straight out.
- Roll weight up by curling right hand over and down, then left hand over and down.
- Keep arms parallel to floor.
- Continue curling right to left hand until weight touches bar.
- Lower weight to starting position by reversing movement.

Standing Palms-Up Barbell-Behind-Back Wrist Curl
Inside Forearms

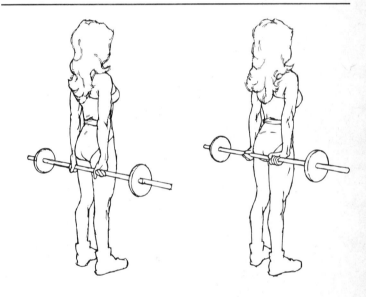

- Put barbell behind buttocks at arms' length, palms back, hands 20" apart.
- Curl hands as high as possible.
- Keep arms straight, elbows locked.
- Lower bar to starting position.
- Inhale up, exhale down.

Standing Olympic-Plate Hand Squeeze
Inside Forearms

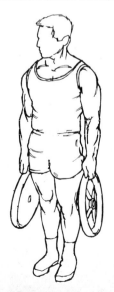
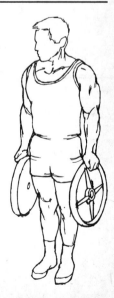

- Hold Olympic plate by ridge in each hand.
- Stand erect, plates at arms' length at sides of thighs, palms in.
- Lower plates until fingers are nearly extended but can still hold weights.
- Close hands, raising plates a few inches.
- Continue raising and lowering weights until grip gives out.
- You can do both hands at same time, alternate, or do one hand at a time.

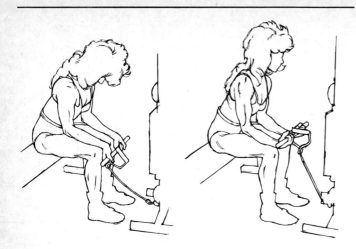

Seated Two-Arm Palms-Up Low-Pulley Wrist Curl
Inside Forearms

- Put stool in front of low wall pulley.
- Move stool far enough away to support weight stack.
- Hold handles with both hands, palms up.
- Step back, sit on stool with feet about 16" apart.
- Lean forward, place forearms on upper thighs.
- Place backs of wrists over knees.
- Lower handles as far as possible, keeping tight grip.
- Curl handles up as high as possible.
- Do not let forearms raise up.
- Inhale up, exhale down.

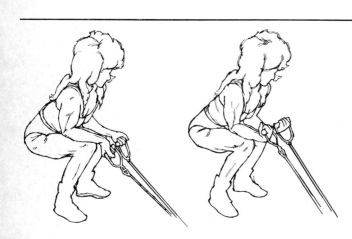

Squatting Two-Arm Palms-Up Low-Pulley Wrist Curl
Inside Forearms

- Stand in front of wall pulley, hold handles with both hands, palms up.
- Stand back far enough to support weight stack.
- Squat until upper thighs are parallel to floor, feet 16" apart.
- Place backs of wrists over knees.
- Lower handles as far as possible, keeping tight grip.
- Curl handles as high as possible.
- Do not let forearms raise up.
- Inhale up, exhale down.

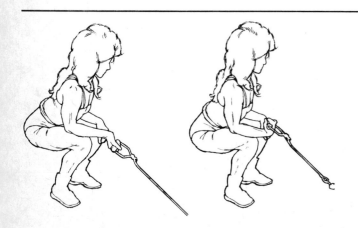

Squatting One-Arm Palms-Up Low-Pulley Wrist Curl
Inside Forearms

- Stand in front of wall pulley, hold handle with right hand, palm up.
- Stand back far enough to support weight stack.
- Squat until upper thighs are parallel to floor, feet 16" apart.
- Lean forward, place right forearm on right upper thigh.
- Place back of wrist over knee.
- Lower handle as far as possible, keeping tight grip.
- Curl handle as high as possible.
- Do not let forearm raise up.
- Inhale up, exhale down.
- Reverse position and repeat with left arm.

Squatting One-Arm Palms-Down Low-Pulley Wrist Curl
Outside Forearms

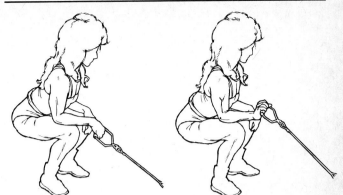

- Stand in front of wall pulley, hold handle with right hand, palm down.
- Stand back far enough to support weight stack.
- Squat until upper thighs are parallel to floor, feet 16" apart.
- Lean forward, place right forearm on right upper thigh.
- Place wrist over knees.
- Lower handle as far as possible, keeping tight grip.
- Curl handle as high as possible.
- Do not let forearm raise up.
- Inhale up, exhale down.
- Reverse position and repeat with left arm. □

NECK

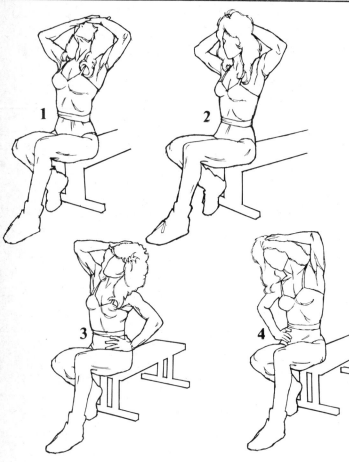

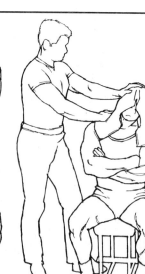

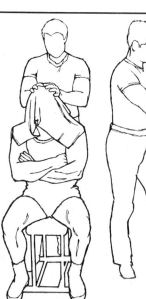

Seated Freehand Neck Resistance
Front, Side and Rear Neck Muscles

- Sit on bench with back straight, head up.
- Place both hands on forehead (1).
- Push head back in semicircular motion as far as comfortable.
- Resist with neck muscles.
- At low position, push head back up in semicircular motion as far as comfortable.
- Resist with neck muscles.
- Do prescribed number of reps.
- Then place both hands on back of head and repeat movement (2).
- Then place palm of right hand on right side of head and resist from side to side (3).
- Then repeat with left hand to complete exercise (4).

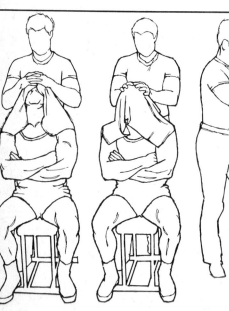

Seated Buddy-System Neck Resistance
Front, Side and Rear Neck Muscles

- Sit at end of flat bench.
- Cross arms or hold end of bench for support.
- Keep back straight, head up.
- Have training partner place towel over your head to keep head from slipping.
- Partner stands to rear, straddling bench, with hands on your forehead.
- Pull your head down as partner provides resistance.
- Partner then smoothly and evenly pulls head back to a comfortable position.
- Resist with neck muscles.
- Do prescribed number of reps.
- Do same up and down movement with partner's hands on back of neck.
- Partner now shifts to right side.
- Repeat up and down movements.
- Then shift to left side and repeat.
- Do not let partner push or pull head far enough to cause discomfort.

Lying Flat Bench Buddy-System Neck Resistance
Front, Side and Rear Neck Muscles

- Lie face down on flat bench, top of shoulders even with bench.
- Have training partner place towel over your head to keep head from slipping.
- Partner stands in front with both hands on back of your head.
- Raise head up as high as possible.
- Partner provides even resistance with hands as head is raised.
- Partner then smoothly and evenly pushes head down to comfortable position.
- Resist with neck muscles.
- Do prescribed number of reps.
- Then lie on your back on bench, top of shoulders even with bench.
- Do same up and down movements with partner's hands on your forehead.
- Shift to right side and repeat movements.
- Shift to left side and repeat.
- Do not let partner push or pull head far enough to cause discomfort.

Standing Towel Neck Resistance
Front, Side and Rear Neck Muscles

- Stand erect, back straight, head up.
- Place middle of rolled-up towel against back of head.
- Hold each end of towel.
- Pull head down as low as possible by applying pressure with arms against towel.
- At low position, pull head up and back in semicircular motion as far as comfortable.
- Do prescribed number of reps.
- Shift towel to right side of head, repeat movement.
- Shift towel to left side and repeat.

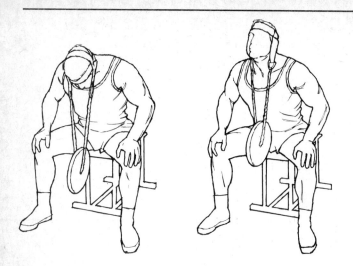

Seated Head-Harness Barbell-Plate Neck Resistance
Side and Rear Neck Muscles

- Place desired amount of weight on rope or chain attached to head harness.
- Put on head harness.
- Sit at end of flat bench.
- Lean slightly forward so plate hangs free.
- Place hands on upper knees.
- Raise head up and back in semicircular motion as far as comfortable.
- Continue going up and back for prescribed number of reps.
- Now draw head over to right side and raise head up and over in semicircular motion as far left as comfortable.
- Continue from right to left until reps are completed.

Standing Head-Harness Barbell-Plate Neck Resistance
Side and Rear Neck Muscles

- Place desired amount of weight on rope or chain attached to head harness.
- Put on head harness.
- Bend slightly forward so plate hangs free.
- Place hands on upper thighs.
- Raise head up and back in semicircular motion as far as comfortable.
- Continue going up and back for prescribed number of reps.
- Now draw head over to right side and raise head up and over in semicircular motion as far as comfortable.
- Continue from right to left until reps are completed.

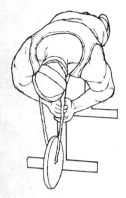
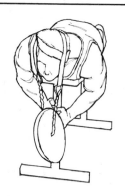

Lying Head-Harness Barbell-Plate Neck Resistance
Side and Rear Neck Muscles

- Place desired amount of weight on rope or chain attached to head harness.
- Lie face down on flat bench, top of shoulders even with end of bench.
- Put on head harness, weight hanging straight down.
- Raise head up and back in semicircular motion as far as comfortable.
- Continue going up and back for prescribed number of reps.
- Now draw head over to right side and raise head up and over in semicircular motion as far left as comfortable.
- Continue from right to left until reps are completed.

Lying-Face-Down Barbell-Plate Neck Resistance
Rear Neck Muscles

- Lie face down, shoulders about even with end of bench.
- Place flat barbell plate on back of head, hold in place with hands.
- Raise head up and back in semicircular motion as far as comfortable.
- Continue going up and back for prescribed number of reps.
- Now draw head over to right side and raise head up and over in semicircular motion as far left as comfortable.
- Continue from right to left until reps are completed.

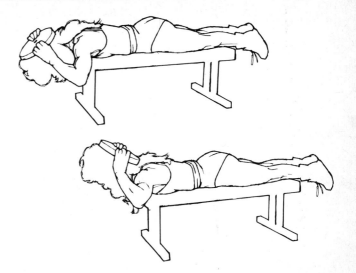

Lying-Supine Barbell-Plate Neck Resistance
Front Neck Muscles

- Lie on your back, shoulders about even with end of bench.
- Place flat barbell plate on forehead and hold in place with hands.
- Raise head up in semicircular motion as far as comfortable.
- Continue up and down for prescribed number of reps.

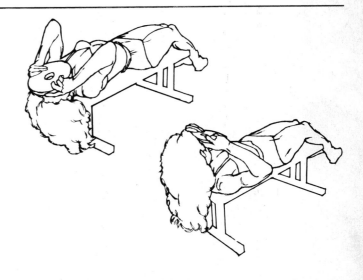

Wrestler's Bridge
Front, Side and Rear Neck Muscles

- Kneel and place top of head on mat or pad.
- Cross arms on chest, raise body to a pyramid position, legs as straight as possible.
- All body weight should be distributed between head and feet.
- Roll top of head frontward and backward causing neck muscles to take bulk of work load.
- Do prescribed number of reps.
- Repeat movement from side to side.
- Then rotate body so chest and midsection are facing up.
- Repeat movements, front and back and side to side.

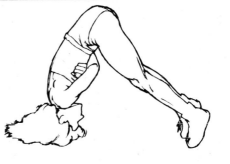

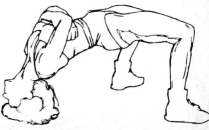

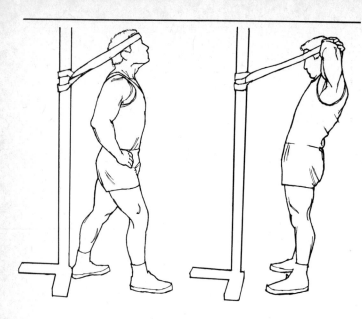

Standing Rubber-Inner-Tube Neck Resistance
Front, Side and Rear Neck Muscles

- Use bicycle inner tube or portion of automobile inner tube.
- Tie tube around post.
- Place inner tube over head against forehead.
- Step forward to stretch tube.
- Pull head forward as far as comfortable.
- Continue forward and backward for prescribed number of reps.
- Turn around, place inner tube against back of head.
- Draw head back to furthest comfortable position.
- Continue going backward and forward for prescribed number of reps.
- Place inner tube against right side of head just above ear and go from side to side.
- Switch to left side and complete reps.

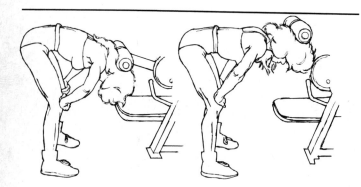

Leg-Extension-Machine Neck Resistance
Rear Neck Muscles

- Bend forward at waist, knees slightly bent.
- Place back of head under one pad of leg extension machine.
- Place hands on upper thighs.
- Lower head to lowest comfortable position.
- Raise head up and back in semicircular motion as far as comfortable.
- Continue up and down for prescribed number of reps.

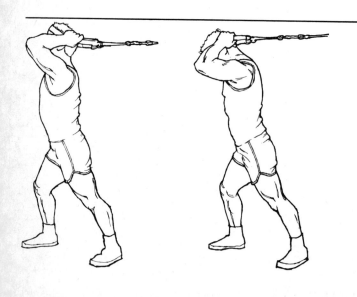

Standing Head-Harness High-Pulley Neck Resistance
Front and Rear Neck Muscles

- Attach upper cable to rope or chain of head harness.
- Put desired weight on head harness.
- Stand erect, back straight, far enough away from pulley to support weight.
- Lower head to lowest comfortable position.
- Raise head up and back in semicircular motion as far as comfortable.
- Continue forward and backward for prescribed number of reps.
- Turn around and place head harness against back of head.
- Continue forward and backward for prescribed number of reps.
- Place head harness against right side of head just above ear and go from side to side.
- Switch to left side and complete reps.

Standing Head-Harness Neck Resistance on Universal Leg-Extension-Machine
Rear Neck Muscles

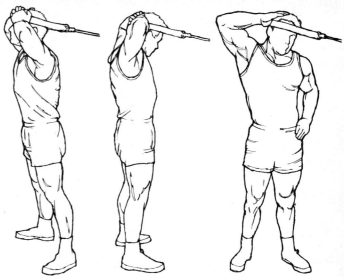

- Place head strap on neck resistance unit of Universal leg extension machine.
- Stand away from machine, place head strap on forehead.
- Step forward, putting tension on spring.
- Draw head back to furthest comfortable position.
- Now bring head up and down in semicircular motion as far as comfortable.
- Continue up and back for prescribed number of reps.
- Turn around and place strap on back of head, repeat movement.
- Next turn to right side and finally left side.

Seated Neck Resistance on Paramount Neck Machine
Front, Side and Rear Neck Muscles

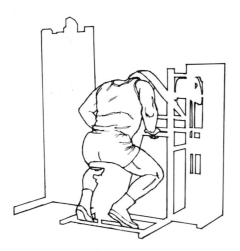

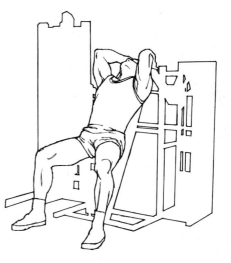

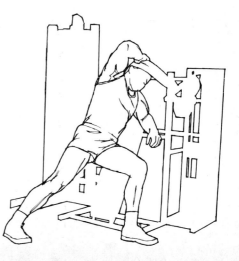

- Select desired weight on neck machine.
- Sit with back against machine.
- Put strap against forehead.
- Hold strap with both hands.
- Draw head back to furthest comfortable position.
- Pull head forward and down as far as comfortable.
- Once in lowest position, push head up and down in semicircular motion as far as comfortable.
- Now turn, put strap against back of head and repeat.
- Next turn to right side and finally left side. □

SHOULDERS

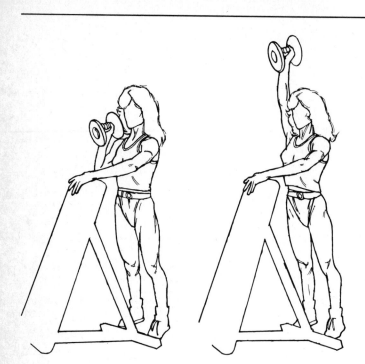

Standing Palm-In One-Arm Dumbbell Press
Front and Outer Deltoids

- Raise dumbbell to shoulder height.
- Hold onto something with free hand.
- Lock legs and hips.
- Keep elbow in, palm in.
- Press dumbbell straight up to arm's length.
- Return to shoulder.
- Repeat movement with other arm.
- Inhale up, exhale down.
- Can also be done seated.

Standing Palms-In Dumbbell Press
Front and Outer Deltoids

- Raise dumbbells to shoulder height.
- Lock legs and hips.
- Keep elbows in, palms in.
- Press dumbbells straight up to arms' length.
- Return to shoulder height.
- Inhale up, exhale down.
- Can also be done seated, or with barbell, seated or standing.

Seated Palms-In Alternated Dumbbell Press
Front and Outer Deltoids

- Raise dumbbells to shoulder height.
- Sit at end of bench, feet firmly on floor.
- Press one dumbbell straight up to arm's length, palm in, elbow in.
- Lower dumbbell to starting position and press other dumbbell up.
- Keep body rigid.
- Do all work with shoulders and arms.
- Do not lean from side to side.
- Inhale up, exhale down.
- Can also be done with palms facing out.
- Can also be done standing, with palms facing in or out.

Standing Palms-In Alternated Dumbbell Press
Front and Outer Deltoids

- Raise dumbbells to shoulder height.
- Lock legs and hips.
- Keep elbows in, palms in.
- Press dumbbell in right hand to arm's length overhead.
- Lower dumbbell to starting position and press dumbbell in left hand up.
- Keep body rigid.
- Do all work with shoulder and arms.
- Do not lean from side to side.
- Inhale up, exhale down.
- Can also be done seated.

Seated Palms-Out Dumbbell Press
Front and Outer Deltoids

- Raise dumbbells to shoulder height.
- Sit at end of bench, feet firmly on floor.
- Keep elbows out, thumbs facing in.
- Press dumbbells to arms' length overhead.
- Lower weights to starting position.
- Inhale at start of press, exhale at finish.
- Can also be done with palms facing in.
- Can also be done standing, with palms facing out or in.

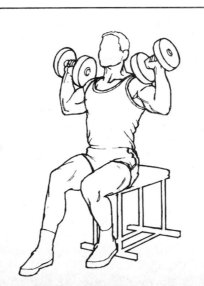

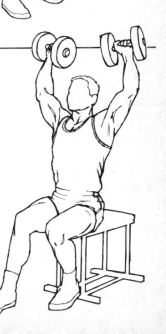

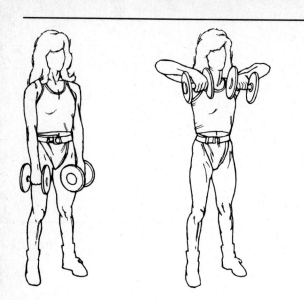

Standing Dumbbell Upright Rowing
Front Deltoids and Trapezius

- Hold dumbbells, hanging, against upper thighs.
- Keep dumbbells 10" apart, thumbs facing.
- Pull dumbbells straight up until nearly even with chin.
- Keep elbows out.
- At top position dumbbells are in line with ears.
- Keep weights close to body, pause at top.
- Concentrate on shoulders as you lower weights.
- Inhale up, exhale down.
- Can also be done with barbell, using close grip.

Lying Rear Deltoid Raise
Rear Deltoids

- Lie face down on fairly tall flat bench.
- Hold dumbbells, palms facing, arms hanging down.
- Keep elbows locked, arms straight.
- Raise dumbbells in semicircular motion to shoulder height, in line with ears at top of lift.
- Lower to starting position using same path.
- Inhale up, exhale down.

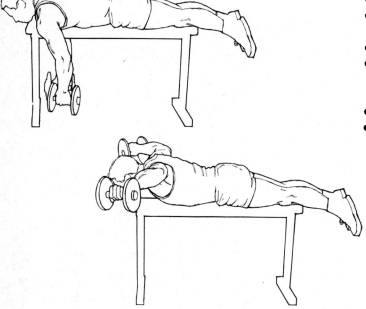

Seated Bent-Over Rear Deltoid Raise
Rear Deltoids

- Hold dumbbells.
- Sit at end of bench, feet firmly on floor, fairly close together.
- Bend forward until chest nearly touches upper thighs.
- Hang dumbbells between lower legs and bench.
- Keep arms straight, elbows locked.
- Raise dumbbells out in a semicircular motion until parallel to floor, even with ears.
- Lower in same path.
- Inhale up, exhale down.

Lying on Floor Across-Body Rear Deltoid Raise
Rear Deltoids

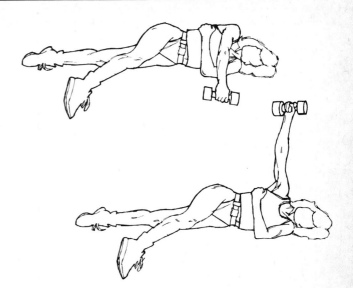

- Lie on left side on floor, legs crossed.
- Hold dumbbell with right hand, palm down.
- Keep arm straight, in line with shoulder.
- Raise dumbbell in semicircular motion until vertical to shoulder.
- Lower weight to starting position using same path.
- Inhale up, exhale down.

Bent-Over Head-Supported Dumbbell Rear Deltoid Raise
Rear Deltoids

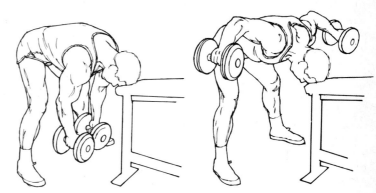

- Rest forehead on comfortable, not quite waist-high object.
- Hold dumbbells, arms straight down, elbows locked.
- Raise dumbbells out to shoulder height, even with ears.
- Hold position momentarily, contract rear deltoids.
- Do not swing dumbbells up.
- Keep body rigid, head on object.
- Do the work with rear deltoids, upper back muscles.
- Inhale up, exhale down.
- Can also be done without head support.

Seated Side Lateral Raise
Front and Outer Deltoids

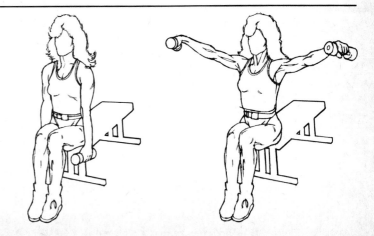

- Sit at end of bench, feet firmly on floor.
- Hold dumbbells, palms in, arms straight down at sides.
- Raise dumbbells in semicircular motion a little above shoulder height.
- Pause, then lower to starting position using same path.
- Keep arms straight.
- Inhale up, exhale down.
- Can also be done standing.

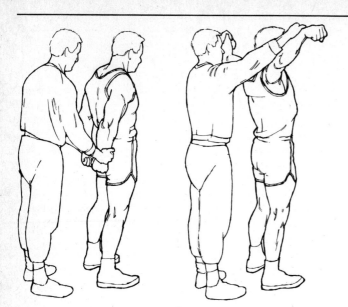

Standing Deltoid Pump
Outer Deltoids

- Stand erect, feet 16" apart.
- Place hands behind back against middle of buttocks, palms facing.
- Have partner provide resistance by holding your upper wrists as you raise your arms in semicircular motion, elbows locked, just above parallel with shoulders.
- Resist as partner pulls your arms back to starting position.
- Keep wrists and elbows locked.
- Inhale up, exhale down.

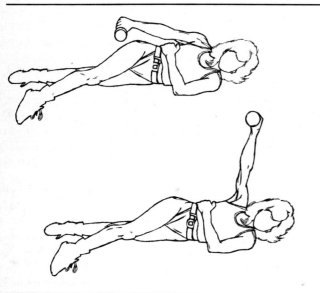

Lying Floor Side Lateral Raise
Outer Deltoids

- Lie on left side, legs crossed.
- Hold dumbbell in right hand, palm facing thigh, arm extended.
- Raise dumbbell in semicircular motion until vertical to right shoulder.
- Lower to starting position using same path.
- Do not turn wrist, keep arm straight.
- Reverse position and repeat with left arm.
- Inhale up, exhale down.

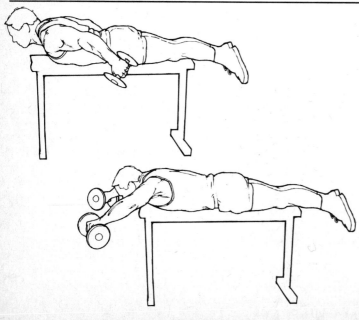

Lying Rear Deltoid Circle
Rear Deltoids

- Lie face down on flat bench.
- Hold dumbbells, arms directly at sides, elbows locked, palms at sides of upper thighs.
- Bring dumbbells out past torso until they touch at arms' length in front of head.
- Return dumbbells in same path.
- Inhale out, exhale back.

Lying Floor Dumbbell-Held-to-the-Side Lateral Raise
Outer Deltoids

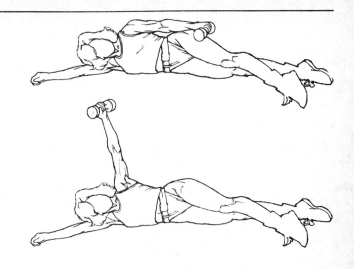

- Lie on right side on floor, legs crossed.
- Hold dumbbell in left hand, arm straight, elbow locked, even with right thigh, palm down.
- Raise dumbbell straight up until vertical.
- Lower in same path.
- Change sides and repeat with right arm.
- Inhale up, exhale down.

Medium-Grip Barbell Upright Rowing
Front Deltoids and Trapezius

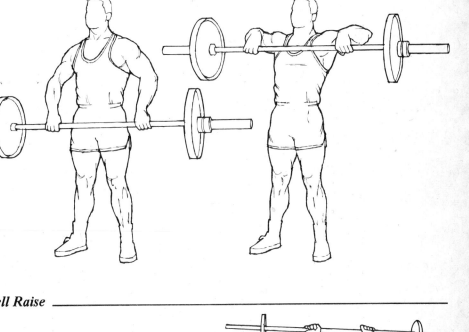

- Hold barbell, palms down, hands 18" apart.
- Start with bar at arms' length.
- Pull bar straight up until nearly under chin.
- Keep elbows out to side, as high as ears.
- Keep bar close to body.
- Pause momentarily at top before lowering to starting position.
- Inhale up, exhale down.
- Concentrate on deltoids as you lower weight.
- Can also be done with wide grip.

Standing Medium-Grip Front Barbell Raise
Front Deltoids

- Stand with feet about 16" apart, back straight, legs and hips locked.
- Use shoulder-width grip.
- Start with bar at arms' length against upper thighs.
- Raise bar in semicircular motion until directly overhead.
- Do not unlock elbows.
- Lower bar to starting position using same path.
- Inhale up, exhale down.
- Can also be done with close or wide grip.

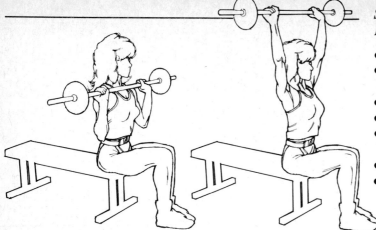

Seated Barbell Military Press
Front and Outer Deltoids

- Raise barbell to shoulders.
- Sit at end of bench, feet about 16" apart, firmly on floor.
- Keep chest high, back straight.
- Press bar to arms' length overhead.
- Use slow, steady motion, keeping tension on muscles.
- Lower to starting position.
- Inhale up, exhale down.

Standing Low-Pulley Deltoid Raise
Outer Deltoids

- Stand with left side facing wall pulley.
- Hold bottom handle of pulley with right hand.
- Stand erect, far enough from machine to create tension on cable.
- Right hand should be in line with groin area of left side.
- Raise pulley in semicircular motion, arm straight, elbow locked, until arm is just above parallel to right shoulder.
- Lower to starting position using same path.
- Inhale up, exhale down.
- Reverse position and repeat with left arm.
- Can also be done with pulley handle to rear.

Standing Barbell Press Behind Neck
Front and Rear Deltoids

- Place barbell on upper back.
- Stand, feet about 16" apart.
- Keep hands 4"-6" wider than shoulders.
- Press bar overhead to arms' length.
- Lower back to shoulders.
- Pause at shoulders on each rep.
- Keep legs straight, hips flexed.
- Inhale up, exhale down.
- Can also be done seated.

Lying Close-Grip Straight-Arm Barbell Rear Deltoid Raise
Rear Deltoids

- Lie face down on high flat bench.
- Hold light barbell at arms' length, not touching floor.
- Keep head over end of bench and up.
- With hands 6" apart, arms straight, elbows locked, raise bar in semicircular motion until parallel to floor.
- Lower to starting position using same path.
- Inhale up, exhale down.
- Can also be done with medium or wide grip.

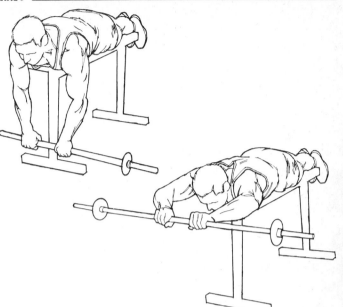

Bent-Over Close-Grip Straight-Arm Barbell Front Raise
Rear Deltoids

- Hold barbell, palms down, hands 12" apart.
- Bend until torso is parallel to floor.
- Keep knees slightly bent.
- With bar at arms' length below shoulders, raise bar in semicircular motion until even with top of head.
- Lower in same path.
- Keep back parallel to floor at all times.
- Inhale up, exhale down.
- Can also be done with medium or wide grip.

Standing Military Press
Front and Outer Deltoids

- Raise barbell to chest, hands shoulder width apart.
- Lock legs and hips solidly.
- Keep elbows in, slightly under bar.
- Press bar to arms' length overhead.
- Lower to upper chest.
- Be sure bar rests on chest and is not supported by arms between reps.
- Hold chest high.
- Inhale up, exhale down.

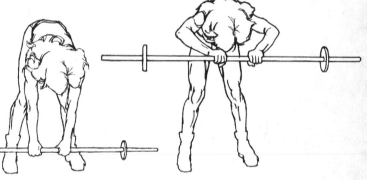

Bent-Over Low-Pulley Rear Deltoid Raise
Rear Deltoids

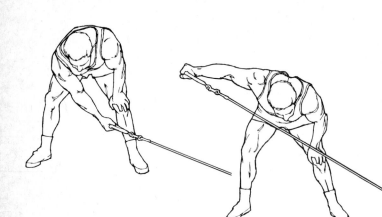

- Stand with left side facing wall pulley.
- Hold bottom handle of pulley with right hand.
- Stand erect, far enough from machine to create tension on cable.
- Bend until torso is nearly parallel to floor.
- Place left hand on left thigh just above knee.
- Keep right elbow locked, arm straight.
- Pull weight up and out in semicircular motion until right hand is as high as shoulder, in line with ear.
- Inhale up, exhale down.
- Reverse position and repeat with left arm.

Bent-Over Low-Pulley Side Lateral
Rear Deltoids

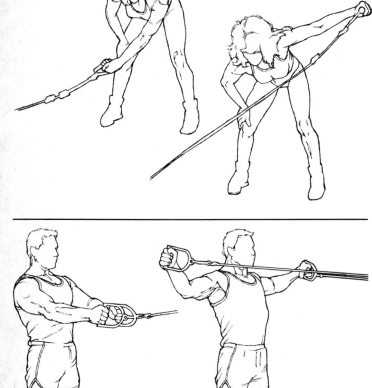

- Hold handle with left hand.
- Stand far enough from machine to create tension on cable.
- Bend until back is nearly parallel to floor.
- Legs slightly bent, right hand on lower right thigh, left arm hanging from shoulder.
- Raise left arm, elbow locked, until parallel to floor, in line with left ear.
- Lower to starting position.
- Inhale up, exhale down.
- Reverse position and repeat with right hand.

Standing High-Pully Rear Deltoid Lateral Pull
Rear Deltoids

- Stand facing wall pulley.
- Hold left upper handle with right hand, right upper handle with left hand, crossing cables.
- Step back with arms straight out, creating tension on cables.
- Pull arms back toward outside of shoulders.
- Keep arms parallel to floor, elbows locked.
- Inhale as you pull, exhale as you return to starting position.

Flat-Footed Wide-Stance Barbell Half-Squat
Inner Thighs

- Place barbell on upper back.
- Use comfortable hand grip.
- Head up, back straight, feet about 30" apart.
- Squat until upper thighs are halfway parallel to floor.
- Head stays up, back straight, knees wide.
- Return to starting position.
- Inhale down, exhale up.

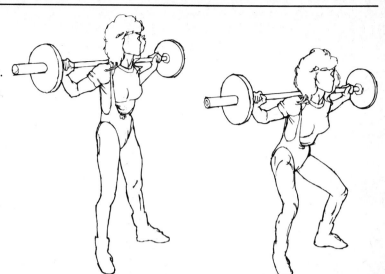

Heels-Elevated Medium-Stance Barbell Front Squat
Upper Thighs

- Put a 2x4 piece of wood on floor for heel support.
- Place barbell on upper chest, resting on front deltoids and upper thorax.
- Place right hand on bar even with left deltoid, left hand on bar even with right deltoid.
- Keep upper arms slightly above parallel to keep bar from sliding.
- Head up, back straight, feet about 16" apart.
- Squat until upper thighs are parallel to floor.
- Head stays up, back straight, knees slightly out.
- Return to starting position.
- Inhale down, exhale up.
- Can also be done with close stance (8-10" apart).

Heels-Elevated Wide-Stance Barbell Front-Squat
Inner Thighs

- Put a 2x4 piece of wood on floor for heel support.
- Place barbell on upper chest, resting on front deltoids and upper thorax.
- Place right hand on bar even with left deltoid, left hand on bar even with right deltoid.
- Keep upper arms slightly above parallel to keep bar from sliding.
- Head up, back straight, feet about 30" apart.
- Squat until upper thighs are parallel to floor.
- Head stays up, back straight, knees wide.
- Return to starting position.
- Inhale down, exhale up.

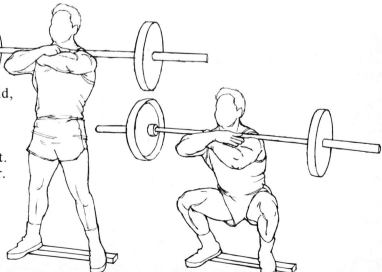

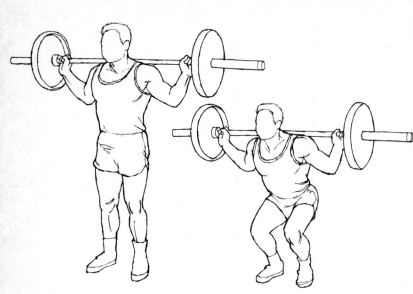

Barbell Breathing Squat
Thighs and Trunk

- Place light barbell on upper back.
- Use comfortable hand grip.
- Head up, back straight, feet about 16" apart.
- Squat until upper thighs are parallel to floor.
- Pause at bottom.
- Return to starting position.
- Pay special attention to breathing.
- Keep chest high, inhale deeply.
- Squat with feet flat on floor or heels raised.
- On first 5 reps, take 2 deep breaths before each squat.
- On second 5 reps, take 3 deep breaths before each squat.
- On third 5 reps, take 4 deep breaths before each squat.
- Take full breaths, keeping chest high.
- Leave bar on shoulders for 15 reps.
- Take 45 breaths for a set of 15 reps.

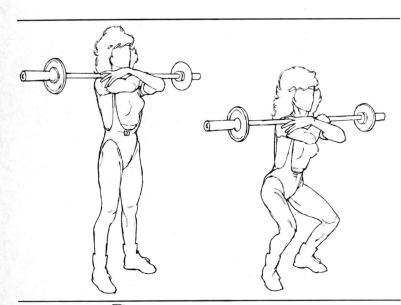

Flat-Footed Medium-Stance Barbell Front Half-Squ
Upper Thighs

- Place barbell on upper chest, resting on front deltoids and upper thorax.
- Place right hand on bar even with left deltoid, left hand on bar even with right deltoid.
- Keep upper arms slightly above parallel to keep bar from sliding.
- Head up, back straight, feet about 16" apart.
- Squat until upper thighs are halfway parallel to floor.
- Head stays up, back straight, knees slightly out.
- Return to starting position.
- Inhale down, exhale up.
- Can also be done with close stance (8-10" apart).

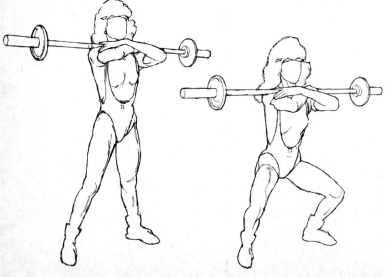

Flat-Footed Wide-Stance Barbell Front Half-Squat
Inner Thighs

- Place barbell on upper chest, resting on front deltoids and upper thorax.
- Place right hand on bar even with left deltoid, left hand on bar even with right deltoid.
- Keep upper arms slightly above parallel to keep bar from sliding.
- Head up, back straight, feet about 30" apart.
- Squat until upper thighs are halfway parallel to floor.
- Head stays up, back straight, knees out.
- Return to starting position.
- Inhale down, exhale up.

Heels-Elevated Wide-Stance Barbell Front Squat to Bench
Inner Thighs

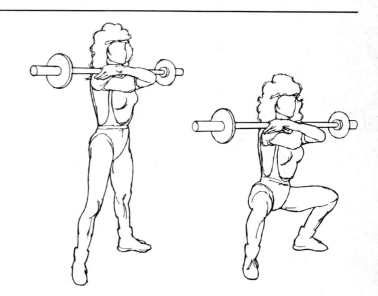

- Put a 2x4 piece of wood on floor for heel support in front of 16" high bench.
- Place barbell on upper chest, resting on front deltoids and upper thorax.
- Place right hand on bar even with left deltoid, left hand on bar even with right deltoid.
- Keep upper arms slightly above parallel to keep bar from sliding.
- Head up, back straight, feet about 30" apart, heels on 2x4.
- Squat until buttocks touch bench.
- Keep tension on thighs, do not rest on bench.
- Head up, back straight, knees out.
- Return to starting position.
- Inhale down, exhale up.
- Can also be done with close or medium stance.

Flat-Footed Wide-Stance Barbell Front Squat
Inner Thighs

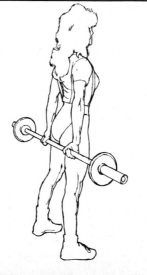

- Place barbell on upper chest, resting on front deltoids and upper thorax.
- Place right hand on bar even with left deltoid, left hand on bar even with right deltoid.
- Keep upper arms slightly above parallel to keep bar from sliding.
- Head up, back straight, feet about 30" apart.
- Squat until upper thighs are parallel to floor.
- Head stays up, back straight, knees out.
- Return to starting position.
- Inhale down, exhale up.
- Can also be done with close or medium stance.

Flat-Footed Wide-Stance Barbell Back Squat
Inner Thighs

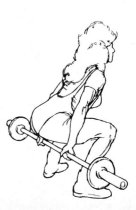

- Hold barbell behind you at arms' length.
- Keep bar tucked against buttocks and upper thighs.
- Palms up, facing back, hands as wide as hips.
- Turn wrists up to lock bar solidly.
- Bar stays this way at all times.
- Head up, eyes up at 45° angle.
- Feet firmly on floor, about 22" apart.
- Squat until upper thighs are parallel to floor.
- Return to starting position.
- Inhale down, exhale up.
- Can also be done with medium (16" apart) stance.

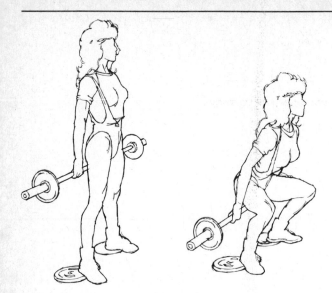

Heels-Elevated Wide-Stance Barbell Hack Squat
Inner Thighs

- Hold barbell behind you at arms' length.
- Put heels on plates about 30" apart.
- Keep bar tucked against buttocks and upper thighs.
- Palms up, facing back, hands as wide as hips.
- Turn wrists up to lock bar solidly.
- Bar stays this way at all times.
- Head up, eyes up at 45° angle.
- Squat until upper thighs are parallel to floor.
- Return to starting position.
- Inhale down, exhale up.
- Can also be done with close or medium stance.

Close-Stance Sissy Squat
Thighs

- Place a 24" strap chest-high around a piece of pipe away from wall.
- Put feet about 3" apart on each side of pipe.
- Hold strap with both hands.
- Support body with outstretched arms and strap.
- Squat while raising toes, thrust hips forward, arch back forward.
- Squat in semicircular motion until thighs are parallel to floor.
- Keep back arched, knees close.
- Return to starting position.
- Inhale down, exhale up.

Jefferson Lift
Inner Thighs

- Straddle barbell on floor, feet about 24" apart.
- Bend and hold front of bar with right hand, palm down, rear of bar with left hand, palm down.
- Squat until upper thighs are parallel to floor.
- Keep back nearly vertical, head up.
- Rise with bar at arms' length until legs are straight, knees locked.
- Keep bar at arms' length, elbows locked.
- Do all lifting with thighs and lower back.
- Return to starting position.
- Inhale up, exhale down.

Freehand Front Lunge
Thighs and Hamstrings

- Stand erect with hands on hips.
- Back straight head up, feet about 12" apart.
- Step forward as far as possible with right leg until upper right thigh is almost parallel to floor.
- Keep left leg as straight as possible.
- Step back to starting position.
- Inhale out, exhale back.
- Repeat with left leg.

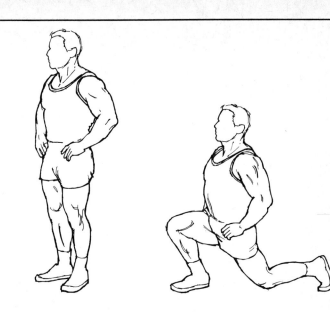

Freehand Side Lunge
Inner Thighs and Hamstrings

- Stand erect with hands on hips.
- Back straight, head up, feet close together.
- Step to side as far as possible with left leg until upper thigh is almost parallel to floor.
- Keep right leg as straight as possible.
- Step back to starting position.
- Inhale out, exhale back.
- Repeat with right leg.

Alternated Barbell Front Lunge
Thighs and Hamstrings

- Place barbell on upper back.
- Keep head up, back straight, feet 14" apart.
- Step forward as far as possible with right leg until upper right thigh is almost parallel to floor.
- Keep left leg as straight as possible.
- Step back to starting position.
- Inhale out, exhale back.
- Repeat with left leg.
- Can also be done with dumbbells hanging straight down at sides.

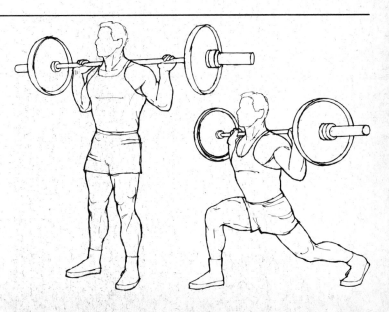

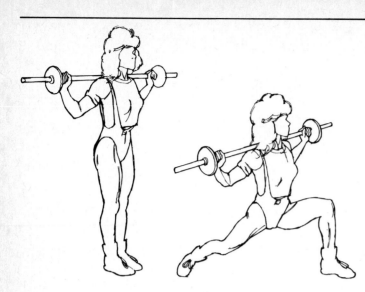

Barbell Front Lunge
Thighs, Hamstrings, Buttocks

- Place barbell on upper back.
- Use comfortable hand grip.
- Keep head up, back straight, feet about 6" apart.
- Step forward as far as possible with left leg until upper left thigh is almost parallel to floor.
- Keep right leg as straight possible.
- Step back to starting position.
- Inhale out, exhale back.
- Repeat with right leg.

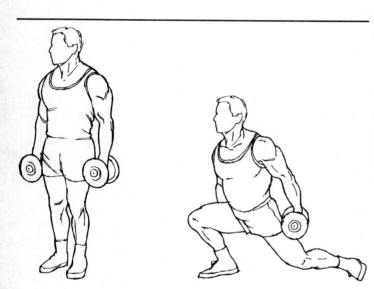

Dumbbell Side Lunge
Inner Thighs and Hamstrings

- Hold dumbbells at arms's length, palms in.
- Keep head up, back straight, feet close together.
- Step to side as far as possible with right leg until upper thigh is almost parallel to floor.
- Keep left leg as straight as possible.
- Step back to starting position.
- Inhale out, exhale back.
- Repeat with left leg.
- Can also be done with barbell held behind neck.

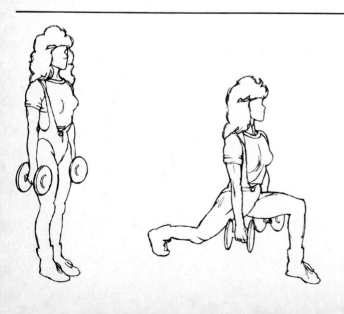

Dumbbell Front Lunge
Thighs and Hamstrings

- Hold dumbbells at arms' length, palms in.
- Head up, back straight, feet about 6" apart.
- Step forward as far as possible with left leg until upper left thigh is almost parallel to floor.
- Keep right leg as straight as possible.
- Step back to starting position.
- Inhale out, exhale back.
- Repeat with right leg.

Freehand Jump Squat
Thighs and Calves

- Stand erect, arms crossed over chest.
- Head up, back straight, feet about 16" apart.
- Squat until upper thighs are parallel, or lower, to floor.
- Keep head up, back straight, knees slightly out.
- Jump straight up in air as high as possible, using thighs like springs.
- Immediately squat and jump again.
- Inhale up, exhale down.
- Can also be done with barbell held on upper back or with dumbbells hanging at sides.

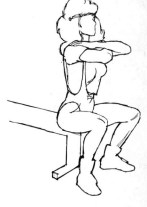

Flat-Footed Medium-Stance Freehand Squat to Bench
Upper Thighs

- Stand erect, arms crossed over chest.
- Head up, back straight, feet 16" apart, with 16" high bench behind you.
- Squat until buttocks touch bench.
- Keep tension on thighs, do not rest on bench.
- Head stays up, back straight, knees slightly out.
- Return to starting position.
- Inhale down, exhale up.
- Can also be done with close or wide stance.

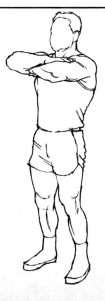

Flat-Footed Medium-Stance Freehand Squat
Upper Thighs

- Stand erect, arms crossed over chest.
- Head up, back straight, feet 16" apart.
- Squat until upper thighs are parallel to floor.
- Keep head up, back straight, knees slightly out.
- Return to starting position.
- Inhale down, exhale up.
- Can also be done with close or wide stance.

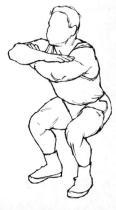

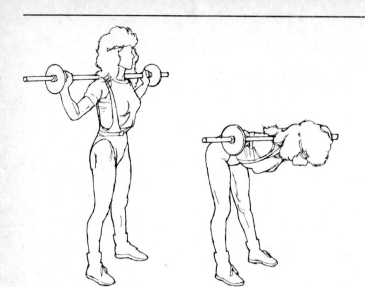

Stiff-Legged Barbell Good Morning
Lower Back

- Place barbell on upper back with comfortable hand grip.
- Keep head up, back straight, feet 16" apart.
- Bend forward until back is nearly parallel to floor.
- Start with legs straight and as you bring weight forward, bend knees into half-squat as weight is at lowest point.
- Return to starting position.
- Inhale down, exhale up.

Dumbbell Hyperextension
Lower Back and Hamstrings

- Position body on special waist-high bench as shown.
- Bend over so head is down.
- Hold dumbbell with both hands behind head or against upper chest.
- Raise torso straight until slightly past parallel.
- Return to starting position.
- Inhale up, exhale down.
- To make easier, do not use dumbbell.

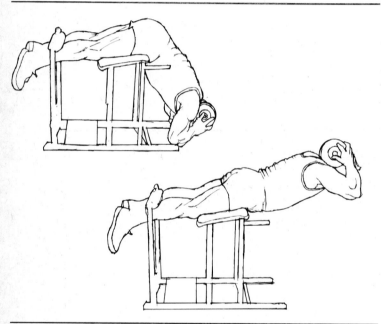

Thigh Biceps Curl on Leg Extension Machine
Hamstrings

- Lie face down on machine.
- Place heels under top foot pad.
- Hold front of machine for support.
- Curl legs up until calves touch biceps.
- Return to starting position.
- Inhale up, exhale down.

One-at-a-Time Thigh Extension on Leg Extension Machine
Lower Thighs

- Sit on right end of machine.
- Place left foot under lower right foot pad as shown.
- Have end of seat against rear of knee.
- Hold seat with left hand behind buttocks.
- Point toes slightly down.
- Raise weight until leg is parallel to floor.
- Return to starting position.
- Inhale up, exhale down.
- Reverse position and repeat with right leg.

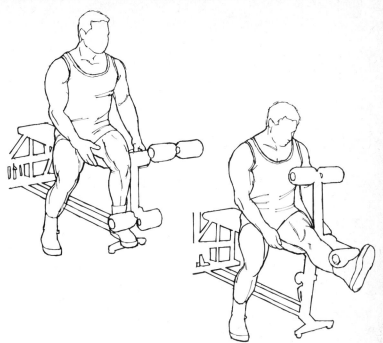

Thigh Extension on Leg Extension Machine
Lower Thighs

- Sit on machine with feet under lower foot pads as shown.
- Have seat against back of knees.
- Hold seat behind buttocks.
- Point toes slightly down.
- Raise weight up until legs are parallel to floor.
- Return to starting position.
- Inhale up, exhale down.

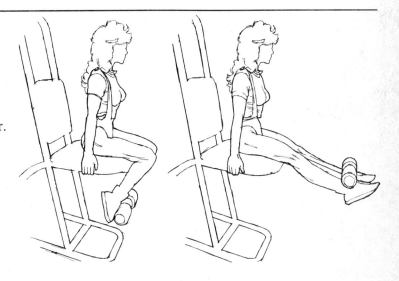

One-at-a-Time Biceps Curl on Leg Extension Machine
Hamstrings

- Lie face down on machine.
- Place heels under top foot pad.
- Hold front of machine.
- Curl right leg up until calf touches biceps.
- Return to starting position.
- Inhale up, exhale down.
- Repeat with left leg.

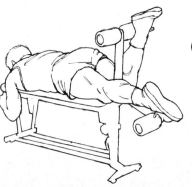

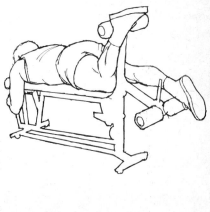

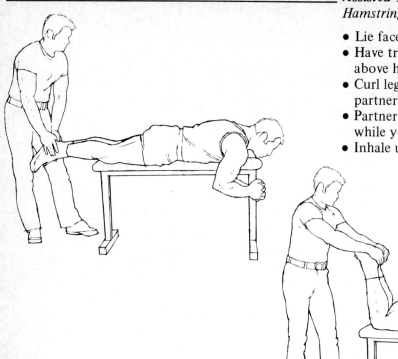

Assisted Thigh Biceps Curl
Hamstrings

- Lie face down on floor or wide bench.
- Have training partner place hands just above heels.
- Curl legs up until calves touch biceps with partner providing resistance.
- Partner forces legs back to starting position while you resist.
- Inhale up, exhale down.

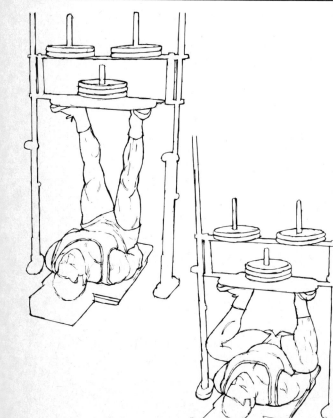

Wide-Stance Leg Press on Wall-Type Leg Press Machine
Inner Thighs

- Lie on support pad under machine.
- Place hips directly under foot pad.
- Place feet on foot pad, 18" to 20" apart.
- Press weight rack up until legs are straight, knees locked.
- Release safety stops.
- Place hands under buttocks, palms down.
- Lower weight rack until upper thighs are away from outer sides of torso.
- Keep knees pointing out.
- Keep hips down.
- Do not rotate lower back.
- Return to starting position.
- Inhale down, exhale up.

Wide-Stance Half-Squat on Thrust Machine
Inner Thighs and Buttocks

- Face machine.
- Place shoulders under pads.
- Plant feet on slanted platform about 18" apart.
- Stand erect, head up, back straight.
- Release safety stops.
- Squat until upper thighs are parallel to machine.
- Keep head up, back straight, knees pointing out.
- Return to starting position.
- Inhale down, exhale up.
- Can also be done to half-squat position.

Medium-Stance Hack Squat on Ram Thrust Machine
Upper Thighs

- Back into machine.
- Place shoulders under pads.
- Plant feet on slanted platform about 14" apart.
- Stand erect, head up, back straight.
- Release safety stops.
- Squat until upper thighs are parallel to machine.
- Keep head up, back straight, knees pointing out.
- Return to starting position.
- Inhale down, exhale up.
- Can also be done with close or wide stance or to half-squat position.

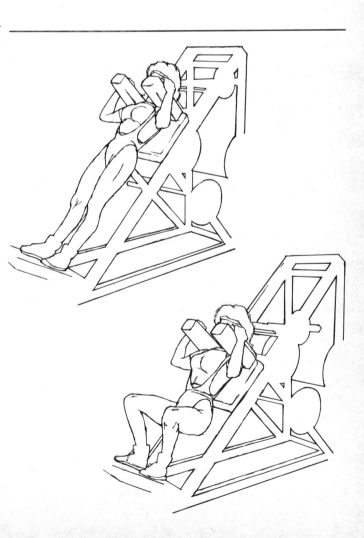

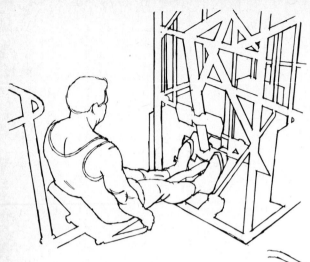

Medium-Stance Lower-Pad Leg Press on Universal Machine
Upper Thighs

- Adjust seat so upper thighs are nearly vertical to floor in contracted position.
- Hold hand rails under buttocks.
- Place feet on lower pads.
- Press out until thighs are straight, knees locked.
- Let weight stack down until it nearly touches remaining plates.
- Keep knees slightly out.
- Inhale down, exhale up.

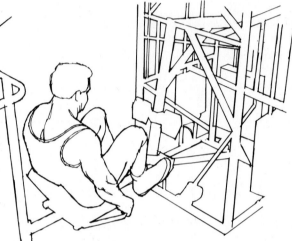

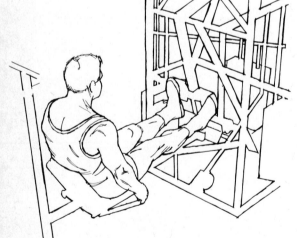

Medium-Stance Top-Pad Leg Press on Universal Machine
Upper Thighs

- Adjust seat so upper thighs are nearly vertical to floor in contracted position.
- Hold hand rails under buttocks.
- Place feet on top pads.
- Press out until thighs are straight, knees locked.
- Let weight stack down until it nearly touches remaining plates.
- Keep knees slightly out.
- Inhale down, exhale up.

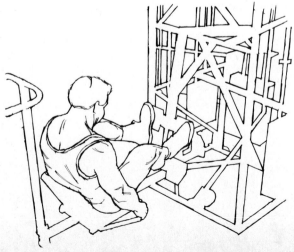

Flat-Footed Medium-Stance Dumbbell Squat to Bench
Upper Thighs

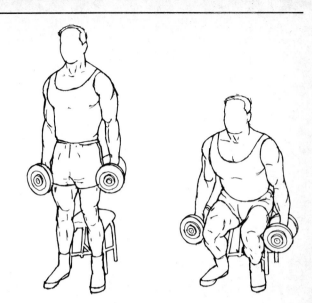

- With 16" high bench behind you, stand with heels even with end of bench.
- Hold dumbbells at sides, at arms' length, palms in.
- Keep head up, back straight, feet firmly on floor, 16" apart.
- Squat until buttocks touch bench.
- Do not sit on bench, keep tension on thighs.
- Keep knees close together.
- Return to starting position.
- Inhale down, exhale up.
- Can also be done with heels elevated on 2x4.

Barbell Jump Squat
Thighs and Calves

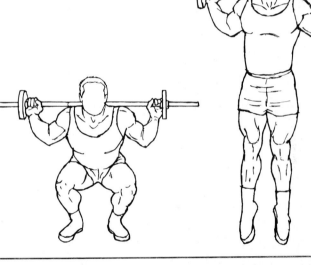

- Place barbell on upper back.
- Head up, back straight, feet 16" apart.
- Squat down until upper thighs are parallel to floor.
- Spring up as high in air as possible.
- Immediately (without rest) squat down and spring up again.
- Continue until all reps are completed.
- Inhale down, exhale up.

Step-Ups With Barbell
Upper Thighs

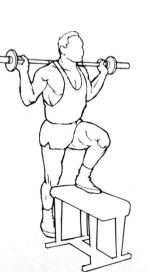
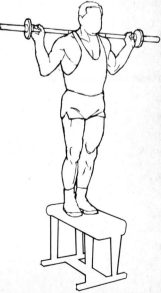

- Place barbell on shoulders.
- Step up with left leg onto flat bench.
- Step up with right leg.
- Step down with left leg first, then right leg.
- Repeat, starting with right leg.
- Inhale down, exhale up.

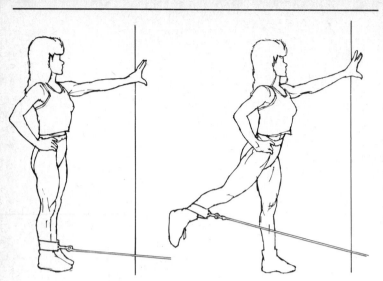

Hip Extension
Hips and Thighs

- Stand erect in front of wall pulley.
- With ankle strap on right ankle, step back far enough from pulley so leg supports weight stack.
- Raise right leg straight back to rear as far as possible.
- Return leg to starting position.
- Keep back as straight as possible.
- Do not bend forward any more than necessary.
- Place ankle strap on left ankle and repeat with left leg.
- Inhale up, exhale down.

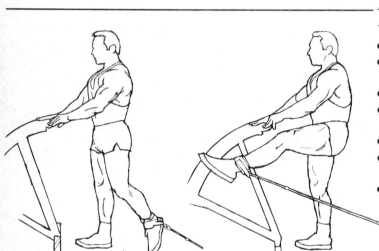

Hip Flexion
Hip Flexors

- Place ankle strap on left ankle.
- Stand with back to wall pulley, far enough away so leg supports weight stack.
- Hold on to waist-high object in front of you.
- Keeping leg straight, knee locked, raise left leg until thigh is parallel to floor.
- Return to starting position.
- Keep back straight, do not bend forward and back.
- Inhale up, exhale down.

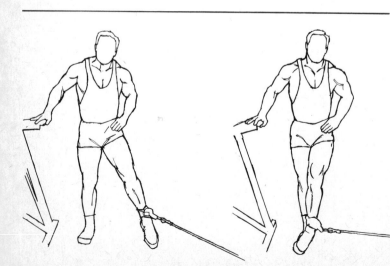

Hip Adduction
Inner Thigh

- Place ankle strap on left ankle.
- Stand with left side to wall pulley, far enough away so leg supports weight stack.
- Hold on to waist-high object with right hand.
- Start with left leg extended to side.
- Pull left leg across, in front of right leg, keeping knee locked.
- Return to starting position.
- Keep back straight, do not swing body from side to side.
- Inhale pulling, exhale returning.
- Repeat with right leg.

Hip Abduction
Hips

- Stand erect, left side facing wall pulley.
- With ankle strap on right ankle, step back far enough from pulley so leg supports weight stack.
- Stand with legs together.
- Raise right leg up and out to side as far as possible.
- Return leg to starting position.
- Keep back straight, do not swing body from side to side.
- Face right side to wall and repeat with left leg.
- Inhale up, exhale down. □

TRICEPS

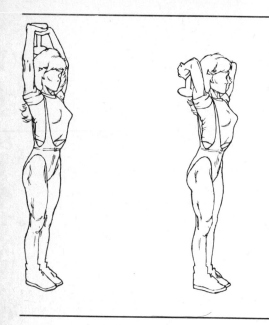

Standing Dumbbell Triceps Curl
Triceps

- Hold dumbbell with both hands, raise overhead to arms' length.
- Stand erect, head up, feet 16" apart.
- Rotate hands while raising dumbbell so top plates of dumbbell rest in palms, thumbs around handle.
- Keep upper arms close to head.
- Lower dumbbell in semicircular motion behind head until forearms touch biceps.
- Return to starting position.
- Inhale down, exhale up.

Seated Dumbbell Triceps Curl
Triceps

- Hold dumbbell with both hands and raise overhead to arms' length.
- Rotate hands while raising dumbbell so top plates of dumbbell rest in palms, thumbs around handle.
- Sit at end of bench, feet firmly on floor, back straight, head up.
- Keep upper arms close to head.
- Lower dumbbell in semicircular motion behind head until forearms touch biceps.
- Return to starting position.
- Inhale down, exhale up.

Seated Bent-Over One-Arm-Dumbbell Triceps Extension
Triceps

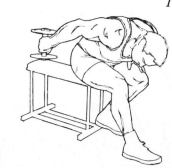

- Hold dumbbell in right hand, palm in.
- Sit at end of bench, feet firmly on floor.
- Bend over as far as possible.
- Draw right upper arm to side, keeping lower arm vertical.
- Press dumbbell back in semicircular motion until entire arm is parallel to floor.
- Hold dumbbell at top momentarily.
- Lower slowly to starting position.
- Inhale up, exhale down.
- Repeat with left arm.

Standing One-Arm Dumbbell Triceps Curl
Triceps

- Hold dumbbell in right hand and raise overhead to arm's length.
- Stand erect, head up, feet 16" apart.
- Keep upper arm close to head.
- Lower dumbbell in semicircular motion behind head until forearm touches biceps.
- Return to starting position.
- Inhale down, exhale up.
- Repeat with left arm.
- Can also be done seated.

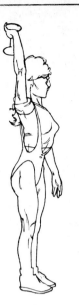 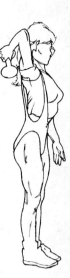

Lying Floor One-Arm Dumbbell Triceps Curl
Triceps

- Lie on back on floor.
- Hold dumbbell in right hand at arm's length above shoulder.
- Lower dumbbell in semicircular motion to side of head, bending arm at elbow, keeping upper arm vertical.
- Return to starting position.
- Inhale down, exhale up.
- Repeat with left arm.
- Can also be done on flat or incline bench.

Lying-Supine Two-Arm-Dumbbell Triceps Curl
Triceps

- Lie on back on bench.
- Hold dumbbells at arms' length above shoulders.
- Lower dumbbells in semicircular motion, bending arms at elbows, keeping upper arms vertical until forearms touch biceps.
- Return to starting position.
- Inhale down, exhale up.
- Can also be done on floor, or on seated or standing incline bench.

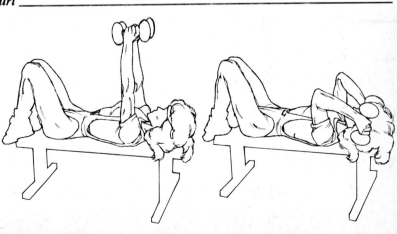

Standing Bent-Over One-Arm-Dumbbell Triceps Extension
Triceps

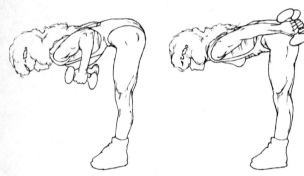

- Hold dumbbell in right hand, palm in.
- Bend over until upper body is parallel to floor.
- Place left hand on left knee.
- Draw right upper arm to side, keeping lower arm vertical.
- Press dumbbell back in semicircular motion until entire arm is parallel to floor.
- Hold dumbbell at top momentarily.
- Lower slowly to starting position.
- Inhale up, exhale down.
- Repeat with left arm.

Standing Bent-Over Two-Arm-Dumbbell Triceps Extension
Triceps

- Hold dumbbells, palms in.
- Bend over until upper body is parallel to floor.
- Draw upper arms to sides, keeping lower arms vertical.
- Press dumbbells back in semicircular motion until entire arm is parallel to floor.
- Hold dumbbells at top momentarily.
- Lower slowly to starting position.
- Inhale up, exhale down.

Seated Bent-Over Two-Arm-Dumbbell Triceps Extension
Triceps

- Hold dumbbells, palms in.
- Sit at end of bench, feet firmly on floor.
- Bend over as far as possible.
- Draw upper arms to sides, keeping lower arms vertical.
- Press dumbbells back in semicircular motion until entire arm is parallel to floor.
- Hold dumbbells at top momentarily.
- Lower slowly to starting position.
- Inhale up, exhale down.

Incline Close-Grip Barbell Triceps Curls
Triceps

- Hold barbell with hands 6" apart, palms down.
- Lie back on incline bench, keeping head off bench.
- Press bar overhead to arms' length.
- Lower bar in semicircular motion behind head until forearms touch biceps.
- Keep upper arms close to head.
- Return to starting position.
- Inhale down, exhale up.
- Can also be done with medium grip or with 2 dumbbells, palms facing in.

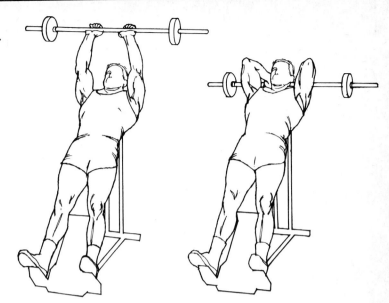

Standing Close-Grip Barbell Triceps Curl
Triceps

- Hold barbell with hands 6" apart, palms down.
- Stand erect, head up, feet 16" apart.
- Raise bar overhead to arms' length.
- Lower bar in semicircular motion behind head until forearms touch biceps.
- Keep upper arms close to sides of head.
- Return to starting position.
- Inhale down, exhale up.
- Can also be done with medium grip or with 2 dumbbells, palms facing in.

Seated Close-Grip Barbell Triceps Curl
Triceps

- Hold barbell with hands 6" apart, palms down.
- Sit at end of bench, feet firmly on floor, back straight, head up.
- Raise bar overhead to arms' length.
- Keep upper arms close to head.
- Lower bar behind head in semicircular motion until forearms touch biceps.
- Return to starting position.
- Inhale down, exhale up.
- Can also be done with medium grip, seated or standing.

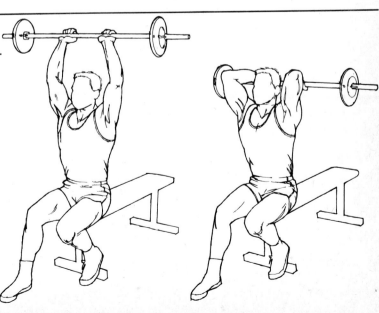

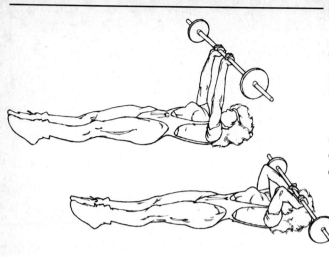

Lying Floor Close-Grip Barbell Triceps Curl to Forehead
Triceps

- Lie on back on floor.
- Hold barbell with hands 6" apart, palms up.
- Press bar to arms' length above shoulders.
- Lower bar in semicircular motion to forehead, bending arms at elbows, keeping upper arms vertical.
- Return to starting position.
- Inhale down, exhale up.
- Can also be done with medium grip, or 2 dumbbells, palms facing in.

Lying-Supine Close-Grip Barbell Triceps Curl to Forehead
Triceps

- Lie on back with head on bench.
- Hold barbell with hands 6" apart, palms up.
- Press bar to arms' length above shoulders.
- Lower bar in semicircular motion to forehead, bending arms at elbows, keeping upper arms vertical.
- Return to starting position.
- Inhale down, exhale up.
- Can also be done with medium grip.

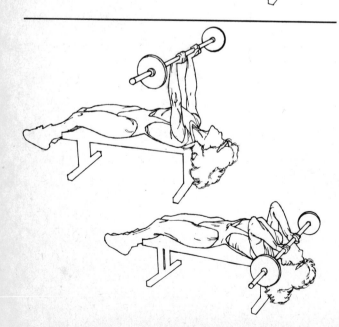

Lying-Supine Close-Grip Barbell Triceps Curl to Chin
Triceps

- Lie on back with head off end of bench.
- Hold barbell with hands 6" apart, palms up.
- Press bar to arms' length above shoulders.
- Lower bar in semicircular motion to chin, bending arms at elbows, keeping upper arms vertical.
- Return to starting position.
- Inhale down, exhale up.
- Can also be done with medium grip.

Lying-Supine Close-Grip Barbell Triceps Kick Back
Triceps

- Hold barbell with hands 8" apart, palms down.
- Lie on back with head close to end of bench.
- Position bar behind head.
- Keep upper arms close to head and parallel to floor, lower arms vertical to floor.
- Push bar up in semicircular motion until lower arms are parallel to floor.
- Hold bar at top momentarily.
- Lower slowly to starting position.
- Inhale up, exhale down.
- Can also be done with medium grip.

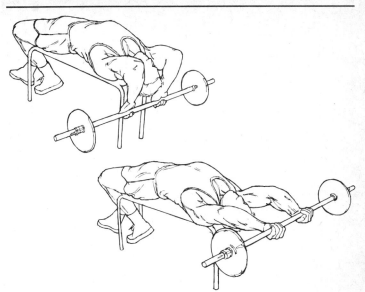

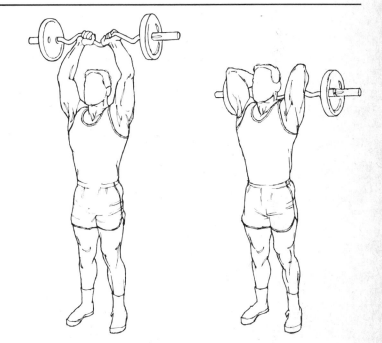

Standing Close-Grip Easy-Curl-Bar Triceps Curl
Triceps

- Use closest hand grip spacing possible on easy-curl bar, palms down.
- Stand erect, head up, feet 16" apart.
- Raise bar overhead to arms' length.
- Lower bar behind head in semicircular motion until forearms touch biceps.
- Keep upper arms close to head.
- Return to starting position.
- Inhale down, exhale up.
- Can also be done with medium grip, seated or standing.

Incline Close-Grip Easy-Curl-Bar Triceps Curl
Triceps

- Use closest hand grip spacing possible on easy-curl bar, palms down.
- Lie back on incline bench, with head over end.
- Press bar overhead to arms' length.
- Lower bar in semicircular motion behind head until forearms touch biceps.
- Keep upper arms close to head.
- Return to starting position.
- Inhale down, exhale up.
- Can also be done seated on incline bench.
- Can also be done with medium grip.

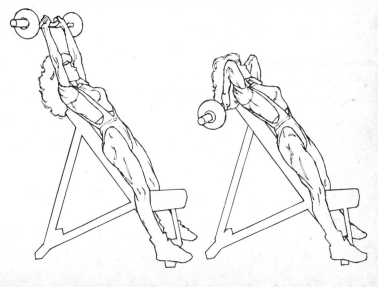

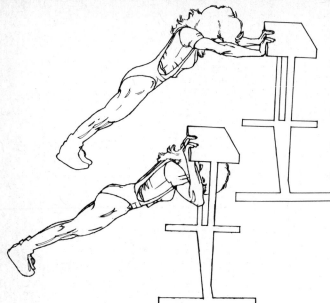

Freehand Triceps Extension
Triceps

- Lean against object slightly lower than waist height, hands 12" apart, palms down.
- Keep back straight, head down, knees locked.
- Bend arms at elbows, lower yourself until head is between hands.
- Forearms and biceps touching, elbows close to head.
- Press back to starting position keeping elbows in.
- Inhale down, exhale up.

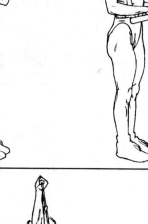

Standing Close-Grip Triceps Press-Down on Lat Machine
Outer Triceps

- Stand erect, head up, feet 16" apart, in front of machine.
- Hold bar with hands 8" apart, palms down.
- Bring upper arms to sides and keep them there.
- Start with forearms and biceps touching.
- Press bar down in semicircular motion to arms' length.
- Return to starting position.
- Inhale down, exhale up.
- Can also be done with medium or reverse grip.

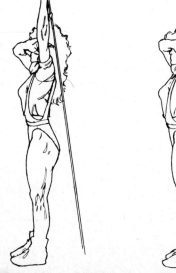

Standing Face-Away Low-Pulley One-Arm Triceps Curl
Triceps

- Hold handle of low pulley with left hand and turn away from machine.
- Raise left hand directly over left shoulder to arm's length.
- Keep upper arm vertical.
- Bend arm at elbow in semicircular motion until forearm touches biceps.
- Press to starting position.
- Keep elbow close to head.
- Inhale down, exhale up.
- Repeat with right arm.

Lying-Supine Close-Grip Easy-Curl-Bar Triceps Curl to Forehead
Triceps

- Use closest hand grip spacing possible on easy-curl bar, palms down.
- Lie on bench with head down, chin pointing up.
- Press bar to arms' length above shoulders.
- Lower bar in semicircular motion to forehead, bending arms at elbows, keeping upper arms vertical.
- Return to starting position.
- Inhale down, exhale up.

Lying Floor Close-Grip Easy-Curl-Bar Triceps Curl to Forehead
Triceps

- Use closest hand grip spacing possible on easy-curl bar, palms down.
- Lie on back on floor, head down, chin pointing up.
- Press bar to arms' length above shoulders.
- Lower bar in semicircular motion to forehead, bending arms at elbows, keeping upper arms vertical.
- Return to starting position.
- Inhale down, exhale up.

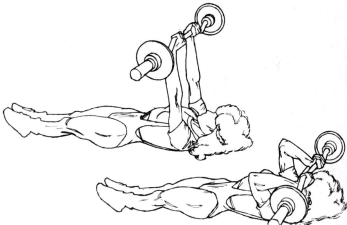

Kneeling Head-Supported Close-Grip Triceps Extension on High Pulley
Triceps

- Place bench sideways in front of high pulley.
- Hold bar with hands 6" apart, palms down.
- Face away from machine and kneel.
- Place head and front of upper arms on bench.
- Keep upper arms close to head.
- Start with forearms and biceps touching.
- Press cable out in semicircular motion until elbows are locked, arms parallel to floor.
- Return cable to starting position.
- Inhale out, exhale back.
- Can also be done with medium grip.

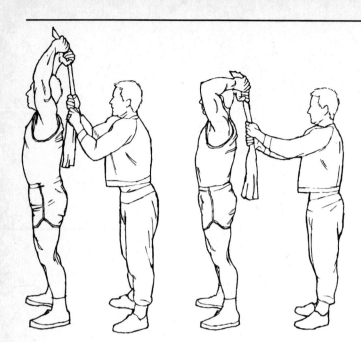

Standing Towel Triceps Curl
Triceps

- Hold one end of towel, or rope, with both hands.
- Stand erect, head up, feet 16" apart.
- Raise arms overhead.
- Have training partner hold other end of towel and apply controlled pressure, pulling arms back in semicircular motion until forearms touch biceps while you resist.
- Upper arms must remain close to head.
- Press arms back to starting position while partner resists.
- Inhale down, exhale up.

Kneeling Concentrated Triceps Curl on High Pulley
Triceps

- Hold handle of high pulley with right hand.
- Kneel on left knee, left side toward machine.
- Keep right knee bent, upper thigh parallel to floor.
- Keep right upper arm against right thigh.
- Extend down in semicircular motion until arm is vertical.
- Return to starting position.
- Inhale down, exhale up.
- Reverse position and repeat with left arm.

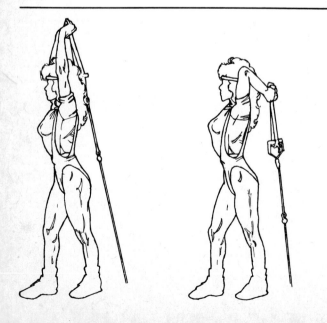

Standing Towel Triceps Curl on Low Wall Pulley
Triceps

- Wrap a towel, or rope, around low pulley handle.
- Hold ends with both hands and turn away from machine.
- Stand away from machine so arms can support weights through full range of motion.
- Straighten arms overhead above shoulders.
- Lower arms in semicircular motion behind head until forearms touch biceps.
- Press back to starting position.
- Upper arms must remain close to head.
- Inhale down, exhale up.

Standing Face-Away Two-Arm Bar Triceps Extension on High Pulley
Triceps

- Attach a short bar to top cables of wall pulley.
- Hold bar with hands 8" apart, palms down.
- Stand away from machine so arms can support weights through full range of motion.
- Straighten arms in front of you, parallel to floor.
- Draw arms back in semicircular motion until forearms touch biceps.
- Press back to starting position.
- Upper arms must remain parallel.
- Inhale back, exhale out.

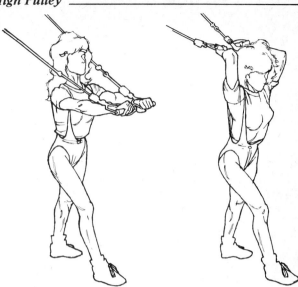

Triceps Curl on Nautilus Machine
Triceps

- Sit in machine and place clenched hands on pads, palms facing.
- Rest upper arms, or elbows, on pads.
- Press arm of machine out in semicircular motion, until arms are straight, elbows locked.
- Keep elbows on pads.
- Keep arms extended momentarily.
- Return arm of machine to starting position.
- Inhale out, exhale back.

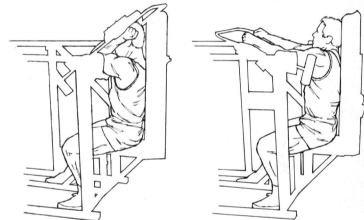

Reverse Medium-Grip Triceps Bench Press
Triceps

- Lie on flat bench, barbell at arms' length above shoulders, reverse grip, hands 16" apart.
- Lower bar until it touches 1" below nipples.
- Press bar back to starting position.
- Keep elbows in close to sides.
- Inhale down, exhale up.
- Can also be done on Smith machine or wall-type leg press.

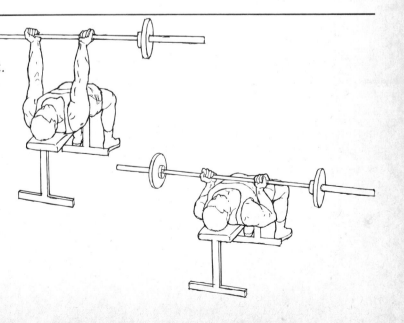

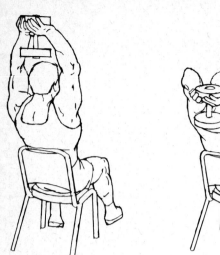
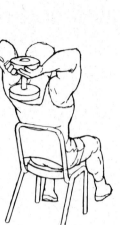

Seated Back-Supported Dumbbell Triceps Curl
Triceps

- Sit on straight-back chair, head up, feet firmly on floor.
- Hold one dumbbell with both hands overhead at arms' length, vertical to floor.
- As you are raising, rotate hands up and over until top plates are resting in palms of hands, thumbs around handle.
- Keep upper arms close to sides at all times.
- Lower dumbbell behind head in semicircular motion until forearms touch biceps.
- Return to starting position using same path.
- Inhale down, exhale up.
- Can also be done using close grip on barbell or easy-curl bar.

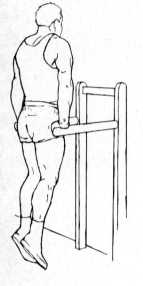
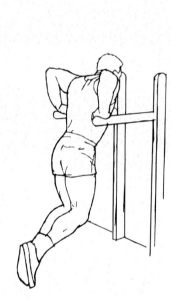

Reverse Grip Dip
Lower Pectorals and Triceps

- Hold yourself erect on bars, reverse grip.
- Lower body by bending arms, elbows out to sides.
- Lower until forearms touch biceps.
- Pause, then press back to arms' length, elbows locked.
- Do not swing body back and forth.
- Inhale down, exhale up.
- Can also be done with weight hanging from waist. □

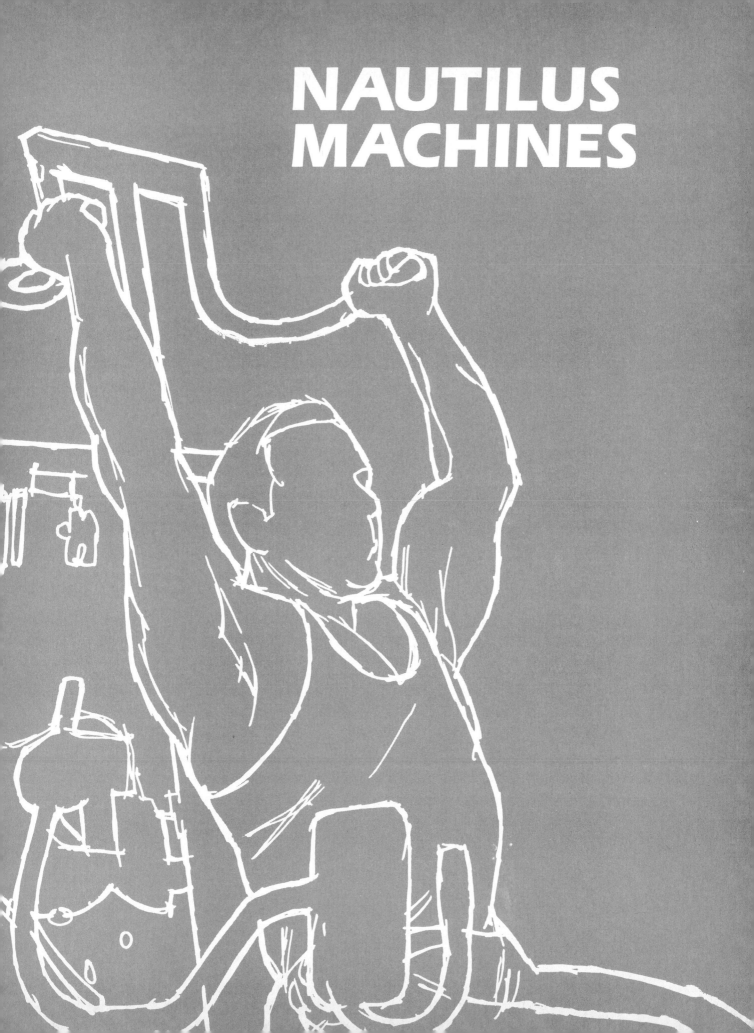

NAUTILUS
MACHINES

EXERCISES FOR NAUTILUS MACHINES

18 Rules for Nautilus Training

Nautilus Sports/Medical Industries, Inc. makes the following recommendations for use of Nautilus equipment:

1. Perform one set of 4-6 exercises for the lower body; and 6-8 exercises for the upper body; and no more than 12 exercises in any single workout.
2. Select a resistance on each exercise that allows you to do between 8-12 repetitions in smooth, steady form, through the full range of motion. If 8 repetitions cannot be performed properly, the resistance is too heavy. If 12 or more repetitions can be performed properly, the resistance is too light.
3. Continue each exercise until no additional repetitions are possible in good form. When 12 or more repetitions are performed properly, increase the resistance by approximately 5% at the next workout.
4. Make certain that the rotational axis of the cam of all rotary exercises is in line with the joint axis of the body part that is being moved.
5. Position your body in a straight, aligned manner. Avoid twisting or shifting your weight during the movement.
6. Maintain a loose, comfortable grip. Never squeeze the handgrips tightly as this results in elevated blood pressure.
7. For overall growth stimulation, select exercises that isolate and work the largest muscle groups first, then proceed down to the smaller muscle groups. Example: hips, thighs, back, shoulders, chest, arms and neck.
8. Accentuate the lowering portion of each repetition. Lift resistance or perform positive work to the count of two ... pause ... lower the resistance or perform negative work slowly and smoothly while counting to four.
9. Use as much of your range of motion as possible on each machine to develop full-range strength and flexibility. Concentrate on flexibility by slowly stretching during the first 3 repetitions.
10. Breathe normally. Try not to hold your breath while training.
11. Move slower, never faster, if in doubt about speed of movement.
12. Walk quickly from machine to machine. The longer the rest between machines, the less effective the cardiovascular conditioning. Do not, however, sacrifice form for speed.
13. Move very quickly—less than 3 seconds—from the primary exercise to the secondary exercise in all double Nautilus machines.
14. Follow the routine as the exercises are numbered on your workout sheet; however, any time the machine you are to do next is being used, go to another exercise and then return to the machine that was in use.
15. Finish your entire workout in 20 to 30 minutes.
16. Rest a minimum of 48 hours and not more than 96 hours between successive workouts.
17. Keep accurate records—date, resistance, repetitions, and overall training time—for each workout.
18. Vary the workouts often.

On the following seven pages are instructions and drawings for Nautilus exercises.

Duo Hip and Back
Buttocks and Lower Back

- Lie on back, legs over movement arms.
- Fasten seat belt, hold handles.
- Keeping left leg fully extended, bend right leg as far as possible.
- Push right leg down until even with left leg.
- Pause, arch back, contract buttocks.
- When contracted, keep legs straight, knees together, toes pointed.
- Repeat with left leg.

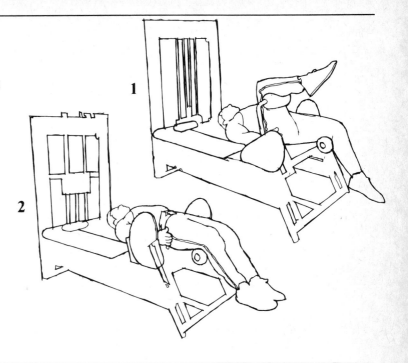

Leg Extension
Quadriceps

- Sit with feet under pads, fasten seat belt.
- Straighten both legs slowly.
- Pause, then return slowly to starting position.

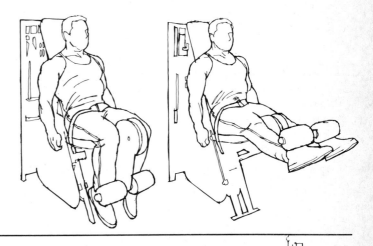

Leg Curl
Hamstrings

- Lie face down, knees just over edge of bench.
- Place feet under pads, hold handles.
- Curl legs, bring heels as close to buttocks as possible.
- Pause, then lower legs slowly to starting position.

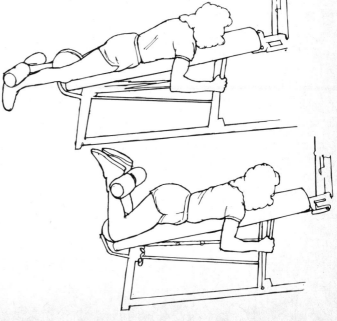

Hip Adduction
Inner Thighs

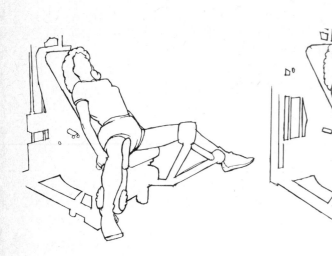

- Sit, legs spread, knees and ankles on movement arms.
- Pull knees and thighs together slowly.
- Pause with knees together, then return to starting position.

Behind Neck
Lats

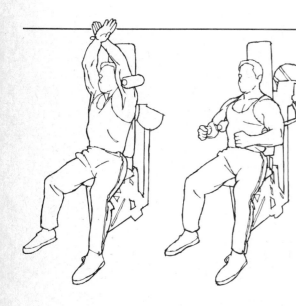

- Sit, fasten seat belt.
- Cross forearms behind neck.
- Place back of upper arms against pads.
- Move both arms down until pads touch torso.
- Do not bring arms or hands to front of body.
- Slowly return to starting position.

70° Shoulder
Deltoids and Trapezius

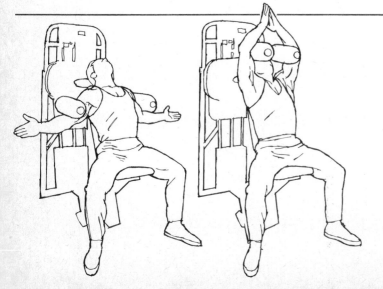

- Sit, fasten seat belt.
- Place arms so pads are in crooks of elbows.
- Rest head on pad behind shoulders, look at ceiling.
- Move both arms in semicircular motion until pads touch over face.
- Pause, then return slowly to starting position.

10° Chest
Pectorals

- Lie on back, head higher than hips, pads in crooks of elbows.
- Move both arms in semicircular motion until pads touch over chest.
- Pause, then return slowly to starting position.

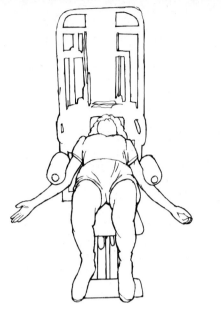
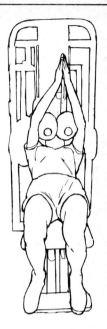

Triceps Extension
Triceps

- Sit with arms bent, elbows on pad, hands palms in against pads on extension bar.
- Straighten arms smoothly.
- Pause, then return slowly to starting position.

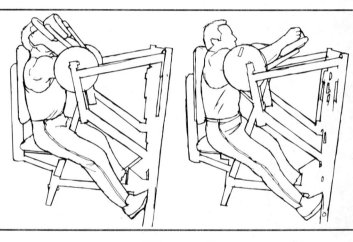

Torso Arm
Lats and Biceps

- Sit so hands are barely able to grasp over-head bar.
- Fasten seat belt, lean forward, hold bar, palms in.
- Pull bar behind neck.
- Keep elbows back.
- Pause, then return slowly to starting position.

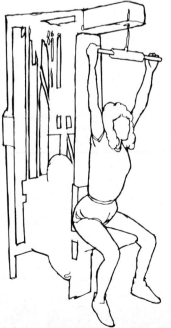
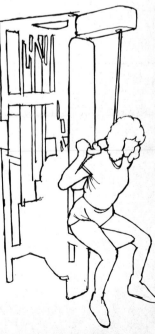

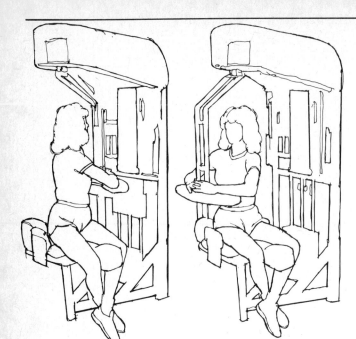

Rotary Torso
Obliques

- Straddle seat on right side, cross ankles securely.
- Turn to right, place forearms on sides of pads.
- Do not turn hips or legs.
- Keep right palm firmly against middle bar of movement arm.
- Rotate torso from right to left by pushing with right palm.
- Move head with torso by focusing between parallel bars of movement arm.
- Pause in contracted position; rotation will be less than 180°.
- Return slowly to starting position.
- For left to right torso rotation, straddle seat on left side and reverse position.

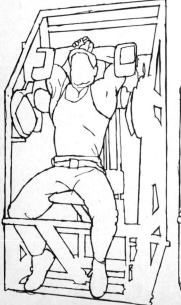

Abdominal
Abdominals

- Sit, hold bars at sides of head, palms in.
- Hook feet under pads.
- Move upper body forward and down.
- Pause in contracted position, then return slowly to starting position.

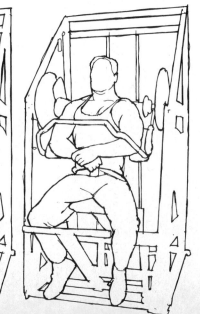

Pullover
Lats

- Sit, fasten seat belt, elbows on pads, one hand holding opposite wrist above and behind head.
- Driving with elbows, bring pullover bar to where it is resting against waist.
- Pause, then return slowly to starting position.

Leg Press
Thighs and Buttocks

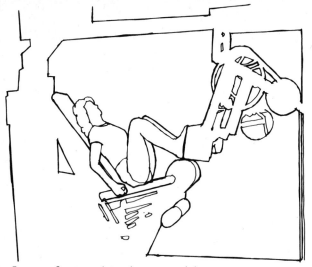
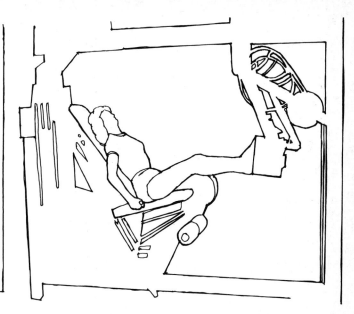

- Lower foot pad to down position.
- Sit with arches of feet on center of leg press pedals, hold hand grips.
- Extend legs to near "lockout."
- Pause, then return slowly to starting position.

Bent Arm Fly
Pectorals

- Sit with forearms behind pads, thumbs hooked under top handgrips.
- Move forearms forward until pads touch.
- Pause, then return slowly to starting position.

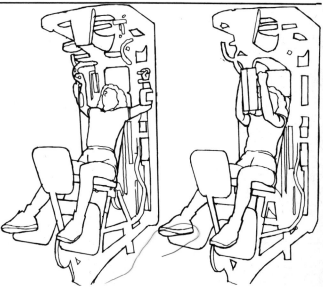

Decline Press
Pectorals, Deltoids, Triceps

- Sit, fasten seat belt, extend arms, hands holding grips.
- Press bar forward slowly.
- Pause, then return slowly to starting position.
- Keep elbows wide.

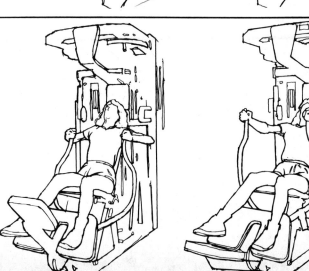
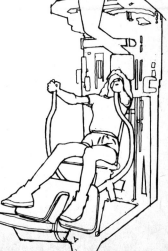

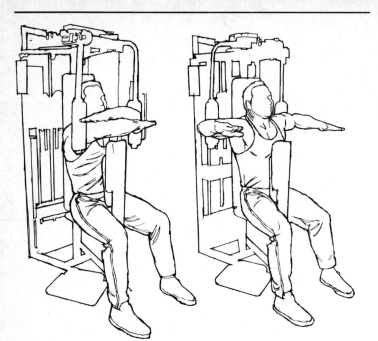

Rowing Torso
Deltoids, Rhomboids, Trapezius

- Sit with arms between pads, then cross arms.
- Bend arms in rowing fashion as far back as possible.
- Keep arms parallel to floor.
- Pause, then return slowly to starting position.

Side Lateral Raise
Deltoids

- Sit, fasten seat belt, hold handles.
- Make sure elbows are slightly behind torso and against pads.
- Raise elbows slowly until at chin level.
- Pause, then return slowly to starting position.

Overhead Press
Deltoids and Triceps

- Sit, fasten seat belt, hold handles above shoulders.
- Press handles overhead.
- Do not arch back.
- Pause, then return slowly to starting position.

Heel Raise
Calves

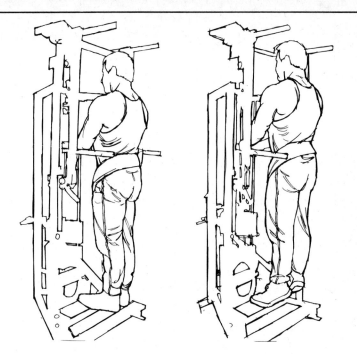

- Stand on first step of multi-exercise machine.
- Lean forward, body straight, heels lower than toes.
- Raise heels until calves have contracted completely.
- Pause, then return slowly to starting position.

Neck Extension
Neck

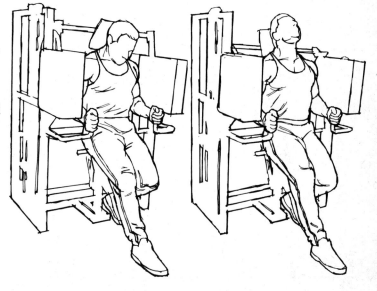

- Sit, torso erect, head against pad.
- Look down, placing neck in stretched position.
- Extend head backwards until looking toward ceiling.
- Pause, then return slowly to starting position.
- Do not lean forward and back when raising and lowering head.

Note: Every Nautilus club has different machines, some newer, some older than those shown here.□

UNIVERSAL
MACHINES

UNIVERSAL AEROBIC SUPER CIRCUIT

On the following two pages is a new high intensity program for athletes. It is designed to develop all four elements of fitness: strength, muscular endurance, cardiovascular endurance and flexibility. It can be used for preseason conditioning and is a quick way to get a thorough and balanced workout.

Important Notes:

- Be sure to consult your physician and obtain prior approval before engaging in this or any other strenuous training program.
- Be sure to begin each exercise period by warming up and stretching to warm up the heart as well as the muscles.

The program shown on the following pages is meant to be performed on 12 Universal single-station machines, but can also be performed on a multi-station machine. Follow the general instructions for lifting (p. 14-17) and the techniques on p. 18-19.

This program consists of alternating upper and lower body exercises: the aim is to keep your body in what is called the *target zone.* To find the target zone, you subtract your age from 220, then take 70-85% of that figure. See chart on p. 74.

Key to program: You do 30 seconds of aerobic conditioning (running in place, exercycle, jump rope, etc.) between each exercise station.

Procedures

1. *How many reps?* 15-20
2. *How many sets?* One at each station
3. *How many circuits?* Three to five
4. *How long at each station?* Maximum 30 seconds
5. *Intervals between stations:* 30 seconds of aerobic conditioning (run in place, jump rope, exercycle, etc.)
6. *How much weight?* 40-50% of maximum for average person, 50-70% for conditioned athlete
7. *How to determine working weight?* Find out your maximum for one lift, take % of that for working weight. Reevaluate every six to eight weeks.
8. *Breathing:* Exhale as weight goes up, inhale as weight comes down
9. *Intensity:* Make your muscles contract explosively throughout the full range of motion to simulate natural resistance of athletic events.
10. *Cool-down:* Don't head for the showers until pulse, breathing and perspiration are back to normal. Gradually decrease body movement, reversing the way you warmed up.
11. *Further details:* Ask your gym manager for a copy of the *Universal Workout Record.*

UNIVERSAL AEROBIC

At each of the numbered stations do one set of 15-20 reps. Maximum 30 seconds at each station. *In between* each station, do 30 seconds of aerobic conditioning. Do the circuit 3-5 times. See p. 321 for complete instructions.

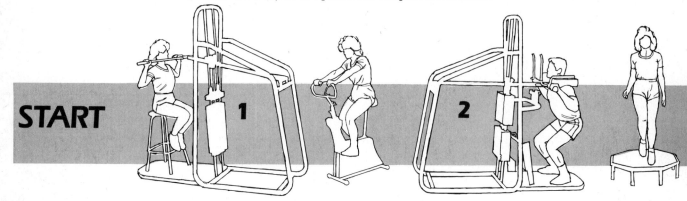

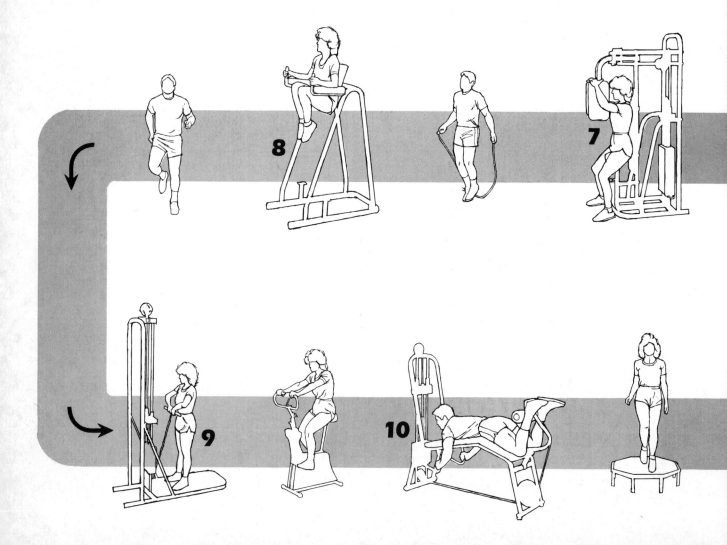

START

SUPER CIRCUIT

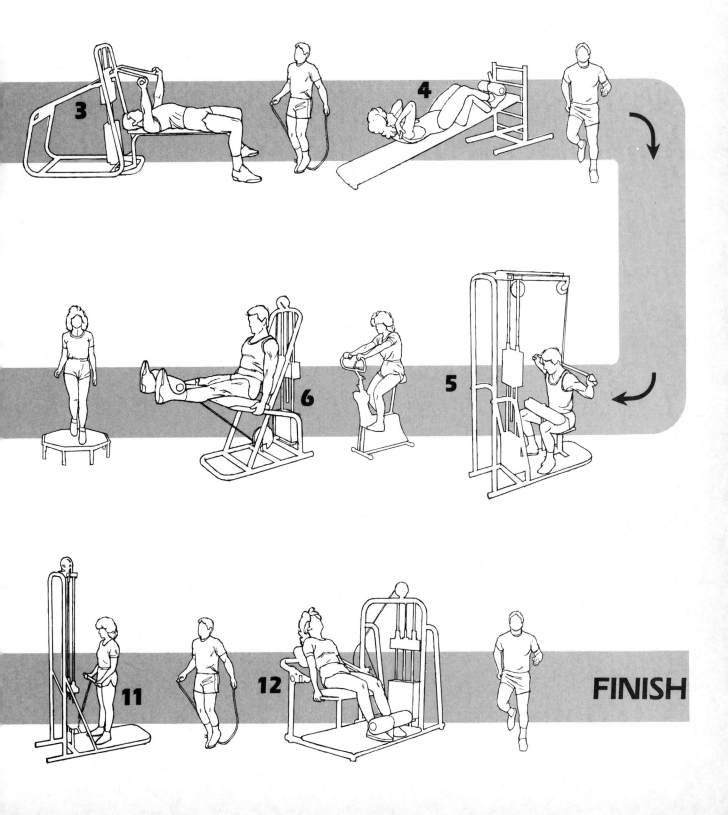

FINISH

The following figures indicate the effectiveness of a similar circuit training program used by the U.S. Navy for its shipboard personnel:

Fitness Changes Following a 10-week Circuit Weight Training Program for Navy Men and Women*

	% Change Men	% Change Women
Upper Torso Dynamic Strength**		
Shoulder Press	+15.5%	+15.6%
Bench Press	+10.3%	+13.9%
Arm Curl	+13.0%	+24.0%
Lat Pulldown	+15.5%	+11.8%
Lower Torso Dynamic Strengh		
Leg Press	+ 10.7%	+15.2%
Knee Extension	+ 24.8%	+30.4%
Muscular Endurance***		
Bench Press	+ 39.6%	+65.7%
Leg Press	+ 28.2%	+44.4%
Stamina		
Maximal Work Capacity on Bicycle Ergometer	+ 3.0%	+ 2.3%

*Sparten: A Hi-tech/Total Body Fitness Program for Health and Physical Readiness. Lt. Edward J. Marcinik, MSC, USN. Naval Research Center, San Diego, California.
**Determined using one repetition maximum strength technique.
***Calculated by determining the maximum number of repetitions performed at 60% of maximum strength for one repetition.□

STRETCHES FOR WEIGHT TRAINING

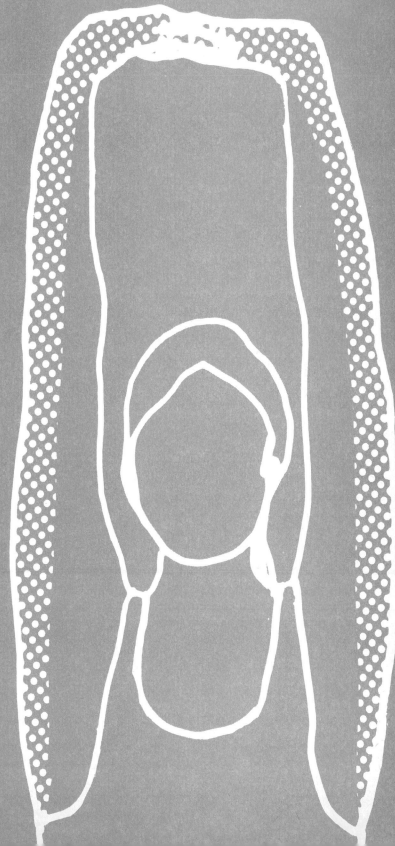

STRETCHES FOR WEIGHT TRAINING

By Bob Anderson
Drawings by Jean Anderson

Bob Anderson, author of *Stretching,* has designed this stretching program for weight training. The stretches should be done before and after working out and can also be done between sets, while you are resting.

The Two Phases of Stretching

The easy stretch: Stretch to where you feel a slight, easy tension. Hold this for 5-30 seconds, and as you do, the tension should diminish. If not, ease off a bit until it feels comfortable. This easy stretch gets the tissues ready for the developmental stretch.

The developmental stretch: After holding the easy stretch, move a fraction of an inch farther into the stretch until you feel the slight tension again. This is the developmental stretch and should be held for 5-30 seconds. This is an excellent way to increase flexibility and get the muscles ready for a workout.

Basic Stretching Rules:

- Stretch slowly and with control.
- No bouncing.
- No pain.
- Don't compare your flexibility with others.
- The key is to *relax.*
- Breathing should be slow, rhythmical. Don't hold breath.
- Hold only stretch tensions that *feel* good.

1

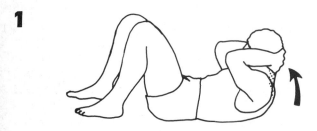

Bring knees together and rest feet on floor. Interlace fingers behind head and rest arms on the mat. Using the power of your arms, *slowly* bring head, neck, and shoulders forward until you feel a slight stretch. Hold easy stretch for 5 seconds. Repeat 3 times.

2

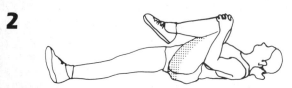

Next, straighten both legs and relax, then pull left leg toward your chest. Keep back of head on the mat, if possible, but don't strain. Hold an easy stretch for 30 seconds. Repeat, pulling right leg toward chest.

3

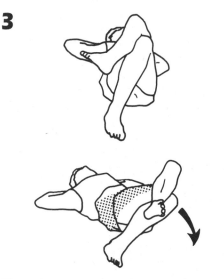

From bent knee position, interlace fingers behind head and lift left leg over right leg. Use left leg to pull right leg toward floor until you feel a stretch along the side of your hip and lower back. Stretch and relax. Keep upper back, shoulders, and elbows flat on floor. You don't have to touch the floor with your right knee, just stretch within *your* limits. Hold for 30 seconds. Repeat stretch for other side.

4

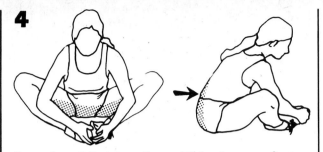

Put soles of feet together with heels a comfortable distance from groin. Now, put hands around feet and slowly pull yourself forward until you feel an easy stretch in the groin. Bend forward from hips and not from shoulders. If possible, keep elbows on outside of lower legs for stability. Hold comfortable stretch for 30-40 seconds.

5

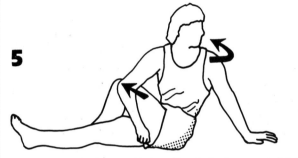

Sit with right leg straight. Put left foot outside of right knee, with left knee bent. Bend right elbow and rest it on outside of upper left thigh, just above knee. During the stretch use elbow to keep this leg stationary with controlled pressure to the inside. Now, with left hand resting behind you, slowly turn head to look over left shoulder, and at the same time rotate upper body toward left hand and arm. As you turn upper body, think of turning hips in the same direction (though hips won't move). This should stretch lower back and side of hip. Hold for 15 seconds. Do both sides.

6

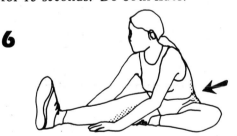

Next, straighten right leg. The sole of left foot will be resting next to inside of straightened leg. Lean slightly forward *from hips* and stretch hamstrings of right leg. Find an easy stretch and relax. If you can't touch your toes comfortably, use a towel to help. Hold for 50 seconds. Do not lock your knee. Right quadricep should be soft and relaxed. Keep right foot upright with ankle and toes relaxed.

7

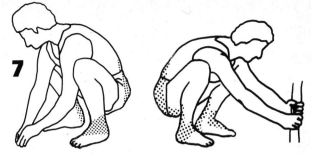

With feet shoulder width apart and pointed out at about 15° angle, heels on ground, bend knees and squat down. If you have trouble staying in this position hold onto something for support. A great stretch for ankles, Achilles tendons, groin, lower back and hips. Hold for 30 seconds. *Be careful if you have had any knee problems. If pain is present, stop.*

8

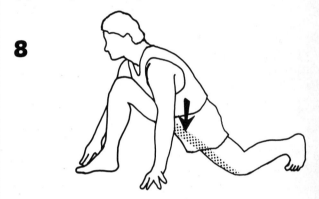

Move one leg forward *until knee of forward leg is directly over ankle.* Other knee is resting on floor. Now, without changing the position of knee on floor or forward foot, lower front of hip downward to create an easy stretch. This stretch should be felt in front of hip and possibly in hamstrings and groin. This helps relieve tension in lower back. Hold for 30 seconds. Do both legs.

9

Opposite hand to opposite foot—quad and knee stretch. Hold top of left foot (from inside of foot) with right hand and gently pull, heel moving toward buttocks. Knee bends at natural angle and creates a good stretch in knee and quadriceps. Pulling opposite hand to opposite foot does not create any adverse angles in the knee and is especially good for knee rehab and problem knees. Hold for 30 seconds. Do both legs.

10

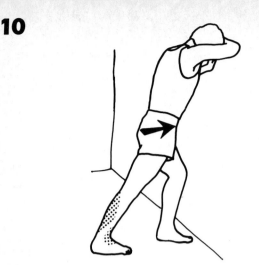

To stretch calf, stand a little way back from a solid support and lean on it with forearms, head resting on hands. Bend one leg and place foot on ground in front of you, leaving other leg straight. Slowly move hips forward until you feel a stretch in calf of straight leg. Be sure to keep heel of foot on ground and *toes pointed straight ahead.* Hold easy stretch for 30 seconds. Do not bounce. Stretch both legs.

11

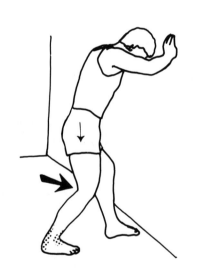

To stretch the soleus and Achilles tendon, slightly bend back knee, keeping foot flat. This gives a much lower stretch—also good for maintaining or regaining flexibility. Hold for 15 seconds, each leg.

12

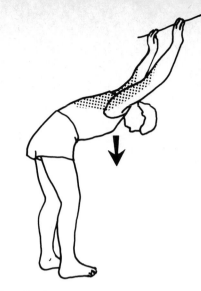

Place both hands shoulder width apart on fence or ledge and let upper body drop down as you keep knees slightly bent (1 inch). Hips should be directly above feet. To change the area of the stretch, bend knees just a bit more and/or place hands at different heights. Find a stretch that you can hold for at least 30 seconds. This will take some of the kinks out of a tired upper back. The top of the refrigerator or a file cabinet are good to use for this stretch. *(Remember to always bend knees when coming out of this stretch.)*

13

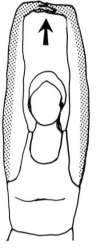

In standing or sitting position, interlace fingers above head. Now, with palms facing upward, push arms slightly back and up. Feel the stretch in arms, shoulders, and upper back. Hold for 15 seconds. Do not hold breath. Good to do anywhere, anytime. Excellent for slumping shoulders.

14

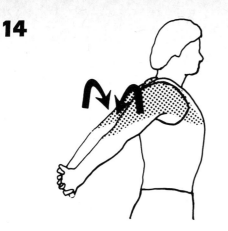

The next stretch is done with fingers interlaced behind back. Slowly turn elbows inward while straightening arms. An excellent stretch for shoulders and arms. Good to do when you find yourself slumping forward from your shoulders. Hold for 5-15 seconds. Do twice.

15

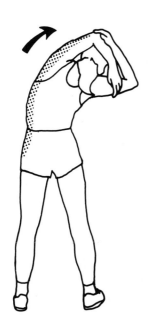

With arms overhead, hold elbow of one arm with other hand. Keeping knees slightly bent (1 inch), gently pull elbow behind head as you bend from hips to side. Hold easy stretch for 10 seconds. Do both sides. Keeping knees slightly bent will give you better balance.

SUMMARY OF STRETCHES FOR WEIGHT TRAINING

See previous pages for instructions.

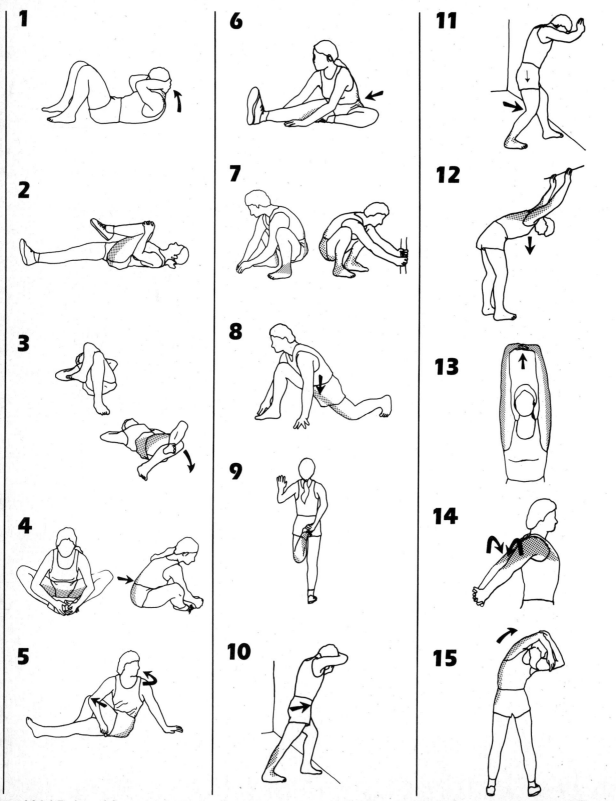

FIT FOR
WORK

FIT FOR WORK

What is the use of health, or of life, if not to do some work therewith?
Thomas Carlyle, 1836

Most of the books, articles, TV and radio shows on fitness these days focus on fitness for play. How to run a faster 10K, how to stay uninjured in aerobics classes, how to play better tennis, etc. But little attention is paid, either in the literature or by the media, to the importance of fitness at the workplace. In this chapter we discuss the most common type of work-related injury—lower back pain—and suggest weight training programs for both white collar and blue collar workers.

- *Blue-collar* refers to workers doing physical or industrial labor.
- *White-collar* refers to workers who sit at desks most of the day.

Requirements of Blue-Collar and White-Collar Workers

There are actually more similarities than differences between the two. Everyone needs to work on:

- Cardiovascular endurance to improve the functioning of the heart, lungs and circulation
- Muscular strength to withstand daily stresses and to prevent injuries

Lower Back Pain

Seventy-five percent of all people in the U.S. will go to a physician at some time in their lives for lower back pain. Workers' Compensation and health plan insurance carriers spend untold millions each year dealing with bad backs. There are two factors here that may surprise you:

1. This problem affects not only people doing physical labor. White-collar workers often injure their backs bending over to pick something up, doing weekend chores, or participating in sports.
2. More people get hurt picking up light than heavy objects. A carpenter gets hurt reaching for the tool box. A mother or father gets hurt bending over for (before even reaching) the baby sitting on the floor.

Why is this such a common injury? Because most people have weak abdominal muscles. Picture a skeleton from the side. There is continuous support along the back (the spine) and the rib cage in front, but no skeletal support in the abdominal area. Structural support there has to be maintained by strong abdominal muscles.

The Most Important Exercise for Workers

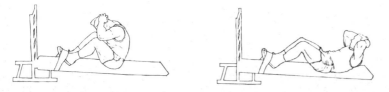

- Knees bent! Bend your knees so there is a 90° angle at the knees.
- Hook feet under a strap or a couch. This allows you to pull up gradually without jerking.
- Do as many as you can, working your way up to 50 a day.

If You Can't Do Sit-Ups

If you haven't exercised your abdominal muscles for awhile (or for years) you may have difficulty doing bent-knee sit-ups. Don't strain at doing them, but rather work your way up to the full sit-ups in this order:

1. Head up

2. Shoulders up

3. Half-up

4. Full sit-up

This will gradually increase the strength of your abdominal muscles.

How to Lift

One type of weightlifting is not covered elsewhere in this book, or in any other books on weightlifting. That is, the lifting of "real"—if you'll excuse the expression—weights. Picking boxes up off the floor or lumber off the ground, lifting sacks of cement, bales of straw or tool boxes, reaching into the back seat of the car to get the bag of groceries, moving a box in the warehouse. It's in such everyday situations—at work or in the home—that most back injuries occur. Following this advice on how to lift properly will reduce chances of injury.

Good Biomechanical Position. Getting in good biomechanical position to lift something means getting your body in a position so the stresses of lifting fall along the lines most favorable to your skeletal-muscular structure. Lift so your body is in a position to get the best possible leverage, posture and balance, thereby minimizing strain.

Do's and Don'ts of Lifting

Do:

- Stand with feet shoulder width apart.
- Position your hands a little wider than shoulder width apart (if possible, depending on object lifted).
- Keep your head up (helps keep back straight).
- Bend knees and lift primarily with legs (saves back).
- Keep object close to body.
- Tighten stomach muscles as you lift (supports low back).
- Squeeze buttocks together as you lift (gets gluteal muscles into the act).
- Wear workboots with a heel lift (aids in balance) and a steel toe (prevents foot injuries).
- When lifting something from a height above your chest, limit yourself to a light load and/or stand on a sturdy platform to bring your shoulders to a height above the object.

Don't:

- Jerk as you lift.
- Lift with your back.
- Reach out as you lift.
- Twist either head or spine as you lift. If you must turn, turn with your feet, not your back.
- Try to lift more weights than you can handle. Test the weight by pushing against it before lifting it.

Lifting Light Objects. Follow the same "do's" and "don'ts" for lifting heavy objects, as above. Practicing good lifting techniques with light objects will help you train for the right way to lift heavy objects.

How to Lower Objects. Keep good form when lowering objects as this is when people often hurt their backs. Follow the same "do's" and "don'ts" for lifting. *Squat* when lowering a weight and keep your back straight, using your leg muscles, rather than back muscles.

Further Reading. An excellent book on the subject is *Maggie's Back Book* by Maggie Lettvin (Houghton Mifflin Company, New York, 1976).

When to Train. The best time to train is when there is available time, and this varies for different people. For example, I work fairly normal hours (9-5) and I train early in the morning. Others with the same hours find it easier to train *after* work in the evening. Train at a time that is most convenient for you, when there is the least chance of being interrupted, and when you can make it into a regular routine. If a shower is available, you might train at your lunch break. (Noon for 9-5'ers, 2:00 a.m. for 11-7 a.m. workers, etc.) This usually makes people more productive at work.

White-Collar Workers Program

- This is a very simple weight training program for people who spend most of their working days sitting at desks. This workout can be done in 30 minutes.
- In addition, it is very important for white collar workers to get some aerobic training, at least 30 minutes a day, 3 times a week.
- Try to do abdominal exercises 6 days a week, even on days when you do not train. As your abdominal muscles get stronger, increase the number of reps.
- *Days per week:* M-W-F or T-Th-Sat

exercises	sets	reps	exercises	sets	reps
1 p.190 middle	1	10 to 30	**4** p.202 bottom	1-2	10 to 15 per set ea. arm
2 p.198 bottom	1	10 to 30 ea. leg	**5** p.218 middle	1-2	10 to 15 per set
3 p.244 top	1-2	10 to 15 per set	**6** p.289 top	1-2	10 to 15 per set ea. leg

GETTING STRONGER ©1986 Bill Pearl & Shelter Publications, Inc.

Blue-Collar Workers Program

- This is a weight training program for people who must do some physical labor each day. It is designed to strengthen upper and lower body muscle groups and thereby help protect against the most common workers' injury: lower back pain.
- In addition, it is very important for blue collar workers to get some aerobic training, at least 30 minutes a day, 3 times a week.
- Try to do abdominal exercises 6 days a week, even on days when you do not train. As your abdominal muscles get stronger, increase the number of reps.
- *Days per week:* M-W-F or T-Th-Sat

exercises	sets	reps	exercises	sets	reps
1 p.191 top	1	10 to 20	**6** p.206 top	1-2	10 to 12 per set
2 p.194 top	1	15 to 25	**7** p.252 top	1-2	10 to 20 per set
3 p.193 bottom	1	15 to 30 ea. side	**8** p.225 middle	1-2	10 to 12 per set
4 p.248 top	1-2	10 to 12 per set	**9** p.288 top	1-2	10 to 15 per set
5 p.251 top	1-2	10 to 12 per set			

GETTING STRONGER ©1986 Bill Pearl & Shelter Publications, Inc.

Chin Up

A Lutheran minister had been training in my Sacramento gym for some time. He stayed on the same program, never changed the sets, or reps or weights, year after year. One day he came up to me. "Bill, I've been training here for ten years. Something must be wrong, because I'm not making any progress. I'm the same as I was ten years ago."

"Al," I said, "You started when you were 40 and now you're 50 and you're in the same shape?"

"Yes," replied Al, still disgruntled.

"That's wonderful," I told him, "In ten years you haven't lost any of your physique or any conditioning. You've turned back the clock ten years. That isn't progress?"

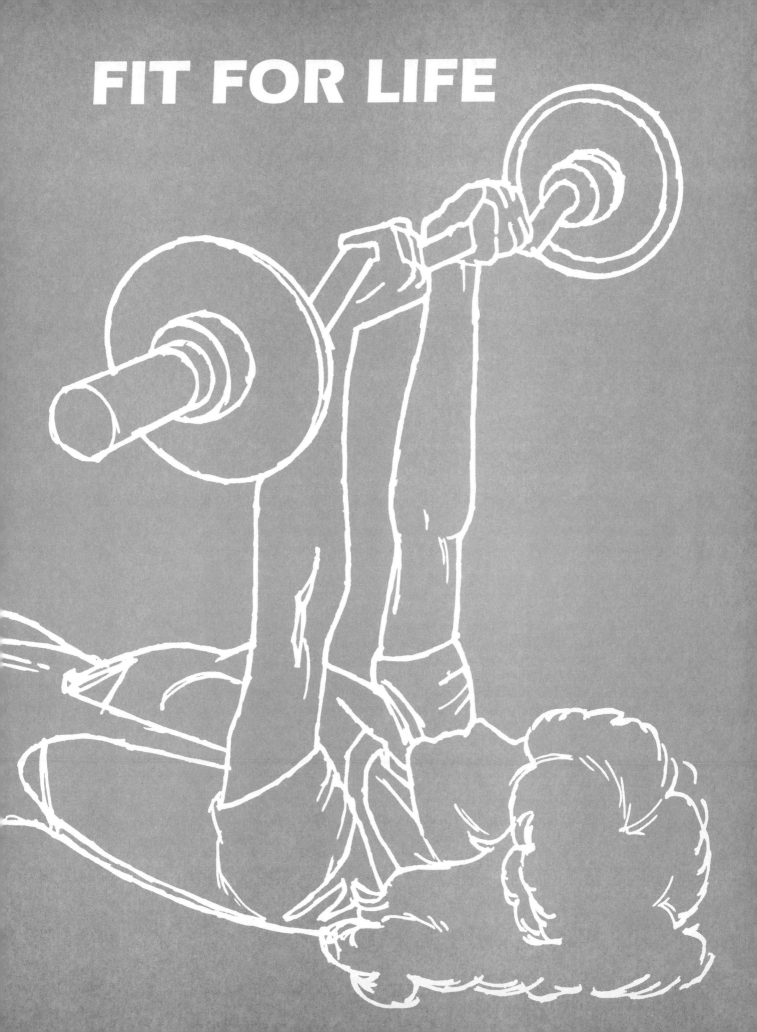

FIT FOR LIFE

SHOULD KIDS LIFT?

Parents often came into my gym in Pasadena with their sons or daughters and asked me to devise a weight training program. Their motives varied: they wanted their children to gain weight, have better posture, get stronger, gain self-assurance, or be able to defend themselves.

I'd first point out two major requirements:

1. Children should be mentally mature enough to know why they are training. Concentration is important, as is the reason for training—it has to be more than the parent's desire.
2. Children should be physically mature, beyond puberty. I instinctively felt that a child would not benefit from weight training prior to physical maturity.

The Importance of Team Sports

Then I'd lay out one other condition: that if I were going to train the children, they would also have to participate in team sports at school. Why? Because team sports help the child evolve as an individual and a member of a larger community. With weight training you don't really depend upon others—it's not a team effort. If children are already introverted, it may make them even more so.

But if they play basketball, soccer or another team sport, they'll have to get along with others and cooperate. They'll learn that the team is only as good as its worst player; this knowledge will carry over to other aspects of life. Then, when they get to an age where they can't find others to play basketball or baseball, they'll still have weight training as an excellent form of general conditioning.

Recent Findings on Children's Weight Training

My attitudes towards prepubescent weight training were based upon physicians' and physiologists' generally-held opinions then that children could not make strength gains because they lacked adequate levels of circulating testosterone. Weight training was considered dangerous for them.

Two studies conducted in 1985 and reported in the *The Physician and Sports Medicine* (February, 1986) cast a different light on that opinion. In one study, a test group which trained for 30 minutes three times a week exhibited a mean strength increase of 42.9% compared to the control group's 9.5% increase. In the other study, children showed significantly increased performances in high jumping and broad jumping after weight training.

The contention that weight training is dangerous for children is still, I believe, a valid one. Prepubescents should never engage in Olympic lifting or power lifting (these are competitive sports) and should always have qualified supervision for any kind of weight training. Many injuries have occurred when children are down in the basement, trying to outlift one another and going beyond their ability.

The National Strength Coaches Association (NSCA) has just published a position paper, *Prepubescent Strength Training*, that describes the risks and benefits and offers some guidelines for strength training. It is available for $2.00 from NSCA, Box 8140, Lincoln, NE 68501.

The American Orthopaedic Society for Sports Medicine (AOSSM) hosted a workshop in 1985 that included the American Academy of Pediatrics, American College of Sports Medicine, National Athletic Trainers Association, President's Council on Fitness and Sports, the U.S. Olympic Committee, the Society of Pediatric Orthopaedics and the

NSCA. The workshop group agreed that weight training is safe provided there are well-designed programs, instruction and supervision. They concluded that the benefits outweigh the risks and developed the following guidelines for prepubescent weight training:

Equipment:

1. Strength training equipment should be of appropriate design to accommodate the size and degree of maturity of the prepubescent.
2. It should be cost effective.
3. It should be safe, free of defects, and inspected frequently.

Program considerations:

1. A physical exam is mandatory before participation.
2. The child must have the emotional maturity to accept coaching and instruction.
3. There must be adequate supervision by coaches who are knowledgeable about strength training and the special problems of prepubescents.
4. Strength training should be a part of an overall comprehensive program designed to increase motor skills and fitness.
5. Strength training should be preceded by a warm-up period and followed by a cool-down.
6. Emphasis should be on dynamic concentric contractions.
7. All exercises should be carried through a full range of motion.
8. Competition is prohibited.
9. No maximum lift should ever be attempted.

Prescribed program:

1. Training is recommended two or three times a week for 20- to 30-minute periods.
2. No resistance should be applied until proper form is demonstrated. Six to 15 repetitions equal one set; one to three sets per exercise should be done.
3. Weight or resistance is increased in one to three pound increments after the prepubescent does 15 repetitions in good form.

Kids Are Not Small Adults

Even with these new findings by sports medicine experts, I still have a few reservations, especially if a child is participating in just one sport.

Children cannot take the same kind of stress as adults. Their bones are still growing, and a bone fracture can slow down or halt the growth of that bone or cause one limb to grow shorter than another.

When I went to high school, kids participated in many sports throughout the year—depending upon what sport was in season. These days there is much more specialization and often a child will train only for swimming, gymnastics, or basketball. What's wrong with this? By concentrating on just one activity, the stresses fall repeatedly on the same body parts. Stress fractures—small cracks in the bones that occur over a period of time—appear all too frequently among young athletes specializing in one sport. Little League pitchers may develop elbow problems, gymnasts may have lower back problems, runners knee problems.

I think children should be encouraged to participate in as many sports as possible. Specialized training, especially when backed up by weight training, is powerful stuff. Unless the child is self-motivated (as opposed to parent-motivated) and relatively mature, early specialization can lead to physical injuries, mental "burn-out" and less enjoyment and fun than is possible with a more well-rounded approach to sports.

Early Bloomer

Many of the qualifications and reservations outlined above disappear once a child has passed puberty. But chronological age is not always a reliable factor. Kids mature at different ages. I learned this in the early '70s when 11-year-old Dougie Brignoli walked into my Pasadena gym. Dougie was from South America, his mother was on welfare, and he knew exactly what he wanted to do and what I could do for him.

He didn't come in to see if I approved of him and would allow him to train. He asked me a host of questions to see if *he* approved of *me*. He put the shoe on the other foot! He wanted to know if I qualified as *his* trainer. I told him my background and he seemed satisfied that I was his man. He then told me—he didn't ask—that he would work Saturdays to pay for his training and that he would train each day after school.

I must tell you that I was highly amused—and somewhat touched. This little squirt—who was, by the way, mature for his age—had come in to interview me, a four-time Mr. Universe, and had decided to accept me. He was sincere and showed a drive and clarity of vision that few adults in my gym ever exhibited. And now he was outlining our working relationship.

As an adult I had to take charge of the conversation. "O.K., Dougie," I said, "I want you down here each Saturday morning to clean the gym. You'll earn your week's training in advance . . . ." I laid out a program and he had to train exactly as I said—no deviation from the program.

Dougie was with us for about eight years. He never missed a Saturday, and he went on to win the Mr. Teenage America in 1981 and later Mr. California. I guess part of my fondness for him was because he reminded me of myself at age 11. I had the same drive, but nowhere near the same level of confidence.

Every child is different. Every child has an individual level of desire, outlook on the future, willingness to work and emotional and physical maturity—and it's not necessarily a matter of age. You as an adult—parent, trainer or interested observer—must be careful to allow the child's inclinations, temperament, desires and abilities direct the course of his or her life, in sports or any other endeavor.

Parents Don't Make Good Training Partners

Sometimes a father would come into the gym and say he was going to train with his son. I'd stop him right there and say, "No, you can come in together, but you each have different ideas, goals and strengths. Since you're paying me as a trainer, I'll take care of each of you separately. You can encourage your boy, but not be the trainer."

Too many parents project their (sometimes unreasonable) demands on their children, who may or may not live up to these expectations. I've seen boys in tears as their dads tried to get them to push too much weight. My wife Judy used to run a gym and once had a mother and her daughter, who had learning disabilities, train there. The mother nagged the daughter all the time—criticizing, telling her she wasn't doing the exercises properly. But the girl was doing the best she could. The mother wasn't using proper form herself, yet she'd criticize the daughter for poor form. The daughter ended up crying.

Very often children will give up weight training from then on. They will have lost a valuable form of conditioning because of parents' pushing too hard.

Once a fellow brought his son into my gym. He had four children, and this one was ". . . the worst coordinated, does the poorest in school, is always in trouble and gives me more grief than all the other kids combined." The poor kid—Harold—had to stand there and listen to all this. He was about 17, skinny and kept staring at the ground. His dad went on about how he thought weight training would make him stronger and more coordinated and help him straighten out his life. He said he'd bring Harold down and watch him every day.

Not knowing as much then as I do now about fathers and sons, or mothers and daughters, I agreed. I started Harold on his program and his father came along to watch. The trouble started right away. If his son was supposed to do 10 reps with 110 pounds and he did only eight, his father would say, "You do two more or you can't drive the car." He'd harass Harold—the boy could never do anything right. This went on for a few months and then I saw the light. One day they came in and the father started right in on Harold. I invited the father into my office to talk.

"Look, I finally figured out what's wrong with Harold. It's *you* that's wrong with him. You're going to be lucky if you don't wake up one morning with an axe in your forehead. You've belittled this kid in every way possible in the last few months, you've done everything you could to alienate him and you still demand love and respect. There's no way he's going to respect you if you don't respect him, and without respect there can't be love. So I don't want you coming in with your son anymore."

The father was shocked. "You can't talk to me like that," he said. And he left in a huff. But a few weeks later Harold came back alone. "O.K., Harold," I said. "Let's get started." I set up a program and pushed him to improve, but didn't brow-beat or threaten him. Harold started making progress and as he did, it was wonderful to watch his self-confidence improve. He actually started looking people in the eye. He started to go out with girls for the first time. I'm certain none of this would have happened had his father continued coming into the gym with him.

Of course, this happens with parents and their children in all sports—Little League baseball, tennis, gymnastics, etc. As a parent, if you practice the gentle art of encouragement, it will allow the child's progress to come from within, to unfold at his or her own pace.□

GETTING OLDER

Push on—keep moving.
        —Thomas Morton, 1763-1830

The shock comes when I look closely in the mirror. A few more gray hairs, the small wrinkles around the eyes, the difference in the photos taken four years apart when I last renewed my driver's license.

Even though I'm often complimented on looking younger than my years, *I* know how old I am—56. I know it when I get out of bed early each morning and have to wait for my back muscles to loosen enough for me to stand erect. I know it when I see the difference between the way I feel inside (still age 18) and what the mirror reveals.

I think everyone past 40 knows what I mean, in one way or another. Forty seems to be a watershed, a turning point in life. It can take many forms: a mid-life crisis, a long-standing marriage ending in divorce, a mother whose children are raised starting a business career, a former champion athlete making a comeback, a second childhood. For many it may be a "last ditch stand" before old age sets in.

Doubtless a lot of this behavior is caused by hormonal or metabolic changes within our bodies, but another important contributing factor can be the feeling that life is passing us by, that there must be more out there than we are experiencing.

There are signs of aging, no matter what we do. Yet although the days and years inexorably pass—the *quantity,* so to speak—the *quality* of life from 40, 50 or 60 on is something over which we can exert considerable control. More and more people are discovering that the watershed of age "40" is more a cultural than a biological phenomenon.

In the 1800s, Victor Hugo said, "Forty is the old age of youth; fifty is the youth of old age." Now, in the latter part of the 1900s, this statement no longer seems true.

Age is No Crutch

The other day I was giving a talk on weight training at the opening of a new fitness store in Seattle. An obviously overweight man who looked to be about 50 jumped up and said, "Is there any hope for a guy like me?" "Sure there is," I replied. "As long as there's movement, there's hope."

These days I spend a fair amount of my time traveling and talking to various groups all over the country. Often older people will ask me questions like this. I feel they're hoping I'll tell them, "Yes, you've got to take it easy, you've got to back off because you're getting increasingly fragile." They want to start slowing down. It's as if there's a subconscious voice encouraging them to be more active, but another voice telling them they better back off from physical activity.

Creeping Rigor Mortis

Without movement there is no life. Many of the changes normally associated with aging actually come from "disuse." As we get older we tend to move less; Bob Anderson, author of *Stretching,* calls this syndrome "creeping rigor mortis."

About 15 years ago, Dr. Walter Bortz spent six weeks with his leg in a cast, the result of a skiing accident. When the cast was removed, Bortz, then 39, was shocked at the sight of the leg. "It was miserable, shriveled, discolored ... it was the leg of an old man."

This set Bortz off on an intensive study of the similarity between biological changes generally associated with aging and those that come from disuse. In a long article in the *Journal of the American Medical Association* in 1982, Bortz stated at the outset that he did not believe that physical inactivity was the *cause* of aging or that exercise would "halt the fall of grains of sand in the hourglass."

But he went on. "It is proposed, however, that the dimension of the aperture may be responsive to the toning influence of physical activity, and consequently the sands may drain more slowly. A physically active life may allow us to approach our true biological potential for longevity."

Bortz listed a number of physical changes such as loss of muscle tone, organ deterioration and osteoporosis that are almost indistinguishable whether caused by age or inactivity. He also hypothesized that exercise may well delay the onset of certain conditions generally associated with aging, such as heart disease or arthritis. If this is correct, he said, "at least a portion of the changes that are commonly attributed to aging is in reality caused by disuse and, as such, is subject to correction."

Looking Young

Whereas exercise in general is obviously desirable for people of all ages, weight training in particular may have certain advantages over other types of physical activity in keeping you young-looking. In a recent article on bodybuilding in *Sports Illustrated*, Terry Todd wrote:

> *Anyone who has spent much time in what is sometimes called the Iron Game has, of course, seen weight trainers over 40 whose physiques were . . . surprisingly youthful. Apparently there is something about the act of regularly stressing the body with heavy exercise that gives it the wherewithal to resist the visual manifestations of advancing age, which such sports as distance running, cycling or swimming, whose cardiovascular benefits are unquestioned, clearly do not. Consider the way aging ironfolk look, compared to, say, middle-aged runners, who sometimes appear to be older than their years. What else could account for the proud sweep of a veteran lifter's haunch—the first part of the body to slacken—compared to the dwindling thews of most men beyond 40, or even 30?*
>
> *The limited research in this area suggests that men and women of middle age will respond to systematic progressive resistance with weights by becoming more powerful and more flexible, with more endurance and less fat. The reasons why this is true are rather complicated, having to do with the body's biochemical goings-on following stressful exercise of this sort. Some of the studies indicate that one of the reasons workouts with weights cause middle-aged men to gain more power and muscular shape than workouts on the jogging track or handball court may be that the stress of progressive resistance weight training causes the body to produce more than the normal amount of the male hormone, testosterone, whereas the stress of the other exercises doesn't.*
>
> —Sports Illustrated, July 18, 1983

The Best Age to Start

I remember my father once saying, "When the day comes I can no longer make even the smallest changes for the better, that's the day I no longer care about living." My father is now 83 and still uses this as one of his daily golden rules. I think this attitude has been instilled in me, for I haven't given up or slowed down. I plan to keep exercising and watching my diet for the rest of my life.

These days, I see more and more people past 40 and 50 who look and act years younger because of a positive attitude, dietary consciousness and regular exercise. In fact, the middle years may be the *best* age to start an exercise program. Any increase in physical activity for a sedentary person generally produces remarkable and inspiring changes in vitality and spirit—more noticeable changes than during younger years.

Training Program for Those Over 50

As long as you are in reasonably good health, you can benefit from weight training. You needn't start out training like an 18-year-old world-class athlete or be intimidated by younger and/or more fit people. This is why there are 2-lb. dumbbells and 100-lb. dumbbells. You may have to start with the lightest weights, but if you stick with the program, you'll progress to heavier weights and start feeling much better.

If you are over 35, you should have an exercise stress test. Weight training raises the blood pressure (more so than running) and in a sense is more dangerous than endurance activities like swimming, cycling or running. (See the risk factor questionnaire on p. 72).

Once you have the green light from your doctor, start with the exercise program below. First read the chapters "Getting Started" and "Techniques of Lifting" on pp. 14-19. Recovery time for the muscles is especially important as you get older, so be sure to rest 1-2 days between workouts.

If you find you can do the exercises in this program with ease and want to move on to a different or a more strenuous program, look at the "General Conditioning" programs or the "Beginning Bodybuilding" or "Intermediate Bodybuilding" programs.

Over 50 Program

This is a beginning training program for men and women over 50. Be sure to have a physical and read the "Getting Started" and "Techniques of Lifting" chapters before starting this program. Once you are doing these exercises easily, you can elect to move on to any of the "General Conditioning" programs, the "Beginning Bodybuilding" or "Intermediate Bodybuilding" programs.

Days per week: 2 or 3, with 1-2 days rest between workouts. Do *not* skip rest days.

exercises	sets	reps	exercises	sets	reps
1 p.193 middle	1	10 to 25	6 p.272 top	1-2	10 to 12 per set ea. arm
2 p.190 middle	1	10 to 30	7 p.206 middle	1-2	10 to 12 per set
3 p.193 bottom	1	15 to 30 ea. side	8 p.300 top	1-2	10 to 12 per set
4 p.196 bottom	1	10 to 30	9 p.220 bottom	1-2	10 to 12 per set
5 p.244 top	1-2	10 to 12 per set	10 p.291 bottom	1-2	10 to 20 per set

HARDWARE

FREE WEIGHTS VS. MACHINES

"How do you train, Bill, with free weights or machines?" I am asked at almost every bodybuilding seminar I give. "I use both, but if I had to make the choice between the two I'd choose free weights." Why? Because free weights develop balance, coordination and a degree of strength not possible in training on machines. In this chapter we'll list the characteristics of free weights, then machines, and make a brief comparison.

Free Weights

Free weights are the most commonly used type of weightlifting equipment in the world. They are inexpensive, will last forever with no maintenance, take up very little floor space and are thus ideally suited for a home gym. For a few hundred dollars you can equip a home gym with enough equipment so you can get a complete workout for every muscle group in your body. Adequate Universal or Nautilus equipment for an equivalent work-out would cost many times as much and take up much more space.

Let's take a close look at the two major pieces of free weight equipment: barbells and dumbbells.

Barbells. A revolution in weight training came with the invention of the adjustable plate-loading barbell in the United States in 1902. Instead of having a different piece of equipment for each weight, one barbell could quickly be loaded with any amount of weight desired. This was a fantastic innovation that made weight training available to everyone. Like the combustible engine, the design has changed very little since its invention.

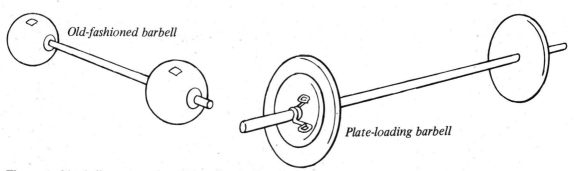

Old-fashioned barbell

Plate-loading barbell

The typical barbell consists of a solid steel or hollow bar, four to six feet long to which you attach flat metal or vinyl-covered concrete discs called plates, by means of collars. Most plates weigh 1¼, 2½, 5, 7½, 10, 12½, 15, 20, 25 or 50 pounds.

In the home gym, barbells are adjustable but in commercial gyms the plates are generally welded or bolted permanently in place. These fixed weights are provided in 5-10 pound increments from 20-150 pounds or more.

In any large commercial gym you will see a longer-than-usual barbell about seven feet long. This is an Olympic barbell. It is an expensive, specially machined, standardized barbell used in national and international competitive weightlifting contests. Olympic bars are also used to load the body with heavy poundages for such exercises as squats, bench presses and dead lifts. They can be loaded to 700 pounds or more, which is enough resistance to accommodate the strongest power lifters in the world.

The weight of Olympic barbells and plates is very precise. In most American gyms, the weights are in pounds and in most other countries of the world, in kilograms.

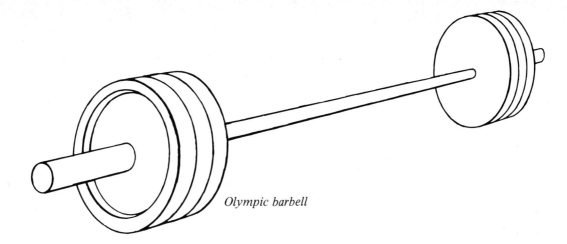

Olympic barbell

Weights of Olympic bars and plates

Pounds		Kilograms
45	Bar	20
5 each	Adjustable Collar	2½ each
2½,5,10 25,35,45	Plates	1¼,2½,5,7½, 10,15,20

Dumbbells. A dumbbell is a shorter version of a barbell—usually about 10-16" long. They are intended for use with one hand, using one or both arms at a time. Dumbbells can be used to exercise all of the major muscle groups of the body. In a home gym you will probably use adjustable dumbbells but in commercial gyms (and in a few serious home gyms) there will be sets of fixed dumbbells ranging from five to as much as 150 pounds.

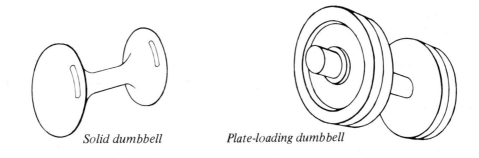

Solid dumbbell   *Plate-loading dumbbell*

Auxiliary Equipment

In any commercial gym there is a wide variety of stationary equipment used along with free weights. The most basic pieces of equipment are flat benches, incline benches, decline benches, and pullover benches. The main purpose of the stationary equipment is to allow you to change your body position so that you can work all the muscles from different angles with the barbells or dumbbells.

Traditional Machines

Some machines have been around for decades: the lat machine, quad pulley, leg extension machine, thigh biceps machine, seated rowing machine, etc. They differ from many of the newer machines in that they are simple, and they are isotonic, not isokinetic. (See pp. 63-64.)

The combination of free weights and these traditional machines make possible many hundreds of exercises. More Mr. Universe and Mr. Olympia physiques have been produced utilizing this type of equipment than any other.

Universal and Similar Type Machines

In the mid-'50s I purchased the first Universal machine to be used in a commercial gym—an eight-station machine I installed in my gym in Sacramento, California. Everyone loved it—from beginners to hardcore bodybuilders. Just prior to this, the UCLA athletic department had acquired several Universal multi-station machines and some of their athletes had been using them. The basic principles of these machines has changed very little in 30 years.

A multi-station Universal Gym machine has "stations" for exercising all the major muscle groups of your body. It is usually built of chrome-plated tubular steel pipe with an adjustable weight stack of 10 to 500 pounds, depending upon the body area to be worked. You can adjust the weight by placing a selector pin at the desired poundage. The weights cannot be removed from the machine so they won't get scattered or lost.

Advantages of the Universal

- The Universal is especially good in schools because up to 14 students can work on the machine at one time. Many of the top bodybuilders and athletes of the mid-'60s and '70s got their first taste of weight training by using a Universal machine at their school's P.E. department. For the number of functions it allows, the Universal is relatively inexpensive.
- Most modern health clubs, spas and gyms are equipped with Universal-type multi-station machines. They are an excellent way for a beginner to start weight training: the concept is simple to understand and the machine is easy to use. Once you become familiar with the machine, little or no supervision is required.
- The machines are safer than free weights in that there is no risk of plates slipping off bars and no risk of being pinned by the weights.
- You can move quickly from one exercise to another, thus making these machines ideal for circuit training.
- You can change weights rapidly (as with all weight-stack machines) by simply changing the pin placement.

Disadvantages of the Universal

- As with other exercise machines, you are limited to a narrow range of individual movements. At most, two or three movements can be done for each body part on a standard Universal without the use of additional benches, accessory handles, etc.
- You cannot work the body from numerous angles, as you can with free weights, since the resistance is on a track or rails.
- The cost is relatively high for the home gym.

Nautilus Machines

Nautilus machines evolved in the late '60s and early '70s and have become so popular that it is said that more money is spent on Nautilus equipment than on all other gym equipment combined.

The Nautilus and other isokinetic machines are said to exercise the muscles evenly throughout the complete range of motion, which free weights do not do. For example, when you do a barbell curl, resistance during the entire lift is not equal. There is a particular part of the lift that is your weakest point. This is called the "sticking point" and it is only at this point that you are getting maximal contraction. The Nautilus machines attempt to provide *accommodating resistance:* perfectly balanced resistance that is constant throughout the entire range of motion, from full stretch to complete contraction. Throughout the entire movement, the resistance is automatically adjusted by an off-center cam, with the aim of maximal resistance throughout.

When Arthur Jones first brought out his line of Nautilus machines, bodybuilders got extremely excited. *Iron Man* magazine was filled with articles and ads touting the advantages of the new machines over conventional weights. There's no better salesman in the world than Arthur. He is one of the most convincing and dynamic men I've ever known. Mike Mentzer, the 1978 Mr. Universe, writes in the forward of *The Nautilus Bodybuilding Book:*

> Arthur Jones is not a relaxing person to be with. He does not lightly exchange words. He spews facts, torrents of them, gleaned from his studies and perhaps more important, from practical application of theory, personal observations and incisive deduction. You don't converse with Arthur Jones, you attend his lectures. He is opinionated, challenging, intense and blunt. He knows more about the physiology of exercise than most people passing themselves off as physiologists at universities.

I could not agree with Mike more! Here's how I felt the influence of Arthur's super-salesmanship when I was training for the 1971 professional Mr. Universe contest: Over the phone Arthur convinced me that things had changed in bodybuilding and that the only way I could win the contest would be to follow his training principles along with the new Nautilus combination triceps-biceps machine and torso pullover machine. It mattered little to him that I'd done quite well with free weights for 25 years.

Arthur shipped me these two machines, free of charge. At the time I was running a gym in Pasadena, California, and I installed them in my living room rather than the gym. I used the machines exactly to Arthur's specifications for a few months but began feeling guilty about not sharing them with members of my health club. I then had them moved to the gym (with my wife's approval!), where they became so popular with the members it was nearly impossible for me to get near them.

Much of the promotional material in the early days of Nautilus was based on the claims that modern plate-loading barbells were obsolete, injury-causing antiques. It was also claimed that Nautilus training would produce top bodybuilders in a fraction of the time taken previously. Neither of these claims has proven to be true. Both methods of training have their advantages and disadvantages. There are so many people now training with weights, for such a variety of reasons, that both systems are used extensively.

Advantages of Nautilus Machines

Nautilus machines can produce some effects that are not possible with free weights:

- They theoretically provide variable resistance that is balanced to conform exactly to the normal strength curve of the working muscles.

- They provide resistance over a full range of motion for each muscle group.
- Because of these features you can get an intense workout quickly. You can make each set so intense that a muscle group can be thoroughly stimulated after only three or four sets.
- They are safer than free weights (they have stretching built into the movement), and you can't drop something on yourself.
- Many people are attracted by the shiny exotic look of Nautilus machines. They're *fun* and provide extra incentive to stick with a training routine.

Disadvantages of Nautilus Machines

- When you lift free weights you must provide the balance with your body. With Nautilus, the machine provides the balance and you don't develop the same tendon or ligament strength in joints.
- Nautilus machines work the muscles in isolation. Free weights involve many more muscles (and the accompanying balance of movement and muscle action).
- Nautilus machines do not teach coordination. By supporting the weights for you, they make things too simple. In providing balance and timing with free weights, you learn to coordinate body movements.
- Only two or three movements can be done for each body part. This can lead to boredom.
- The machines are expensive and take up a lot of space. Of course, this isn't a disadvantage to you if you're going to a gym that already has the machines.
- The Nautilus literature encourages you to train to failure on each set to get maximum training effect. But in most Nautilus studios, the owners do not have members train this way. They've probably found that even though training to failure theoretically produces the best results, the public won't buy it. It's just too painful a process for people who are not highly motivated.

Developing Sports Skills With Free Weights and Machines

There are two primary types of movement in sports: ballistic and tension.

- *Ballistic* — A movement initiated with maximal forceful contraction that continues on its own momentum or less force. Most sports involve ballistic movements (throwing, kicking, running, batting, etc.). Ballistic skills are best improved by isotonic exercises where you must exert the most force at the start of the exercise, such as lifting free weights.
- *Tension* — A movement where maximum force is applied throughout the movement. Wrestlers, football linemen and gymnasts use tension movements. Tension skills are best improved by isokinetic exercises, such as Nautilus, where you must exert maximal force throughout the movement.

Free Weights Are the Foundation of Any Weight Training Program

I believe that beginning weight lifters or bodybuilders should use free weights—barbells and dumbbells—as the best way to build a solid foundation. The exercises should be basic—bench presses, squats, military presses, stiff-legged dead lifts, overhead triceps curls, etc. As you enter the intermediate stage, machines will play a part, maybe an ever-increasing part. They can be used to work certain muscles specifically and this can improve proportion, balance and symmetry. Machines can help in fine-tuning, but *free weights are the fastest way to produce strength and muscle mass.* □

PICKING A GYM

There are four basic types of gyms:

1. Commercial bodybuilding and weightlifting gyms
2. Health clubs, Nautilus facilities or spas
3. School, University or YMCA weight rooms
4. Home gyms

Commercial Bodybuilding Gyms

Most commercial bodybuilding and weightlifting gyms are extremely well equipped with a large variety of free weights and specialized exercise equipment. Their business hours are usually long (10-17 hours on weekdays), and there are often instructors qualified to help you with bodybuilding. But if sports training is your objective, see the programs on pp. 81-175 for guidelines to strength training for various sports.

    If there are several gyms in your area, it's best to try a workout in each before deciding which one to join. You can check the yellow pages under gymnasiums and health clubs. At each gym check:

- Condition of equipment and cleanliness. If the place is dirty, in need of repair or the weights are scattered around the floor, beware. This means poor management.
- Type of people training there. Do they seem like people you'd like to spend time with? You'll be putting in a lot of hours there.
- Management/instructors. Tell them what you want to do, your goals. Are they helpful, knowledgeable?
- The emphasis of the gym. Is it compatible with your goals?

Health Clubs/Nautilus Facilities/Spas

Health clubs differ from bodybuilding gyms in that they have less exercise equipment and are generally set up more for people interested in general conditioning and socializing. Some of the bigger health clubs need the income from a lot of members to support high operating costs. Disadvantages can be overcrowding and lack of supervision; often the program given you is designed to get you through your workout in the shortest time. You can often spot these clubs by their hard-sell advertising. However, a club is a good place to start, and many are improving as the public becomes more knowledgeable about weight training. Most will let you come in for a few trial workouts and you can decide if the equipment, management, members and atmosphere are right for you.

    Spas have been popular in Europe for many years. They are often at fashionable hotels or resorts and generally include hot springs or mineral baths. Spas include a wide range of services designed to rejuvenate guests. In recent years the emphasis has shifted from being merely "fat farms" to providing a wider range of fitness activities, along with typical spa services. Many health clubs now offer spa services, such as massage, tanning beds, skin care salons, Jacuzzis, saunas, hydrotherapy pools, Swiss showers, herbal wraps, etc. but health clubs that have services like these generally do not have the serious weight training equipment that good commercial gyms have.

School, University or YMCA Weight Rooms

School or YMCA weight rooms vary widely. Many of the large universities have excellent facilities for training athletes. This is ideal if you are interested in either training for a specific sport or general conditioning. Also, school weight rooms are often lively and full of enthusiastic and energetic students—it can be catching!

One problem with many school and YMCA gyms though, is lack of respect for equipment. Often weights are scattered all over the floor and nothing is returned to its proper place. Equipment that is broken or needs replacing often has to wait until funds are available from the school budget. This can be frustrating when you are serious about your workouts.

YMCA gyms have made some big strides recently in order to compete with private gyms. Even though many of them still do not come up to the standards set by the private gyms, many have now acquired enough equipment for most people interested in general conditioning or bodybuilding. YMCA gyms are a good place to work out when travelling.

The Home Gym

The home gym can be as good a place to train as a commercial gym if you have the room, equipment and knowledge to train properly. I know of three Mr. Americas who came out of the same small one-car garage gym in Queens, New York: Tony Sansone, Joe Abbenda and Dennis Tinerino. Many champions got their start training at home, including Jack La Lanne.

There are several advantages to working out at home:

- You save time—no travelling to and from the gym, and no waiting for the equipment to be free.
- You can concentrate better. You're not distracted by overcrowded facilities or other people.
- You can work out any time of day or night.
- The whole family (and friends) can get involved.
- You can equip a home gym with free weights for the price of one machine. For example a Nautilus-type abdominal machine sells for about $500 and is designed for only a single movement. The same amount of money can buy you a good bench, with leg extension device and enough free weights to do several hundred movements.

One disadvantage to a home gym is staying motivated. Many people have a hard time staying with it when working out alone. A solution is to find a training partner: a family member, a friend, another athlete. I'd recommend, however, that you don't become *too* dependent on your partner. It can be a big disappointment if he or she drops out. The best way to avoid this is to set an exact time to start each session and to begin whether your partner shows up or not. Your partner will quickly realize how serious you are about training and will be more likely to show up on time.

Getting Equipped. You don't have to spend a lot of money, or wait until you have every piece of equipment you've ever dreamed of, to start your own gym. Watch the papers for good used equipment or shop at a local fitness store. You can also build, or have built, many of the benches and other apparatus you may need.

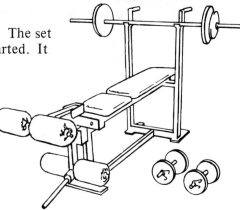

The Standard 110 lb. Barbell/Dumbbell Set: The set (along with a bench) is a great way to get started. It generally consists of:

- One 60" x 1" barbell bar
- Two 14" x 1" dumbbell bars
- Four 10 lb. plates
- Six 5 lb. plates
- Collars for barbell and dumbbells.

Bench with leg extension attachment and adjustable back; standard 110 Barbell/Dumbbell set with two extra 25 lb. plates.

In addition to this it's a good idea to also buy two 25 lb. plates.

There are deluxe versions and cheap versions. I'd advise you to get the best, as it will make your workouts more enjoyable. The plates with the machined holes are of higher quality than those with the cast holes. They slide on and off the bars smoothly and are a pleasure to handle. Chrome bars are the best and will last forever. I also recommend the chrome squeeze grip collars that make changing weights easy and quick.

Chrome squeeze grip collar

Advice in the Home Gym: This book should tell you all you need to know to get started. You can also go into a local gym for advice, or for a supervised training session. The gym manager can critique your form and offer tips on technique. If you train primarily at home, you might return to the gym every so often for some professional help. It may raise your spirits and boost your enthusiasm if you get low in motivation working out alone.

My bodybuilding career started at home and it looks like it will end at home, but the occasional workouts I get at different gyms help me stay up-to-date with the sport. Moreover, I enjoy the spirit and camaraderie of being around other people with similar interests and goals.

Rock Bottom Low Cost Home Gym Workouts. On the following two pages are workout programs specially designed for a home gym with a minimum amount of equipment. One program can be done with two dumbbells and a flat bench, the other with one barbell and a flat bench. You'll be amazed at the thorough workout you can get with the simplest set of free weights.

Home Gym Dumbbell Training Program

Two plate-loading dumbbells with a selection of plates and a flat bench are the only pieces of equipment needed for this training program. Use enough weight so that the last rep of each exercise is fairly difficult. Perform the exercises in the order shown. Do 1, 2 or 3 sets of each exercise, depending on how long and hard a workout you want.

Days per week: M-W-F or T-Th-Sat.

exercises		sets	reps	exercises		sets	reps
1 p. 193 middle		1	10 to 15	**9** p.300 top		1-3	10 to 12 per set
2 p.190 top		1	15 to 50	**10** p.302 bottom		1-3	10 to 12 per set
3 p.191 bottom		1	15 to 50 ea. side	**11** p.218 middle		1-3	10 to 12 per set
4 p.196 bottom		1	15 to 50	**12** p.218 top		1-3	10 to 12 per set
5 p.248 top		1-3	10 to 12 per set	**13** p.258 top		1-3	15 to 20 per set
6 p.250 top		1-3	10 to 12 per set	**14** p.290 bottom		1-3	10 per set ea. leg
7 p.204 middle		1-3	10 to 12 per set	**15** p.290 middle		1-3	10 per set ea. leg
8 p.275 bottom		1-3	10 to 12 per set	**16** p.236 middle		1-3	15 to 20 per set ea. leg

Home Gym Barbell Training Program

One plate-loading barbell with a selection of plates and a flat bench are the only pieces of equipment needed for this program. Use enough weight so that the last rep of each exercise is fairly difficult. Perform the exercises in the order shown. Do 1, 2 or 3 sets of each exercise, depending on how long and hard a workout you want.

Days per week: M-W-F or T-Th-Sat.

exercises		sets	reps	exercises		sets	reps
1 p.191 top		1	10 to 25	**9** p.205 top		1-3	10 to 12 per set
2 p.190 middle		1	15 to 50	**10** p.206 middle		1-3	10 to 12 per set
3 p.193 bottom		1	15 to 30 ea. side	**11** p.304 top		1-3	10 to 12 per set
4 p. 197 middle		1	10 to 50	**12** p.225 middle		1-3	10 to 12 per set
5 p.244 top		1-3	10 to 12 per set	**13** p.305 top		1-3	10 to 12 per set
6 p.277 middle		1-3	10 to 12 per set	**14** p.226 bottom		1-3	10 to 12 per set
7 p.251 bottom		1-3	10 to 12 per set	**15** p.287 bottom		1-3	10 to 12 per set
8 p.279 bottom		1-3	10 to 12 per set	**16** p.290 top		1-3	10 to 12 per set each leg

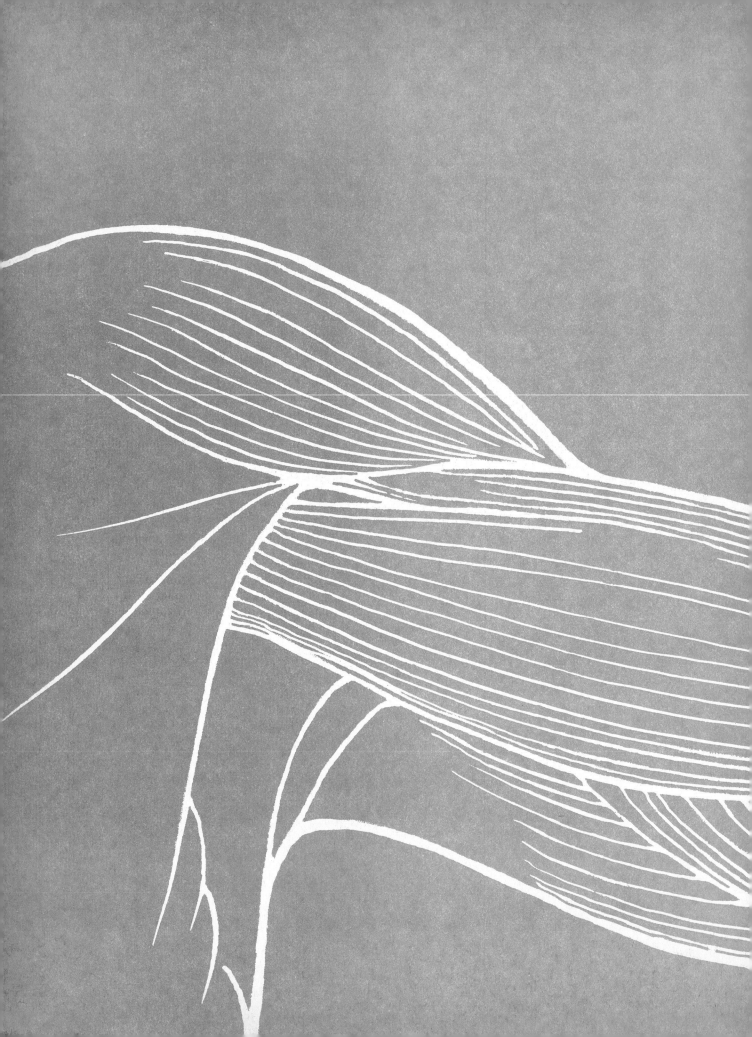

MUSCLES

MUSCLES

The human body is an incomparable instrument, a marvelous
mechanism, truly breathtaking in its intricacy.
                                    Henry G. Bieler, M.D.

The inner workings of the human body are so refined and complex that it is difficult for
the non-scientist to grasp the underlying principles. Yet a basic understanding of some
of the simpler principles can be useful to anyone who lifts weights. You will understand
more about the effectiveness of different training techniques and programs, how to
achieve your individual goals and what takes places *inside* your body that causes you
to get stronger and look better.

Here is a general description of the working systems of the human body:

- *Bones* are the framework of the body. The skeleton provides internal structure and
  in some body parts, such as the skull, external armor.
- *Muscles* control all movement in the human body, and make up 40-50% of the
  body's weight.
- *Connective tissue* of various types, including tendons and ligaments, connects muscles
  to bones and tethers and cushions organs and various body parts.
- The *brain and nervous system* initiate and guide all the body's activities.
- The *digestive system* changes food into energy.
- The *heart, blood vessels* and *lungs* provide oxygen and nutrients to the muscle and
  other cells to sustain them so they can perform their functions.

Of the six systems of the human body listed above, two of them—muscles and connective
tissue—are of most interest to the weight lifter. In this chapter we will explain just what
muscles, tendons and ligaments are, describe the "overload principle" that causes muscles
to grow larger and stronger and present a simplified explanation of what goes on inside
muscle cells when you lift weights. Later in the book we will describe weight training
techniques for developing strength and muscular endurance and for improving specific
body movements used in sports.

What follows is only a very simplified version of what goes on inside muscle cells. If
this interests you and you want to know more about muscle structure and function,
we recommend *Exercise Physiology—Human Bioenergetics and its Applications*, by
George A. Brooks and Thomas D. Fahey (John Wiley & Sons, New York, 1984).

Types of Muscle

There are three types of muscle tissue in the human body:

1. Smooth
2. Cardiac
3. Skeletal

- *Smooth muscle*, also called nonstriated, is found in the internal organs, for example
  in the intestine, stomach and in the walls of the blood vessels. They are involuntary
  muscles—not under conscious control.
- *Cardiac muscle* forms the main part of the heart wall.
- *Skeletal muscle* is the largest group of muscles; they are under conscious control. This
  is the type of muscle we will talk about in these pages.

Inside the Muscle Cells

All movements made by the body or within the body, whether voluntary or involuntary, are produced by muscles. Muscles are the flesh or "meat" of the body. (The meat on a chicken leg is muscle; a steak is a section of a steer's muscle.)

Skeletal muscle is composed of cells, but not the round amoeba or paramecium cells you may remember from your high school biology class. Muscle cells are in the form of *fibers*—long, cylindrical cells bound together by a membrane. In most muscles, the fibers run the entire length of the muscle.

The fibers are bound together by a membrane in *bundles*. To visualize a bundle of muscle fibers, think of a telephone cord (or a bridge cable) with bundles of wire running along inside.

The Architecture of Muscle

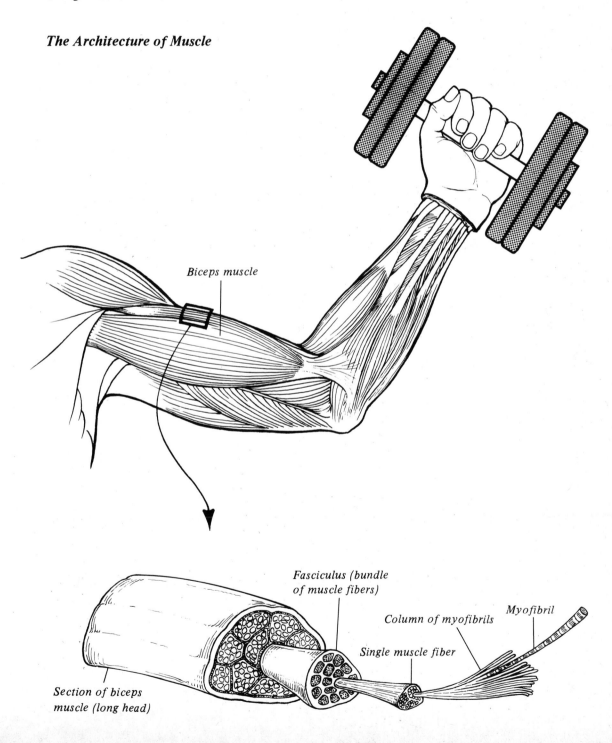

Biceps muscle

Fasciculus (bundle
of muscle fibers)

Column of myofibrils

Myofibril

Single muscle fiber

Section of biceps
muscle (long head)

Inside the muscle fibers are *myofibrils*. The myofibrils contract—shorten—when chemically stimulated by the nervous system. The myofibrils extend—lengthen—as soon as the nerve stimulus stops. *Muscle tone* is the gentle interplay of these forces—a slight yet constant contraction of the muscles. This ability to contract is unique among muscle cells—no other cells do this.

Just how does this contraction occur? Under an electron microscope, the myofibrils are shown to consist of thin and thick *myofilaments*. The thin myofilaments contain the protein *actin*, the thick myofilaments contain the protein *myosin*. When you decide to move a body part, for example your arm, a nerve impulse travels from your brain along the *motor nerve* circuit to the *motor end plate* attached to the fibers of the appropriate arm muscles. This causes a chemical and mechanical link to occur between the actin and myosin filaments. The two types of filaments then slide across one another, contracting (shortening) the muscle—as when you interlace your fingers and then slide them together.

What Happens Inside the Muscles with Weight Training?

1. The contracting elements—the actin and myosin myofilaments—increase in size (hypertrophy).
2. The myofibrils increase in size.
3. The motor nerves and the motor end plates that stimulate muscles may increase in number.
4. The amount of connective tissue within muscle cells may increase.
5. The amount of blood circulation to and through the muscles increases and the number of capillaries within the fiber may increase.

This is how muscles grow in response to the high intensity stress of weight training.

- The first four types of growth listed above—hypertrophy or increase in size—are associated with strength training: low repetitions, high weights.
- The fifth type of growth—vascularization or increase in blood supply and capillaries— is most enhanced by endurance training: high repetitions, low weights. *See pp. 59-61 for more details.*

Hyperplasia: Another possible result of weight training is an increase in the number of muscle fibers (cells), called *hyperplasia.* Some recent tests have shown fiber splitting (subdivision of the fibers to form new muscle cells) to occur in the fast-twitch fibers of cats and rats as a result of intensive training. However, other researchers have criticized the manner in which these studies were conducted and hypothesize that the split fibers could be damaged, not new, fibers. Also, there have as yet been no human tests that have demonstrated an increase in the number of muscle cells. Thus hyperplasia is an unresolved question right now.

Tendons and Ligaments

Tendons connect muscles to bones. They are made up of tough, cordlike tissue. They do not stretch and do not contract as do muscles. Their function is to respond to muscle contraction and pull the bones into action. Frederick C. Hatfield, in his *Complete Guide to Power Training*, describes tendons:

> *Picture a piece of raw steak. It has little white lines running through it, separating the muscle fibers into bundles. The connective tissue enclosing each bundle ultimately narrows down to form tendon, which joins muscle to bone. The force generated by the contracting muscle fibers is transmitted via the connective tissue and tendon to the skeleton, causing movement.*

Ligaments connect bone to bone. Like tendons, they are a tough, fibrous material. They prevent dislocation of bones and limit the range of motion.

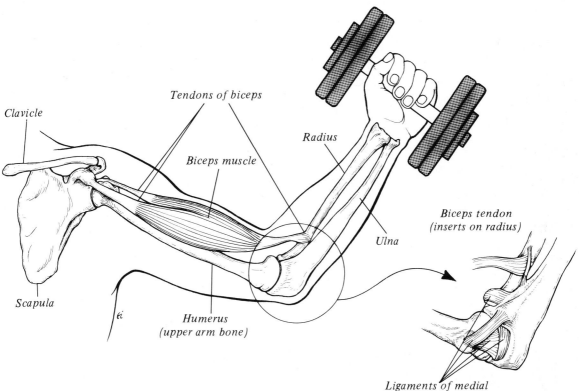

Clavicle

Tendons of biceps

Biceps muscle

Radius

Ulna

Scapula

Humerus
(upper arm bone)

Biceps tendon
(inserts on radius)

Ligaments of medial
aspect of elbow

One very important reason for an athlete or anyone training with weights to understand the difference between tendons and ligaments is in treating an injury. See "Injuries", pp. 365-72.

Why Muscles Get Bigger and Stronger

> *The human body is the magazine of inventions, the patent office, where are the models from which every hint is taken. All the tools and engines on earth are only extensions of its limbs and senses.*
>
> R.W. Emerson, 1870

In many ways the human body is a machine. To describe how it works, you could compare it to a car. The body uses food for fuel, as a car uses gas. Both have pumps, circulating liquids, cooling mechanisms, electrical systems, waste disposal systems, filters and joints. Both convert chemical energy to mechanical energy to provide power for movement through space. This is admittedly a simplistic analogy, and when you follow it through—though you can list many more similarities—you eventually get to the point where you run out of comparisons.

Then you ask the obvious (and exciting) question: Just what can the human body do that the machine cannot? First, obviously we have a brain which controls and directs our functions. And our bodies are made out of living tissue, which is continually changing, regenerating and *adapting* throughout our lifespan. It is this adaptation of living tissue to the different demands placed upon it that is the foundation of weight training.

Stress and Response

The word *stress* is generally considered to mean nervous tension, or "distress." Yet stress can be a positive as well as a negative force. In pioneering research done in the 1930s, Dr. Hans Selye developed his revolutionary concept of stress. In his book *The Stress of Life*, first published in 1956, Selye described a three-stage response to stress, the *general adaptation syndrome (GAS)*:

1. *Alarm:* When the body is stressed, it puts its defense mechanisms into gear—the "flight or fight" syndrome of an increased pulse rate, elevated blood sugar, redistribution of blood flow.
2. *Adaptation:* As the stress continues, many of the effects of the alarm stage are reversed and the body begins to build up its reserve, make repairs and increase its capacity to perform.
3. *Exhaustion:* If the stress continues too long, the body begins to break down. According to type, intensity and duration of the stress, this can result in either exhaustion, injury, disease or even death.

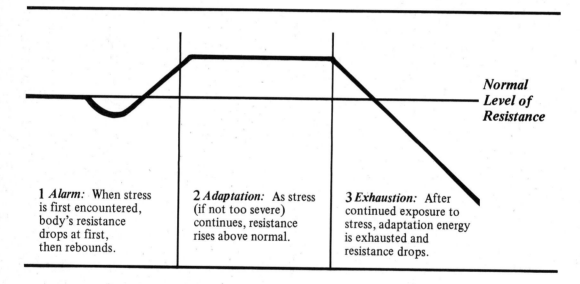

Normal Level of Resistance

1 *Alarm:* When stress is first encountered, body's resistance drops at first, then rebounds.

2 *Adaptation:* As stress (if not too severe) continues, resistance rises above normal.

3 *Exhaustion:* After continued exposure to stress, adaptation energy is exhausted and resistance drops.

The Overload Principle

What Selye calls stress, athletes call "overload." They know that *for gains in strength or endurance, you must overload the muscle.* This is probably the most important principle to understand in any sport, but especially in weight training.

To "overload" a muscle means simply that you stress the muscle in intensity or duration *beyond* the demands of previous activity. This is then followed by a rest period during which the muscle rebuilds with greater strength and endurance. The cells are programmed to rebuild stronger so they can handle greater stress the next time. The following table illustrates the principle:

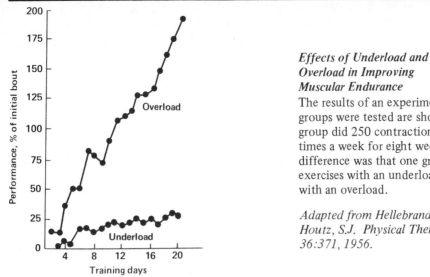

Effects of Underload and Overload in Improving Muscular Endurance

The results of an experiment in which two groups were tested are shown at left. Each group did 250 contractions a day, three times a week for eight weeks. The only difference was that one group did the exercises with an underload, the other with an overload.

Adapted from Hellebrandt, F.A. and Houtz, S.J. Physical Therapy Review, 36:371, 1956.

In overload training you progressively increase the amount of work performed.

- *For a gain in strength* increase the resistance (the weight).
- *For a gain in muscular endurance* increase repetitions and lower the resistance.

As your muscles adapt to the increased stress you must overload them even more for further gains.

In 300 B.C., Milo of Croton demonstrated this principle—now called *progressive resistance* training—by carrying a calf every day until it became a full grown bull.

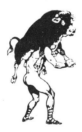

Physiological Benefits of Weight Training

Physiology is the science of essential life processes. With all the attention that has been focussed on health and fitness in recent years, scientists have come a long way in their understanding of the benefits of exercise. We now know that weight training can provide the following physiological benefits:

There will be an increase in:

- Muscular strength
- Muscular endurance
- Bone and ligament strength
- Cartilage thickness
- Capillary density in the muscles

- Muscle mass (hypertrophy)
- Stamina: longer duration of effort before exhaustion
- Flexibility
- Speed and power
- Blood volume and hemoglobin
- Muscle enzyme levels

There will be a decrease in:

- Body fat
- Stress and tension
- Resting heart rate

Additional Benefits of Weight Training

Weight training can also:

- Improve your overall health
- Make you feel better
- Help you to maintain your desired weight
- Make you look better
- Help prevent or rehabilitate injuries
- Improve coordination and balance
- Develop greater speed and stamina
- Improve circulation
- Improve elimination
- Help flush lactic acids and toxins out of your system
- Improve digestion □

INJURIES

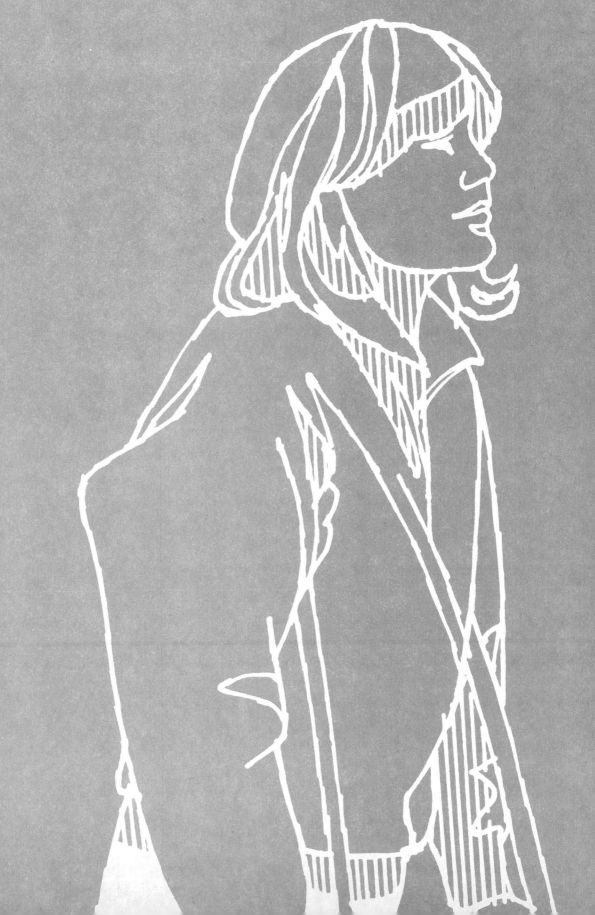

INJURIES

The single greatest cause of improvement is remaining injury-free.
Jeff Galloway
1972 Olympian
10,000 meter run

As the benefits of your weight training program quickly become apparent, you'll feel great. You'll want to do more—more reps with more weight. Beginners often try to do too much too soon, and find themselves getting injured. If you're injured, you can't work out. If you can't work out, you can't improve. That's a simple concept, and a very important one to remember.

Your muscles, tendons and ligaments need rest. An important equation is stress + rest = improved strength and muscular endurance. Rest is equally important to stress in this equation.

Muscles, Tendons, Ligaments

Muscle: A body tissue consisting of fibers that are organized into bands and bundles that contract (shorten) to cause bodily movement. Muscle fibers run in the same direction as the action they perform. Muscles have a large supply of blood circulating through them. This facilitates intake of oxygen and nutrients as well as removal of waste products. For this reason muscles recover, heal and repair relatively quickly.

Tendon: A band or cord of strong fibrous tissue that connects muscles to bones. Tendons are tough, do not stretch, and do not contract as do muscles. Many sports injuries are due to torn fibers in a tendon. There is very little blood flow in a tendon, so they can take a long time to heal.

Ligament: A strong, fibrous band of connecting tissue connecting two or more bones or cartilages or supporting a muscle, fascia or organ. Like tendons, ligaments have a poor blood supply and can be slow-healing.

Note: See the drawing that shows muscles, tendons and ligaments on p. 361.

Types of Lifting Injuries

The main types of lifting injuries are:

- Strains and sprains
- Tendinitis
- Bursitis
- Dislocations and fractures

Strains and Sprains. The most common lifting injuries are:

- *Strains:* stretch or tear of a muscle and/or tendon
- *Sprains:* stretch or tear of a ligament

Both strains and sprains are commonly caused by:

- Not warming up properly
- Twisting or jerking during the lift
- Lifting too much weight too fast or with too little rest
- Putting too much strain on an old injury before it has healed

Strains and sprains are grouped by degrees:

- *1st degree:* Tearing of a few fibers, mild tenderness, some swelling
- *2nd degree:* Partial disruption of the tissue, more tenderness and swelling
- *3rd degree:* Complete tearing of tissue, significant pain and swelling. Joint may be difficult to move or the torn muscle may exhibit a bulge.

Common strains in lifting:

- Chest and back muscles (shoulder girdle)
- Arm muscles (shoulder girdle)
- Hamstrings
- Quadriceps

Common sprains in lifting:

- Shoulder
- Knee
- Wrist
- Ankle

Tendinitis. This is an inflammation of the tendon caused by a tearing of some of its fibers. There is swelling and tenderness. It is usually caused by too many repetitions of the same lift. Tendinitis commonly occurs in the Achilles tendon, the patella tendon of the knee, tendons in the shoulder and elbow, and tendons in the wrist and hand.

Bursitis. *Bursitis* is an inflammation of the *bursa.* The bursa is a sac strategically located in or near a joint and containing a fluid that acts to reduce friction between tendons and bones or tendons and ligaments. Sometimes the bursa becomes inflamed and painful from abrasion or pinching. The shoulder is the most common site of bursitis for lifters. Other sites of bursitis are elbows, knees and hips.

Dislocation and Fractures. A *dislocation* is the displacement of a bone from its normal position in a joint. Dislocations most commonly occur in the shoulder, elbow, wrist, knee and vertebrae. In many sports these injuries are caused by a collision or fall, such as heavy contact in football or a fall in gymnastics.

In weight training, a dislocation can occur when there is misalignment of a body part during a lift, such as twisting the neck or back while lifting, or by a severe strain or sprain from lifting. Some people, because of their joint structure, are more vulnerable to dislocation than others. If you are in this category, make sure you have correct body position and when possible, have a spotter around to help.

A dislocation is usually quite painful; there is swelling and tissue damage and it is difficult or impossible to move the injured joint.

A *fracture* is a partial crack or complete break in the bone. Fractures are much less common in lifting than in some other sports, but once in awhile they do occur. The most common sites are the wrist and feet. Overhead lifts like the snatch or clean and jerk put stress on the wrist joint and can cause a crack or break. The other type of lifting-related fractures, sometimes called *fatigue fractures*, are hairline cracks in the bones of the feet. These usually produce tenderness and swelling and are often caused by repeated stress without enough rest in between.

Muscle Soreness. Temporary muscular soreness just after working out is thought to be caused by an excess accumulation of lactic acid in the tissues. This diminishes in one or two days as the lactic acid is carried away in the bloodstream.

Delayed muscle soreness—continuing three days or more after a workout—may be due to small micro-tears in the muscle tissues. This type of damage is an indicator that you should back off on your training program and exercise that body part lightly for several days.

Scar Tissue. This is a thick fibrous material that forms as part of the healing process of torn fibers of a muscle, tendon or ligament. Fibers of a muscle, tendon or ligament run in parallel lines, like telephone wires. When they tear, it would naturally be best for them to heal parallel again. But this often doesn't happen. In healing, the fibers not only rejoin end-to-end, but also stick to those running alongside them, sometimes "gluing" together fibers that are meant to operate independently. Muscles are sometimes "glued together" by adhesions, restricting movement. Scar tissue occurs more often in tendons and ligaments than in muscles and results from repeated, untreated and/or chronic tendinitis. With a chronic injury—an area that you hurt over and over—there is continual tearing and matting together of scar tissue: a vicious cycle.

Treatment of Injuries

If you work out regularly you will probably get injured now and then. But most injuries are minor and can be self-treated. The key is learning when to treat yourself and when to see a trainer, physical therapist or doctor. These questions can best be answered by being attentive to any symptoms and by learning to "listen to your body."

When to see the doctor (or athletic trainer, nurse practitioner, physical therapist):

- If pain is severe or continues
- If you cannot move the injured part
- If the injury does not seem to be healing

What to do when you're first injured:

R.I.C.E.

R = Rest
I = Ice
C = Compression
E = Elevation

Rest. With *severe* injuries—severe strains, sprains, bursitis, tendinitis or fractures—you must rest. Let your doctor be your guide.

If the injury is *not so severe*, however, complete rest may not be necessary. Within a few days after an injury, the tissues begin to repair themselves. Light exercise can speed recovery by increasing blood circulation. This brings blood and nutrients to the injured area and flushes away injury-produced wastes. Movement will help get the injured muscle functioning again and allow a quicker return to your sport.

Gary Moran, my co-author, has a Ph.D. in biomechanics and is one of the most knowledgeable people I know in treating sports injuries. Last year when Gary and I were together in San Francisco, a runner told Gary he'd been nursing along a groin injury for several months. When Gary learned that he had stopped running he said, "Look, there are two things you can do. First, you can stay idle; this won't irritate the injury but it will also probably take forever to get better. Or second, you can start some light activity and begin to strengthen the muscles that caused the injury in the first place." Gary gave the runner some specific exercises to do and he eventually credited his recovery to Gary's advice to "get active" rather than to "lay back."

The sooner you can use the muscles the sooner you will recover. Exercise increases blood circulation, rebuilds strength and improves flexibility. What type of exercise you do will depend upon the type of injury.

How do you judge the amount of activity? Listen to your pain. If the pain is severe or very sharp, stop exercising or moving the injured area. If the pain is tolerable, the movement will probably help the healing process. For more details on rehab exercises, see the next page.

Ice can work wonders, especially if applied right after the injury. Ice constricts the blood vessels and temporarily reduces blood flow to the injured area. Swelling is reduced so you can move the injured part with less pain. Movement is important to maintain flexibility and muscle tone in the newly-forming tissue.

Ice should be applied for 10 minutes on, 10 minutes off, three times. One of the best techniques is to freeze water in a styrofoam cup and then peel the styrofoam off as the ice melts (this keeps your fingers from freezing). Massage the ice on and around the injury. A very effective ice treatment is immersion of the injury in ice water. Some world-class runners treat leg injuries by sitting in a bathtub a foot deep in ice water. Some baseball pitchers immerse their elbows in ice after a game. (Buy a bag of ice at the liquor store.) Or wrap ice cubes in a washcloth and hold them over the injury. Or use a bag of frozen peas—it will conform to the joint.

Never use ice for more than 12-15 minutes at a time. If you notice any redness, stop the icing for a few minutes and try moving the injury or just resting it.

The on-again, off-again ice treatment stimulates blood flow and healing. Circulation is restricted when the ice is on, but when it's removed, blood flushes into the injured area and cleans out wastes.

Compression. Wrapping the injured part with an elastic bandage will compress the area and help reduce swelling. It does this by restricting the flow of fluid to the injured parts of your body. Be careful not to wrap too tightly and cut off the blood supply. It's best to have a broad rather than a narrow bandage. If the injured area becomes blue or numb, loosen the bandage.

Another method is to wrap an ice bag around the injured area with an elastic bandage. You may elevate the body part at the same time.

Elevation. Elevating the injured area also helps reduce swelling. Get the injured part higher than the next nearest joint so gravity can help drain away excess fluid. This, along with compression, can also help limit muscular bleeding. You may want to elevate the injury while sleeping. For example, if your knee is injured, sit (or sleep) with your leg propped up higher than your hip. If it's your elbow, get your elbow higher than your shoulder. If it's your wrist, put your arm in a sling with wrist higher than elbow. And so on.

Other Remedies

Heat. Although ice is the prevalent treatment for sports injuries, heat also has its place. For one, heat *feels* good. It also increases blood circulation to the area and aids healing. Heat should, however, only be used *when swelling has gone down.* It can be applied with hot water bottles, heating pads, hot baths or analgesic balm. A rule of thumb is to ice for one to two days, then apply heat if swelling is gone.

Aspirin reduces swelling and relieves pain. The main drawback is possible stomach irritation or (occasional) bleeding in the gastrointestinal tract. If aspirin upsets your stomach you can try buffered aspirin, such as Bufferin, or take it with milk. Non-aspirin pain relievers containing acetaminophen, such as Tylenol, can reduce pain but are not effective in reducing inflammation.

Cortisone, Butazone. These anti-inflammatory agents are prescription drugs and should be prescribed and administered by a physician. They are usually reserved for severe or chronic cases that do not respond to other treatments.

REHABILITATION OF INJURIES

Weight training can be used to speed recovery of injured muscles, tendons and ligaments. In all cases, you should wait until swelling has gone down and the injured part(s) can be moved through a full range of motion with little or no pain.

Muscle Injuries

Muscles, unlike tendons and ligaments, have a great deal of blood circulation. Thus light or medium to high repetition (10-15), low-weight exercise after swelling has subsided will speed recovery by coursing blood through the injured muscle, rebuilding tissue and flushing out wastes.

Rehab Program for Muscle Injuries. Go through a full range of motion with little or no weight. If you have pain, back off. Try to increase the range of motion each day. If there is little or tolerable pain and swelling has gone down, you are ready to start lifting.

1. *Weeks 1-2:* Do one to three sets of 15 reps with medium weights. Work toward increasing the weights.
2. After this you want to build muscle strength that was lost during the inactive/active period. *Remember!* It's not enough to merely rebuild to your former strength level. Your muscles were not strong enough then to prevent the injury. Now you must make those muscles stronger to prevent further injuries.
3. *Weeks 3-4:* Do three to six sets of 10 (8), 8 (6), 6 (4). Increase the weights to develop strength.
4. After this you can gradually return to your normal program.
5. *Note:* First you rebuild *strength,* then muscular endurance. See pp. 59-60.

Tendon and Ligament Injuries

Tendons and ligaments differ from muscle in that they are tough, fibrous, inelastic tissue with very little blood circulation and thus slower to heal. Tendons, the connective link between muscle and bone, produce some of the most common sports injuries. Tendon and ligament injuries usually consist of tears in the fibers and are accompanied by inflammation (i.e., *tendinitis*). With these injuries, doing many reps usually causes further irritation and should be avoided.

Rehab Program for Tendon or Ligament Injuries. After you can move the injured part through its full range of motion with little or no pain and swelling has gone down:

1. *Weeks 1-2:* Do one to three sets of 8-10 reps with medium weights. Do *not* strain. You should finish the set feeling you could have done another two or three reps.
2. There may be some swelling or tenderness. If it subsides before the next workout, continue with the exercises. If it does *not*, continue with reduced sets and weight once the swelling has gone down.
3. *Weeks 3-4:* Gradually increase amount of weight and number of sets. Do three to six sets of 10 (10), 8 (8), 6 (6). Continue these until there is little or no post-exercise swelling or soreness.
4. *Weeks 5-6:* Strength development stage. Do three to six sets of 10 (10), 8 (8), 6 (4). Increase weights to develop strength and increase effort to where you are working hard to reach the target number of reps for each set.
5. Back to normal: After six week of this rehabilitation, gradually return to your normal program.

PREVENTING INJURIES

I've had very few injuries over my many years of bodybuilding. I learned at an early age that to make progress in any sport, you've got to train consistently—and you cannot do that if you are injured. I've always realized that no one workout was going to take care of all my expectations, hopes and desires. I've always tried to leave a little bit left in the gym so I could come back the next day and pick it up. Hemingway, who used to get up at dawn to write, once said to an interviewer, "You write until you come to a place where you still have your juice and know what will happen next and you stop and try to live through until the next day when you hit it again."*

Many people work so hard in the gym they become exhausted—and that's often when injuries occur. Very often a lifter will hyperventilate during a tough workout. My son Phil was once in a gym and sat down on a bench next to a guy who had been going at it hot and heavy. "We were talking, facing the same way, and this guy started leaning forward, so I leaned with him. I kept leaning until I realized he was going to keep going. He fell flat on the floor. He'd fainted from exhaustion. We propped him up and he fainted again, so we called the paramedics."

Other people take on more than they can handle. Boots was a big, strong (and overweight) man who trained at my gym in Pasadena. He kept trying to get me to buy a set of 120-pound dumbbells (our heaviest were 100). I said, "Boots, if you can handle the 100s on a bent-arm lateral (see p. 248) I'll gladly get the 120s." Boots lay back on the bench and hoisted the 100s overhead at arms' length. He then let them down to the side of his chest. On his first rep he got them 2/3 of the way up, his elbows gave out and they fell back and hit him right in the face. He didn't break anything, but he was bruised for quite a while.

Most injuries are not this spectacular and will heal in time. In fact, if you're injured right now while reading this, try to realize that although it may seem like the end of the world, you *will* recover. Most athletes, when they are out of commission, think they will never recover, but find that with time, care and proper rehab exercises, recovery is possible.

Here, in case you are interested, is a list of injuries I've seen in the gym:

- Biceps muscles torn from insertion
- Pectoralis muscles torn from deltoid insertion
- Latissimus dorsi muscles torn from under upper armpit (insertion)
- Severe headaches caused by pushing head into the bench pad while doing exercises such as a bench press
- Inner thigh strain
- 11-12th ribs extremely tender—from exercises such as leg press with the knees so close they pressed into the chest area; a pain similar to pleurisy
- Stiff neck—one side of the trapezius tightening up caused by heavy overhead pressing
- Shin splints of the anterior edge of the tibia
- Shin splints of the forearms—usually caused by barbell curls or barbell-pullovers off bench
- Irritated sternum caused by pullovers or overhead pressing
- Dislocated vertebrae
- Dislocated shoulders
- Dislocated elbows
- Dislocated knees
- Rise in blood pressure causing headaches
- Hemorrhoids caused by heavy strain and leg work
- Broken blood vessels in the eyes, thighs and forearms, caused by heavy strain

*Writers at Work: The Paris Review Interviews, Second Series. Ed. George Plimpton, 1963, Penguin Books, New York.

To prevent injuries from occurring in the first place, here are some simple rules:

Warmup. A good warmup prepares the muscles, tendons and ligaments for action. It gets the blood circulating, raises body temperature and enhances flexibility of joints. Move each body part through the full range of motion, first without resistance, then with light resistance. (Many lifters use a light first set as a warmup.) Include some calisthenics and stretching as part of your warmup. Warming up is especially important in cold weather.

Lift Progressively. Start with a light weight and progressively add resistance with each set. Never start with your heaviest set first, as the muscles and tendons are not prepared for such sudden exertion.

Bill Starr in *The Strongest Shall Survive*, tells of the importance of starting light, even with champion athletes:

> *I was in the warm-up room that historic night in Columbus, Ohio, when the Russian super heavyweight, Alexeev became the first man to elevate 500 pounds overhead. The giant strongman warmed up with 135 pounds ... he wanted to make sure these ... muscles had a chance to be warmed up thoroughly before attempting a heavier poundage. If the procedure is good enough for the strongest man in the world, it should be good enough for all who train with weights.*

Positioning Yourself. Proper positioning is important in maintaining the correct alignment of the skeletal system and in positioning the exercised muscles for maximum force development. The instructions for each exercise include positioning details.

Muscle Balance. There are two types of muscle groups: the agonist and the antagonist (see p. 70). The agonist, or prime mover muscles are directly engaged in contraction— they make the body part move. The antagonist muscles have to relax at the same time the agonists are working. Ida Rolf, in her book *Rolfing*, writes the following:

> *All body movement is dual action. At any given moment in time, movement is the result of the action of paired muscles: the moving muscle (agonist) and its balancing mate (antagonist). It would be more realistic to look at these as cooperating rather than antagonistic units.*

When you bend your elbow, the biceps brachii is the agonist, the triceps the antagonist. When you work out you do not want to overdevelop one muscle to the detriment of the other. When the natural balance is disrupted by the overdevelopment of one muscle, the opposite muscle is often injured. □

NUTRITION

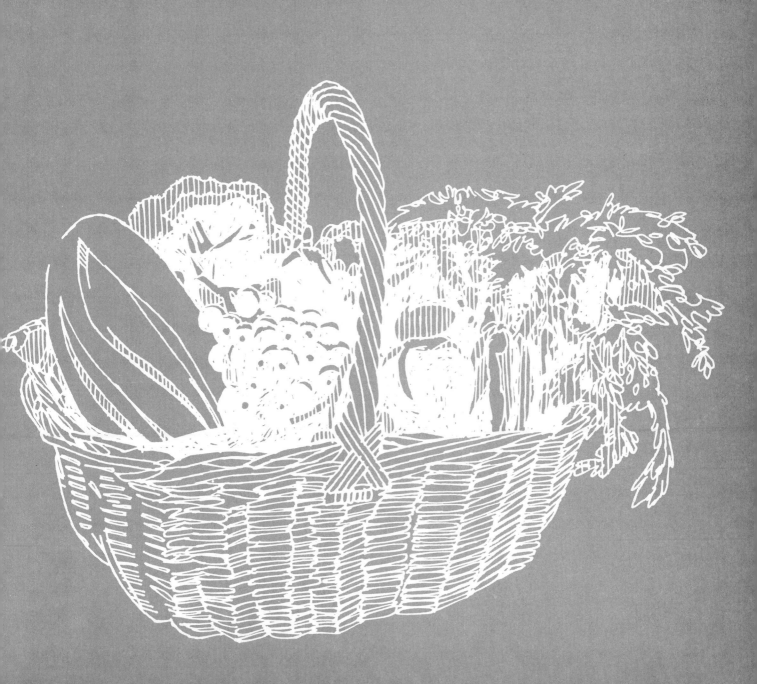

NUTRITION

It is not the horse that draws the cart, but the oats.
—Russian proverb

In the mid-'70s I often ate lunch at a Perry Boy's "all-you-can-eat" restaurant in Pasadena. Bob, a hardcore bodybuilder who worked out in my gym, used to eat there too. Bob believed that ingesting huge quantities of protein was necessary for muscle strength and bulk. In one session he would eat 15 minute steaks, 3-4 heaping platters of chicken, mounds of cottage cheese and a quart of ice cream. One day a girl came in who apparently felt the same way about starches that Bob did about protein. She took a large platter and proceeded to put a heaping mound—about a gallon—of mashed potatoes on it. Then she dug a hole in the middle and filled it with peas, corn and gravy. She sat down, pulled out a novel and commenced to eat and read.

"Bob," I said, "You guys ought to get together. You'd make a perfect couple." Bob wasn't amused. He'd been watching the mashed potato proceedings with no compassion at all and replied, "That makes me sick!"

The bodybuilding world is filled with tales of awesome food consumption. A good friend of mine has been known to eat 32 eggs a day. Bob, living in a glass house and throwing stones, thought the bizarre amount of protein he was consuming was necessary and justified since he was a serious bodybuilder.

I don't believe extremes like this are necessary (or healthy). You don't need a radical diet just because you are lifting weights. Eating a sensible, well-balanced diet and paying some attention to the latest developments in nutritional supplementation are the keys to good health and nutritional soundness, whatever your activities.

NUTRIENTS

Nutritional balance is the foundation of a healthy diet. The six essential components of the human diet are proteins, carbohydrates, fats, vitamins, minerals and water. These nutrients contain chemical substances that function in one or more of three ways:

- They furnish the body with heat and energy.
- They provide material for growth and repair of body tissues.
- They help regulate body processes.

No nutrient acts independently of the others. They must all be present for your body to function well. Everyone needs nutrients, but how much each person requires for good health depends upon physical condition, age, sex, size and amount of physical activity.

The Three Basic Fuels. The body burns three fuels for energy: proteins, carbohydrates and fats.

PROTEIN

Protein is essential for growth and maintenance of all body tissue. It is also the major source of building material for muscle, blood, skin, hair, nails and internal organs, including the heart and brain. Protein is also needed for formation of hormones, including testosterone, enzymes, substances necessary for basic life functions, and for antibodies, which help resist foreign substances in the body.

During digestion, protein is broken down into simpler units called *amino acids*. They are the units from which proteins are originally made and are the end products of protein digestion. Once broken down, the amino acids enter an amino acid "pool" where they are stored along with amino acids from previous meals. The body will then draw on this pool 24 hours a day when new protein is needed for tissue growth or repair.

Essential Amino Acids: The body needs approximately 22 amino acids to manufacture new protein. Thirteen of these can be manufactured in the body from almost any source of nitrogen. The nine that cannot be produced in the body are called the *essential* amino acids. They must come directly from what we eat. For the body to properly synthesize protein, all the essential amino acids must be present at the same time and in the proper proportion. If any one of these is missing, protein synthesis will fall to a very low level or cease completely. The result is that all the amino acids present are reduced in proportion to the amino acid that is low or missing.

Complete Protein: Protein in foods that contain all the essential amino acids is called *complete protein.* Protein contained in foods that lack or are low in any one of the essential amino acids is called *incomplete protein.* Meats and dairy products are complete protein foods. Starches (except soybeans), vegetables and fruits are incomplete protein foods.

To get complete protein from incomplete protein foods you must combine and balance foods to obtain the right proportion of amino acids. This is especially important for vegetarians. For example, a well-known combination of non-animal and incomplete proteins that forms complete protein is corn and beans—the staples of many South American countries. I won't go into detail here, but two excellent books on the subject of complementary proteins for non-meat meals are *Diet for a Small Planet* by Francis Moore Lappe (Ballentine, New York, 1975) and *Laurel's Kitchen* by Laurel Robertson, Carol Flinders and Bronwen Godfrey (Nilgiri Press, Petaluma, California, 1976).

Protein Deficiency: Too little protein may cause poor muscle tone, low energy levels, poor resistance to infection, slow recovery from wounds and weakening of the nails, hair and skin. A protein deficiency also makes it difficult to "bounce back" from a hard workout. If you suddenly shift to a diet extremely low in protein, your body will burn protein stored in less critical tissues (like the muscles) in order to protect vital organs like the heart and kidneys. During actual starvation, the protein tissues of the muscles are broken down and burned as fuel for the brain and central nervous system. People who have eaten meat all their lives and suddenly switch to a vegetarian diet often fail to get enough protein. It takes the body some time to switch over to synthesizing protein from grains and vegetables.

Another factor to be aware of is that it is not so much the *amount* of protein you take in, but the *type* protein that counts. You could actually be in a protein starved condition while consuming a fair quantity of protein if that protein was incomplete—if it did not have all the amino acids.

Protein Overload: In the '60s most bodybuilders I knew drank about two gallons of milk a day for extra protein. They would chug-a-lug a gallon while training in the gym. Most sedentary Americans get enough protein for building and repairing body tissue. Unlike fats or carbohydrates, protein cannot be stored as such. When you eat too much protein, excess nitrogen is passed out (as urea) in the urine (nitrogen is the element that distinguishes protein from carbohydrates and fats) and the rest is broken down for energy or stored as fat.

The main danger here is kidney overload. Your kidneys have to work double time to process the nitrogen from a protein-heavy diet. This is why people with kidney problems are put on a low-protein diet. Since kidney function decreases with age, it is increasingly important for older people to watch excessive protein intake. It is also important to drink plenty of water to help flush the kidneys.

It's a Complicated Question: Too much protein or too little—both extremes have their hazards. A further complication is that the RDAs (Recommended Dietary Allowances) for protein, as well as for other nutrients, may be based upon questionable testing techniques and therefore be unreliable. Whereas the National Academy of Science's Committee on Dietary Allowances recommends 0.59 grams of first class protein per kilogram of body weight, some nutritionists believe that over twice this amount is needed by people who train intensively. Over the years I've concluded that a good, simple guideline is to divide body weight by two, and the result will be the approximate number of grams of protein required each day. At the same time I am keeping an eye on the latest nutritional research, to see if new findings alter this formula.

CARBOHYDRATES

Carbohydrates are the primary fuel of the human machine. This largest of the food groups includes grains, bread, pasta, potatoes, vegetables and fruits. The smallest molecules of carbohydrates are sugars. There are three types of sugars:

- Single sugars *(monosaccharides):* found in honey and some fruits and vegetables.
- Double sugars *(disaccharides):* found in table sugar, maple syrup, milk and some fruits and vegetables.
- Complex carbohydrates *(polysaccharides):* These are chains of many single sugars linked together, such as in starches found in grains, legumes, vegetables and fruit.

Single sugars are easy to digest. Double sugars require some digestive action, but are not nearly as complex as the starches found in whole grains. Such complex carbohydrates require prolonged enzymatic action to break down into single sugars for digestion.

Once the digestive process has broken carbohydrates into single sugars, they are transported by the bloodstream to the liver, where they are converted to *glucose*—"blood sugar." Most of this glucose is then carried by the bloodstream to provide energy for the muscles and brain. A small amount of it is converted to *glycogen* and stored in the muscles and liver. Any excess glucose is converted to fat, which is stored throughout the body as a reserve source of energy. Glycogen is the single most important fuel for endurance athletes because it is the most readily available energy source.

A diet deficient in carbohydrates rapidly depletes glycogen and makes any kind of physical activity difficult. When you feel fatigue after prolonged exercise, it is often due to low blood sugar and/or depleted glycogen stores. A low-carbohydrate diet, a "liquid protein" diet or water fasts make vigorous exercise extremely difficult. The major dietary change to make when you start exercising is to increase complex carbohydrate intake.

FATS

In a recent interview, *New York Times* health consultant Jane Brody contended that our eating patterns are ". . . upside down and inside out. There's far too much emphasis on animal foods laden with calories and fats, with too little emphasis on foods that were eaten by the evolving human species before processing was invented."*

There are two types of fat: body fat and dietary fat. Body fat can be made by the body even if you eat no dietary fat. It can be made out of excess protein or carbohydrates and stored as energy—to be used when needed.

Dietary fat—that which we ingest—is the most concentrated source of energy in the diet. When oxidized, dietary fat provides more than twice the calories per gram as those furnished by carbohydrates or protein.

San Francisco Chronicle, November 21, 1985

We need fats in our diet. They act as carriers for fat-soluble vitamins such as A, D, E and K. They surround, protect and hold in place the kidneys, heart and liver. Body heat is preserved by a layer of fat.

Dietary fat may be "invisible," such as fat on a steak, butter or creamy dressings. Or it can be less obvious: the butter or oil used in baking cookies or cakes, the oil in avocado or nuts.

More than 40% of the calories in the average American diet comes from fat. While some fat is necessary, the high amount of fat in American diets is now recognized as a leading factor in heart disease. One to two tablespoons of unsaturated vegetable oil daily are said to be nutritionally sufficient.

Fat storage in the body averages about 15% for males and 25% for females. Most of this fat is available for energy, especially during moderate, prolonged exercise. Excess nutrients are readily converted to fat for storage. Fat is thus the major storehouse of excess energy. As with carbohydrates, usage of fat as a fuel "spares" protein for its critical role in tissue synthesis and repair.

Nathan Pritikin has probably been the foremost proponent of a low-fat diet. Although his earlier books were too strict for many people, his current book, *The Pritikin Promise,* is a more moderate approach to reducing fats in the diet. It contains some good low-fat ideas, such as substituting apple juice for most of the oil in salad dressings, making pancakes, muffins or corn bread with no egg yolks and no oil or making "mock sour cream" out of low-fat cottage cheese and low-fat buttermilk.

The Pre-Game Meal

In the not-so-recent past, the traditional football team's Friday night dinner was a protein extravaganza: steak, eggs, milk, ice cream, etc. The thinking in those days was that you needed the meat and other high-protein foods for power and aggressiveness on the field the next day. While the players undoubtedly enjoyed such a high-protein (and high fat) treat, it has more lately been recognized that a pre-game or pre-event meal high in complex carbohydrates is a better approach to optimizing performance. For one thing, carbohydrates are digested and absorbed more rapidly than either proteins or fats; they are converted into energy faster. Further, digesting and assimilating a high-protein meal increases the body's metabolic rate considerably. This generates heat that puts a strain on the body's heat dissipating mechanisms and can impair performance in hot weather. At the same time, the conversion of protein to energy promotes dehydration during exercise, since the by-products of protein breakdown utilize large amounts of water for urinary excretion.

Another good reason for the pre-game meal being predominantly carbohydrates is that this is the nutrient that assures a normal level of blood glucose and enough glycogen "fuel" for endurance activities—provided that the athlete has followed a nutritionally sound diet throughout training.

VITAMINS, MINERALS & WATER

In addition to protein, fats and carbohydrates, the other three essential components of the human diet are vitamins, minerals and water.

In the early '50s my gym in Sacramento was across the street from a veterinarian supply store that sold medicine and supplements for livestock. One day a new Cadillac with an expensive horse trailer pulled up in front of the store. Inside the Cadillac was a fat farmer puffing on a cigar and inside the trailer were two beautiful chestnut horses that looked like they could run in the Kentucky Derby. The farmer went into the store and came out with what looked like $200 worth of supplements for his horses. I remember thinking that he'd be a lot better off if he fed the cigar to the horses and took the supplements himself. Apparently he didn't care about his *own* physical health, but he cared enough to do right by his horses.

As time passed and as I watched the farmers come and go, I started thinking that if these supplements were good enough for these big muscular horses, maybe they'd be good enough for me and my bodybuilding. I finally crossed the street and met the vet and we became friends. Remember, this was in the '50s and health food stores and knowledge about vitamins and supplements (for humans) was practically non-existent.

I started by buying gallons of liquid multi-vitamins for horses and unrefined wheat germ oil, and using them daily. That's how I first started taking vitamins and supplements. (Not too scientific!) I then started reading more about nutrition and eventually decided it would be better to get nutritional products formulated for humans. In 1953 I opened a small health food store in my gym. I sold vitamins, minerals, blackstrap molasses, fertile eggs, local honey and home-baked bread.

Vitamins

Vitamins are essential for life. They are organic food substances, but cannot be made by the body. Each of the 20-odd known vitamins are present in varying quantities in specific foods, and each is essential for growth and health. Their most important role is in acting as catalysts for the processing of proteins, carbohydrates and fats.

The three fuels—protein, carbohydrates and fats—are merely the raw materials for energy production. Vitamins allow the biochemical reactions to take place that convert food into energy and assist in forming bone and tissue. Unlike hormones, vitamins cannot be manufactured inside the body—they must come from what we ingest. Each vitamin has a specific task that no other substance can accomplish, and the absence of all or part of a single vitamin can disrupt biochemical reactions.

Minerals

Minerals comprise about 4-5% of our body weight. All bodily tissues and our internal fluids contain varying amounts of minerals. Minerals are constituents of bones, teeth, soft tissue, muscle, blood and nerve cells. They are important in strengthening bones, maintaining physiological processes and acting as catalysts for a variety of vital functions within the body. Minerals regulate blood and tissue fluid and help maintain the proper acid/alkaline ratio. They also help draw chemicals in and out of the cells and aid in the formation of antibodies.

Minerals in the body are classified as either *macrominerals*—those occurring in large quantities and having known biological functions—and *trace minerals*, those present in minute quantities. The macrominerals are calcium, phosphorus, magnesium, sodium, chloride and potassium. The trace minerals are iron, zinc, iodine, manganese, copper, selenium, molybdenum, chromium and flourine. Most all of these minerals occur freely in nature, mainly in rivers, lakes and the ocean. They are found in the root systems of plants and trees and in the body structure of animals who eat the plants and drink the water.

Water

Water is the most essential ingredient that we consume. You can go far longer without food than you can without water. Water is needed for:

- Digestion
- Absorption
- Circulation
- Excretion
- Transporting nutrients through the body
- Maintaining normal temperature
- Healthy functioning of every living cell

The average adult's body contains about 11 gallons of water. About 50% of our body weight is water. Picture 11 gallon jugs standing side by side and you get an idea of the tremendous quantity of water we carry around all the time. An average adult loses about three quarts each day through perspiration, although environmental conditions and level of physical activity can alter this amount.

Sweating. Vigorous physical activity produces heavy sweating. Evaporation of sweat on the skin is the body's cooling mechanism. In high humidity, this cooling process is seriously hindered. When humidity is 100%, the air is completely saturated with water vapor and evaporation of liquid from the skin into the air is impossible. In humid conditions sweat beads on the skin and rolls off. On dry days evaporation of water from the skin is rapid, and body temperature is more easily regulated.

How Much Water Should You Drink? Most people would benefit from drinking more water. This is especially important if you are undertaking a new exercise program. Since your body loses water throughout the day, it is best to take it in gradually. Small portions of 6-8 ounces are assimilated more easily than larger ones. Try to drink a glass every hour if you're working out hard and/or the day is hot.

The only pure water is distilled water. It is found in nature in the form of rain water and in all fruits and vegetables. (However, rain water may be contaminated by atmospheric pollutants it picks up on its way to the ground.) Artificially distilled water is pure, but all minerals have been removed, along with the impurities, in the distillation process. Many people who drink distilled water take a mineral supplement to insure adequate mineral intake.

In addition to loss of water, those who regularly sweat profusely (such as endurance athletes) must be concerned with loss of *electrolytes.* Electrolytes are ionized salts in the blood, tissue fluids and cells including sodium, potassium and chlorine. If they are depleted, along with water in heavy sweating, certain metabolic functions, as well as transmission of neural signals can be impaired. A few years back, there was a rash of electrolyte replacement drinks for athletes on the market, but in many of these the ratio of electrolytes was off (too much sodium, for example, without adequate potassium, calcium, magnesium, etc.).

THE CASE FOR NUTRITIONAL SUPPLEMENTATION

As we discussed earlier, it is only in comparatively recent times that humans have not had to work physically hard to survive—foraging, hunting, farming, building. This has only changed in the last 100 years or so. These days, with machinery, technology and specialization, little physical labor is needed to produce the necessities of life. If we want food we jump into a car and drive to the market. Or we can go to a restaurant where we not only buy food, but have it prepared for us as well. Shelter is bought or rented, seldom built by inhabitants. Most jobs no longer require arm or leg power, but involve hours of sitting and inactivity each day. One result of this inactive lifestyle is a reduction of food intake. The need is just not there.

Today the intake for middle-aged American women is about 1500 calories a day, for middle-aged American men about 2200 calories a day. This low level of energy exchange has reduced the intake of nutrients so much that many people are not getting the recommended daily averages from the four basic food groups. This is obviously a problem for people who are dieting, those who are too poor to afford good nutrition or for those whose lifestyle is sedentary and must cut down on food intake to avoid obesity. Conversely, other people take in adequate or excess calories, but of the wrong kind of food.

Many nutritionists today claim that a "well-balanced diet," with servings from the four major food groups (1. fruits and vegetables; 2. cereals and grains; 3. chicken, fish, meat, beans; 4. dairy products) will ensure nutritional adequacy. Moreover, it is commonly argued that people who engage in regular, strenuous physical activity burn enough calories so they consume more food—and contained in that extra food are more vitamins, minerals and other elements necessary for good nutrition.

Not so, say others—most notably, Dr. Michael Colgan of the Colgan Institute of Nutritional Science in La Jolla, California. Even if you knew enough to choose a well-balanced diet, says Colgan, these factors and variables in modern day life probably insure that you are *not* getting the vitamins and minerals you need for optimum health:

• Crops are often grown in soil that has been depleted of minerals.
• In processing, storage and cooking, food may lose much of its value.
• Insecticides are often used in the soil and sprayed on foods.
• Modern life is stressful.
• Our air and water often contain pollutants.

In addition, there are startling variations in the vitamin content of common foods. In his book *Your Personal Vitamin Profile* (William Morrow and Co., Inc., 1982), Colgan gives various examples. Some oranges bought from a local supermarket contained no vitamin C at all, probably from being stored a long time, yet "... they looked, smelled and tasted perfectly normal." Other oranges, bought direct from the grower and picked the same day, contained a healthy 180 mg of vitamin C per orange. Similar discrepancies existed in other foods tested. Raw carrots showed a variation of 70 to 18,500 international units of vitamin A and pro-vitamin A per 100 grams.

What Does All This Mean? For one thing, that it has become increasingly difficult in these times to know if your nutritional needs are being met by the foods you eat. For another, if the recommended dietary allowances (RDAs) commonly accepted for years turn out to be wrong, we may see an overhaul of many long-held nutritional concepts in coming years. *This problem is compounded for physically active people, who probably need more nutrients than sedentary people.*

What Can You Do? Whatever your level of activity, you naturally want to be sure you are getting the right quantity and quality of food and nutrients for good health and optimum performance. The ideal solution—and one that will become increasingly available in coming years—will be to have an intelligent professional who is up-to-date on current research analyze your individual background, present biochemical and other conditions, and future needs and prescribe a diet along with supplements (vitamins and minerals) to achieve your nutritional goals.

If you do *not* know of a nutritional consultant you trust, the next best approach, I believe, especially if you are an athlete, is to take a daily combination of vitamins and minerals to help correct any possible deficiencies and hopefully to assist in proper functioning of the body's biomechanical reactions. Here is a list of these elements. *Please note:* Since everyone differs (in age, weight, activities, genetics, environment, eating habits, etc.) this obviously applies only to the mythical "average person."

Vitamin A . . . . .15,000 IU[1]	Vitamin E . . . . .500 IU
or Beta Carotene[2] . . . . . . .15 to 25,000 IU	Calcium . . . . .1000-1600 mg
Vitamin B 1 (thiamine) . . . . .110 mg[3]	Magnesium . . . . .400 mg
Vitamin B 2 (riboflavin) . . . . .110 mg	Phosphorus . . . . .500 mg
Vitamin B 3 (niacinamide) . . . . . . .125 mg	Iron . . . . 18 mg
(niacin) . . . . 25 mg	Copper . . . . .1000 mcg
B 5 (pantothenic acid) . . . . .100 mg	Molybdenum . . . . .100 mcg
B 6 (pyridoxine) . . . . .175 mg	Manganese . . . . 10 mg
B 12 (cyanocobalamin) . . . . . . .200 mcg[4]	Zinc . . . . 25 mg
Folic Acid . . . . .400 mcg	Chromium (GTF) . . . . .200 mcg
Biotin .300 mcg	Silenium . . . . .100 mcg
Choline . . . . .200 mg	Nickel . . . . .50 mcg
Inositol . . . . .150 mg	Vanadium . . . . .75 mcg
PABA (para-amino-benzoic acid) . . .100 mg	Iodine . . . . .150 mcg
Vitamin C . . . . .1000 mg	Potassium . . . . 99 mg
Vitamin D . . . . .300 IU	

[1] IU = International Units
[2] Take either Vitamin A or Beta Carotene, *not* both.
[3] mg = milligrams
[4] mcg = micrograms

NATURAL FOODS

In the last 10 years, the words *natural* and *organic* have been greatly overused and often misused. Yet if anyone asks me what I eat, I reply "natural foods" and might further add, "organic when possible."

Natural foods are those grown without toxic fertilizers or pesticides and which have not been altered by processing or refining. Here are examples of natural foods:

- Wheat grown in fertile soil rich in humus, fertilized with compost and naturally occurring minerals. It is not refined or made into white flour but eaten in the form of whole grain bread or other whole wheat dishes. Such grains are rich in proteins, vitamins, minerals and enzymes. By contrast, white flour has neither the germ and its beneficial oil nor the bran and its essential fiber.
- Natural fertile eggs, laid by hens living outdoors, enjoying fresh air, sunshine, mating with roosters and eating their own share of natural foods—insects, grass, seeds and minerals. Supermarket eggs are produced in egg "factories" by chickens who never see the sun, green grass or a rooster and are confined in square-foot cages. They are fed medicated grain and produce sterile eggs that will not hatch a chick. Such eggs have an altered chemical balance and a lower vitamin content than natural eggs.

- Certified raw milk which provides a very high grade of protein that is easy to absorb (for most people). Pasteurization, in destroying any possible pathogenic bacteria, unfortunately also destroys many vitamins and makes some of the proteins and minerals harder or impossible to absorb.
- Natural cheese (not processed) without added coloring, such as Swiss, Longhorn, Danish or cheddar.
- Organic fruits and vegetables, eaten raw when possible.

More than 90% of the foods most Americans eat today have been tampered with in one way or another. Many of the important nutrients present in natural whole foods have been removed or destroyed. White sugar, white bread, processed cereals, and canned foods are generally devitalized and denatured. (In order to prolong shelf life, the most vital elements of foods are often removed or altered.) Most oils are extracted with high heat or chemical solvents.

The consumption of fresh fruits and vegetables has declined one-third since 1930. At the same time we consume 25 billion dollars worth of baked goods, soda pop, white flour products, confections and other non-nutritive, empty calories that can produce nothing but diminished vitality and disease.

TEN SIMPLE RULES

Here are ten basic rules of nutrition for optimum health:

1. Eat foods that are as natural as possible: whole, unrefined and unadulterated.
2. Eat some raw or "living" foods. If cooking is required, cook as little as possible to preserve enzymes and other nutrients.
3. Eat food that is as "poison-free" as possible. Chemicals in your food, water and air harm your health.
4. Follow a "high-in-complex-carbohydrate, low-in-high-fat-animal-protein" diet. The proteins from grains, vegetables, eggs and milk are as valuable as meat protein when combined correctly.
5. Don't take megadoses of vitamins or minerals.
6. Drink plenty of water.
7. Eat as little fat as possible.
8. Relax during and after eating.
9. Don't be too rigid, whatever your diet. Once in a while, have that piece of cake or ice cream cone, so you're not continually craving a treat. Give yourself a break!
10. Try to stop eating before you are completely full.

> *If thou rise with an appetite, thou are sure never to sit down without one.*
>
> —William Penn, 1693

A VEGETARIAN BODYBUILDER?

At age 39, I was a three-time Mr. Universe winner lying on the couch in my living room, having a hard time clenching my fists and wondering what other medication I could take for the pain in my elbow and knee joints. I also had high blood pressure, high cholesterol and high uric acid. For some time, these problems had been interfering with my weight training, making it hard for me to train the 2-3 hours a day necessary to keep up the image I felt was expected of me in the bodybuilding world.

At the time I was working for Rockwell International in Los Angeles as a physical training consultant for their top executives. Because of this connection I also trained some of the American astronauts, who naturally had to be in good condition for the rigors of their training. For years I'd been eating lots of meat, cheese and dairy products. When my cholesterol read out at 309 (plus high triglycerides), the doctor hired by Rockwell said, "Bill, you could easily drop dead on us. What do you think that would do for the space program?" I then went to my own doctor and he advised me to change my eating habits. He didn't say to give up meat, he just said to cut back on animal fats and sugar.

It took this kind of scare to make me realize what I was doing. You generally think it will happen to the other guy and not yourself, but I realized I was just as vulnerable as anyone. Just because I was Mr. Universe and had a 19" arm didn't mean that I was healthy.

I took things a step further than the doctor's recommendation. My wife Judy and I first gave up red meat, but continued eating chicken and fish. Then one night at a fried chicken take-out place I cracked open a piece of chicken and saw a large growth on the joints. When I found out that this was due to the female hormones they feed the chickens to make them grow faster, I decided I didn't want excess female hormones floating around in my system, so Judy and I gave up chicken.

Then, when we were down to fish as our only animal flesh, the mercury scare came along and we gave up fish as well. Here I was a bodybuilder, expected to eat pounds of meat weekly to build muscle and I'd become a vegetarian. What would I eat? How would I get the protein, nutrients and energy I needed to train and compete?

I replaced the meat with fertile eggs, fresh fruits and vegetables, fresh raw nuts and seeds, whole grains, brown rice, baked potatoes and low-fat dairy products such as cottage cheese, unprocessed cheese, yogurt and kefir. Slowly, I noticed a change in how I felt and how I acted.

With each succeeding year on the diet—it's called lacto-ovo-vegetarianism—I've felt better. I'm more healthy, I can train with more energy, and I'm not as much of a "hard guy" as I used to be. I've become more concerned with my fellow man and the other inhabitants I share the earth with.

Judy and I have now been vegetarians for almost 20 years. We have no fish, fowl or red meat in our diet. Yet I can still carry the same amount of muscle mass at age 56 as I did in winning my four Mr. Universe titles.

People can't believe it. They think that to have big muscles you have to eat meat— it's a persistent and recurring myth. But take it from me, there's nothing magic about eating meat that's going to make you a champion bodybuilder. Anything you can find in a piece of meat, you can find in other foods as well.

What is a Vegetarian?

A vegetarian is someone who, for whatever reasons, does not eat animal, fowl or fish flesh and sometimes other animal products like milk, cheese or eggs. Vegetarians generally eat all other foods, including grains, legumes, vegetables, fruits, nuts and seeds. There are three types of vegetarians:

- *Lacto-ovo-vegetarians*—This is what Judy and I are. We eat all foods associated with vegetarianism plus dairy products and eggs.
- *Lacto-vegetarians*—vegetarian foods plus dairy products, but no eggs.
- *Vegans*—pure vegetarians—eat only plant foods and no animal products whatsoever.

What are the Advantages of a Vegetarian Diet?

- It (usually) contains less fat. A large amount of fat in the diet, especially animal fat, is a known factor in heart disease. Among other diseases and illnesses thought to be at least partially caused by a high-fat diet are breast and colon cancer.

- It contains more complex carbohydrates and fiber (roughage). A diet low in fat and high in starches and fiber helps protect against heart disease and cancer.
- There is less exposure to unnecessary toxins and poisons. Over 200 man-made substances, including antibiotics, growth hormones and other drugs, are allowed in the feed and water of livestock. Animal flesh contains these in concentrated dosages. It also contains pesticides from food they eat. All this is passed along to the consumer.
- It uses less resources. As Frances Moore Lappe has pointed out in *Diet for a Small Planet,* it takes 16 pounds of grain and soybeans to produce just one pound of beef. To produce marbled fat (the texture and flavor desired in beef), feedlot cattle eat a great deal of grain in the last few weeks of their lives. If the demand for meat went down, there would be surplus grain and soybeans available for feeding the poorer countries of the world.

Will I Get Enough Protein?

Protein is important to all living creatures. It is the main source of building materials for your organs, heart, cells, tissues and muscles.

Meat is a unique form of protein, in that it is "complete:" it provides all the amino acids needed for protein synthesis. But by combining different foods to provide all the amino acids, a vegetarian can definitely get enough protein. A glass of milk with a meal usually does the trick, or a serving of beans and rice. For more information about amino acids in a vegetarian diet, see *Diet for a Small Planet* and *Laurel's Kitchen.*

It is often said that all the essential amino acids must be consumed in one meal to properly synthesize protein. This is not true. The body stores the acids and uses them as needed. As long as they are in your digestive tract at the same time, the acids will combine effectively.

Can you get enough protein without meat? Yes! A well-balanced (non-meat) diet can provide adequate protein; even without trying you will often get the right combination of amino acids. Many foods that go naturally with one another are protein-complimentary: beans and corn, bread and milk, or sesame seeds and garbanzo beans.

What About Vitamin B 12?

Vitamin B 12 is the one nutrient that an all-plant or vegan diet does not include. B 12 is essential for the functioning of most body cells and prolonged deficiency can cause anemia or eventual damage to the central nervous system. Sometimes a B 12 deficiency does not show up for several years after one has switched to a vegan diet. This is because the body can store enough of it to last for 3-5 years or even longer.

Meat and fish are good sources of B 12, but for vegetarians, dairy products, except for butter, are the most concentrated sources. *Laurel's Kitchen* recommends two glasses of milk or one glass of milk and an egg daily for adequate B 12. For vegans they recommend a B 12 supplement, and implore, "Please don't court a B 12 deficiency."

Will I Get Enough Calcium?

Calcium is easier to get in a vegetarian diet than B 12. It is important for bones, teeth, transmission of nerve impulses, the heart and other muscles. You probably know that dairy products are rich in calcium. It is also contained in dark green leafy vegetables, cabbage, cauliflower, carob, seaweed and almonds. Calcium is relatively difficult to absorb. Typical calcium supplements are amino acid chelates (the most easily assimilated), calcium lactate, bone meal, calcium carbonate and dolomite.

Calcium is most easily absorbed if there is an equal amount of phosphorus in the diet. The calcium/phosphorus proportion in milk is just about perfect. However, a diet rich in phosphorus will slow down the body's absorption of calcium. Since meat is high in phosphorus, meat eaters are at a disadvantage.

Surviving the Changeover

It took some adjusting for me to settle into a vegetarian diet. It takes a long time for the enzymes to switch over. For months I felt hungry and would eat huge tubs of salad to satisfy the craving. For most people, the sensible route is to first give up red meat but still have chicken and fish—this will make the transition easier.

A good way to start is to get a few good vegetarian cookbooks. For any questions you have about vitamins, minerals, food combinations or minimum daily requirements, see the back section of *Laurel's Kitchen* or *Jane Brody's Nutrition Book.* For some delicious vegetarian recipes, see Mollie Katzen's *The Enchanted Broccoli Forest.* You'll find that a meat-free diet can be full of delicious and satisfying food. The variety of recipes may surprise you and the ease of preparing vegetarian dishes will please you. And there's one final bonus to the vegetarian diet—no greasy pots!

Do I recommend a vegetarian diet for everyone? Yes and no. Yes, if you are motivated to start with, and do some homework and research before jumping in head first. No, if you don't begin with a firm conviction of why you want to make the change and adequate knowledge of what's involved. It's all too easy to slip back into your old habits the first time it becomes an inconvenience and chalk it up as another failure along with losing weight, or exercising regularly.

To be successful with such an important change in your lifestyle you have to stick with it and not make exceptions. In order for a vegetarian diet to pay dividends it must be practiced regularly. As wonderful as your body is, as phenomenal as its recuperative powers are, you still must take enough time to correct the abuses caused by poor eating habits.

I look at my vegetarian diet as money in a savings account, drawing interest. Each year the interest payments are higher. I see no reason to start drawing off these interest payments *now* when there may come a time later in my life when this reserve will be needed to pull me through a major illness so I can continue to make every day of my life happy and productive.

Full Circle

Whereas 10 to 20 years ago most bodybuilders and weight lifters overdid protein in general and red meat in particular, more recent research and common knowledge has reversed the trend. Most bodybuilders I know today are knowledgeable about keeping body fat low and the dangers of protein overload. I know very few bodybuilders who eat more than a small amount of red meat weekly. In fact, since people know I'm a vegetarian I get calls and letters from bodybuilders—about once a day—for information on how to eliminate red meat from their diets. It's a changing world! □

There's More to Life Than Fitness

The main purpose of this book is to help you to become stronger, more physically fit and to improve your appearance. But I hope that the same attitude, the same desire for improvement will carry over into other parts of your life as well. Physical fitness is only a portion of your total life.

Large muscles, strength or achievement in sports will not bring you lasting success or respectability. It's important to understand that along with success will come attention and the higher your profile, the more important it is to treat others with kindness and respect.

I have trained a number of bodybuilding champions over the years and I have talked to every one of them about "conduct becoming a champion," as follows:

- Always try to give more than you receive. This attitude alone will make you a champion in your own right.
- Keep an eye open for helping people out. Lend a hand if anyone needs it or gets into trouble.
- Remember the people who helped you along the way. Try to share your wealth and success with them. Let them know how you appreciate their help.
- There are things in life more important than your physique or sports ability. In time these things will diminish but your ability to get along with others and earn their respect is important as long as you live.

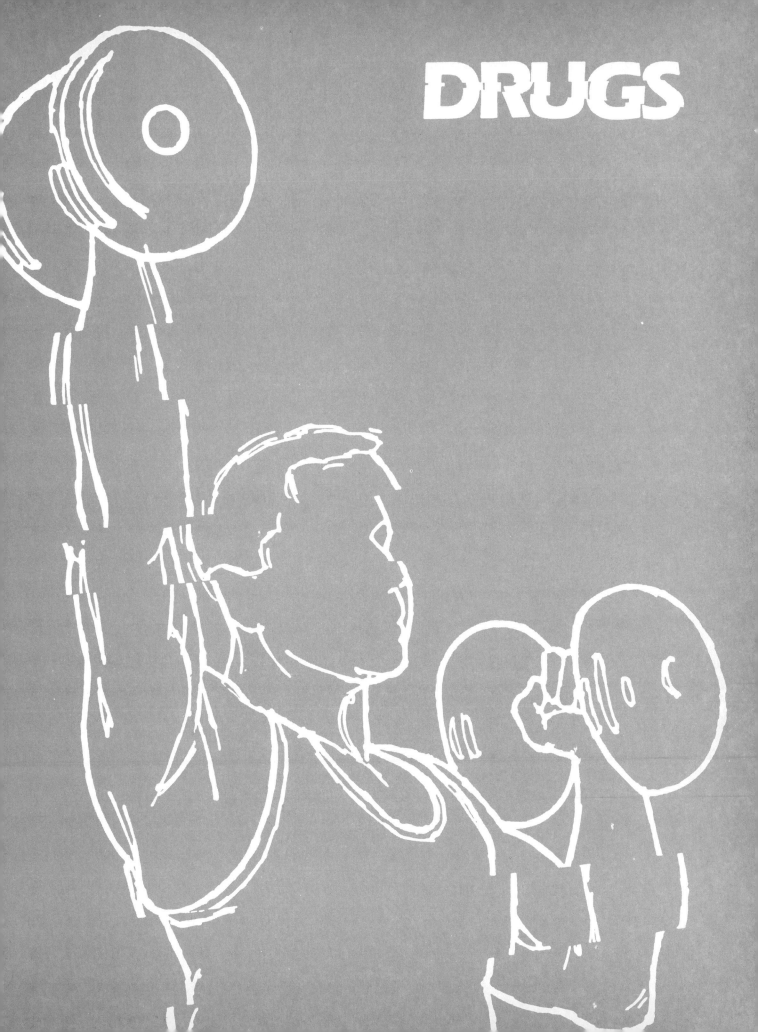

DRUGS

DRUGS

*The strongest people—the strongest athletes—in the world are
all using steroids. They're being used not only in the strength
field, but also in track and field and swimming. So you've got
to be on drugs if you want to survive.*

Steve Courson, 6'1", 285 pounds,
Offensive guard, Tampa Bay Buccaneers*

No subject is more controversial in sports today than the use of drugs for gains in strength
and size. Two hostile camps with diametrically opposing views are fighting it out:

1. Athletes who use anabolic steroids and other "growth" drugs for gains in strength,
   trainers and a few doctors who see the drugs as a means to improved power and
   performance, necessary in today's competitive sports world.
2. Athletes, medical people, officials, sports watchers and concerned citizens who
   are increasingly alarmed about the dangers and long-term health risks, ethical
   considerations and often the alleged uselessness (placebo effect) of steroids and
   related drugs.

These are two extreme positions. The users and advocates deplore the outcry, the
warnings and the accusations. The critics and researchers publish articles, call for tests
of athletes and advocate an outright ban.

At this stage in my career I don't find myself in total agreement with either camp. I
don't agree with the alarmists that every athlete who uses the drugs will suffer irreversible
damage or that the drugs have only a placebo effect. Likewise (or conversely), I don't
agree with the users and coaches who feel the drugs are absolutely necessary and are
certain there can be no damaging side effects. It's a very confusing subject.

Why is this an issue for readers of this book? Because steroid usage is more closely
associated with weight training than with any other athletic activity. Drugs are often
used along with weights to gain muscle mass, either for strength (in sports) or for size
(in bodybuilding).

Further, the use of steroids and related drugs is no longer an issue only for professional athletes and bodybuilders:

*I suppose there are some sports that don't have any drug
problems, but most do—professional and amateurs, from
high school age on up.*

Dr. Irving Dardik, Chairman
U.S. Olympic Committee on Sports Medicine

College players are using them. A surprising number of non-competitive bodybuilders
are using them. These days many of the hardcore women bodybuilders use the drugs.
They have the potential of affecting an increasingly broad spectrum of ages and sports,
so it behooves anyone lifting weights to know something about them.

Many champion bodybuilders and top athletes take steroids under medical supervision
(or with a strength coach's advice). They will stay on a cycle—on for a certain period,
then off. Most of the serious abuse comes from would-be athletes who get them on the
black market and go by hearsay.

*Sports Illustrated, May 11, 1984

Why Do Athletes Use Steroids?

They work. I won't try to tell you they don't. The idea in sports today is to win, to be number one. Everyone wants to be able to stand on the winner's platform with arms raised in victory. There's much less glory in being number two or number five. If you knew about some pills that could take you from number five to number one, wouldn't you be tempted? Athletes see drug-taking as a way to reach their goals—earning a living as a professional athlete, making the college football team or becoming a champion.

My first experience with steroids was in 1958. I had won the Mr. America and Mr. Universe contests and was in Florida making a movie with Arthur Jones, a thoroughly unorthodox and eccentric friend (who would later revolutionize weightlifting with the invention of the Nautilus machines). Arthur told me about a new chemical the Russian weight lifters were using. When I returned to California I did some research.

At the University of California at Davis I met a veterinarian who told me that steroids were being used with good results to develop strength and growth in cattle. The name of the drug was Nilivar and the daily recommended dosage for humans was 10 mg.

Now it might seem extreme for someone with no more information than that to begin using the drug, but that's what I did. Good enough for a bull, good enough for me! It never even occurred to me that there could be anything harmful in the drug or any side effects. I took dosages of 30 mg. a day for three months while training very hard. My weight jumped from 225 to 250 and my strength increased considerably. For example, I could squat with over 600 pounds—my best ever. I'd never experienced so much progress in so short a time, and I knew this was no placebo effect.

But there were problems. I felt heavy and awkward and actually couldn't bend over to tie my shoes. I had always felt limber and flexible, but now I was the proverbial "muscle-bound" bodybuilder. I decided I looked and felt better at a lighter body weight and quit using steroids.

Two years later I decided to enter the 1961 Mr. Universe contest. By then, steroids were out of the experimental stage and well-known to most competitive bodybuilders. They were no longer an underground item. I remembered the fast progress I'd made using them and decided to do so again. Looking back, I think they were a crutch I didn't really need, but at the time it seemed easier to take them—so I did. I won the contest, but something inside me wasn't happy with steroid use, so I quit them again, this time for good.

I gradually began to "listen to my body." I changed my diet, I quit eating red meat and began eating more whole grains, raw milk, fertile eggs, nuts, fruits and vegetables. I won the Mr. Universe contest in 1967 and again in 1971 without the use of steroids, although by then most bodybuilders were deeply into steroid usage.

After I quit, I began to hear stories that made me feel I'd made the right choice. When I was running the Pasadena Health Club, all the serious bodybuilders who worked out there were using steroids, taking triple the daily recommended dosages. (Today many athletes take 10-20 times the daily recommended dosage.) One friend had to have a mammary gland removed. Later two other bodybuilders had the same thing happen. A well-known bodybuilder who'd won both the Mr. America and Mr. Universe earlier in his career, died of cancer at age 38. The autopsy indicated it was probably due to steroid use. Other bodybuilders were having liver and kidney damage. I was lucky in not having to pay such a price.

Most of the old-time bodybuilders will not touch steroids now, but probably used them at one time or another. The young bodybuilders today are aware of the dangers of steroids but many of them still use the drugs. I'm sure that many pro football linemen do the same. And surprisingly large numbers of the people who work out seriously in gyms today, even those not competing, are taking steroids.

Just What Are Steroids?

Both men and women have steroids in their bodies, mostly in the form of testosterone, which is a hormone or chemical messenger that accelerates tissue growth and stimulates blood flow. Men have more testosterone in their bodies than women. Since testosterone is chiefly responsible for increases in muscle size, most women—even if they work out extremely hard—cannot naturally develop large muscle mass.

Building muscle requires not only stress, in the form of exercise, but also protein for growth. Anabolic* steroids (which chemically resemble testosterone) are chemical messengers that tell the muscle cells to increase their synthesis of protein, which in turn builds larger muscles. Larger muscles mean more strength.

Some steroids work better than others and some artificial ones work better than naturally-occurring testosterone. It's important to remember that steroids alone produce no increase in strength. Improvement only comes when steroids are combined with exercise, and the gains are in proportion to the effort expended.

Synthetic steroids were first marketed in 1958 by Ciba Pharmaceutical under the name Dianabol. Their purpose was to stimulate protein synthesis in cases of low hormone production, malnutrition and various surgical situations. By the late 1950s athletes in many countries had discovered them the way I had and many people in "strength sports," like weightlifting, football and some track and field events, were using them. From sample interviews at the 1972 Olympics, it was estimated that 68% of the athletes in track and field were taking them. By 1977, James Wright, author of *Anabolic Steroids and Sports*, estimated that 90% of the athletes in the strength sports were using steroids on a regular basis. In a 1984 article in *Sports Illustrated*, William Oscar Johnson reported that "steroid use also appears to be rapidly increasing among high school athletes ... fueled not only by visions of future collegiate and professional athletic glory but also ... as a way of dealing with the self doubts of young boys about their masculinity."

Every anabolic steroid container has a printed disclaimer stating that the drugs do not enhance athletic performance. The recommended dosages outlined by the manufacturers pertain only to the illness or deficiency that it is intended to treat. No steroid manufacturer has ever recommended dosages for increased athletic performances by healthy people.

What Do Anabolic Steroids Look Like? How Do You Take Them?

Anabolic (or artificial) steroids come in two forms:

1. Oral—a tablet to be swallowed
   Muscle cells make and store an organic molecule called creatine phosphate, or CP. CP is a short-term energy restorer. Without it, everyone would find it hard to do more than one or two repetitions of an exercise. Oral steroids enable you to make, store and use large amounts of CP. This allows you to lift long and heavy, and recuperate more quickly after a workout.
2. Injectible—a liquid to be injected into the muscle
   All steroids promote protein synthesis for growth, but while orals promote CP synthesis, injectibles do not. Injectibles are more gradually released and have fewer side effects.

*Anabolic simply refers to a process that promotes growth, in this case the building up of complex molecules from simple ones (or the conversion of food and other simple substances into living tissue).

How Do We Know That Athletes Are Using Drugs?

For three reasons:

1. Some admit it publicly.
2. Controlled, sanctioned drug testing at major events has attained "positive" results among competitors in numerous sports.
3. Side effects directly related to drug use have been increasingly documented.

> *You can find steroids in every pro locker room. It is not a minute thing. It gets to a point where some guys, especially at the pro level, think they have to do it to make it.*
>
> Kent Hull, Center
> New Jersey Generals

> *Eighty-six U.S. athletes flunked drug tests before the 1984 Olympics when evidence of stimulants or anabolic steroids were found in their bloodstreams, the U.S. Olympic Committee reported.*
>
> Associated Press article
> 1/11/85

> *Anabolics are going to be taken. It's a fact of life.*
> Richard Anthony (Tony) Fitton,
> a former British powerlifting champion,
> after being sentenced to 4½ years in prison
> in California for illegal trafficking in
> anabolic steroids.

There are records of athletes taking various drugs to enhance performance as far back as the late 1800s—mostly stimulants in one form or another—but it first happened on a large scale in the 1950s when amphetamines ("speed") became popular, especially among cyclists who used the drug to mask fatigue. (Of course, when the ultimate crash came, it was more pronounced.) Several deaths prompted the first anti-doping laws in France and Belgium in 1965, but the laws had little effect on drug use except to drive it underground.

The International Olympic Committee (IOC) finally added steroids to the list of banned drugs in 1974, once a test was developed to detect their presence in urine samples. The first real testing for steroids took place at the 1976 Olympic games in Montreal, and several "positives" were recorded. Unfortunately no test for testosterone had been developed by that time, so most athletes used this "loophole" and simply discontinued their use of standard anabolic steroids as a competition approached, and substituted testosterone. Finally in 1981 a test for testosterone was developed and the IOC added it to the list of banned drugs.

In 1983, when some athletes were tested for drugs at the Pan American Games in Caracas, Venezuela, 15 athletes were disqualified (some for testosterone) and stripped of 23 medals. Moreover, 12 American athletes left the games once they realized how accurate the testing had become. Similar rules are now enforced at the Olympics. However, many athletes use the drugs up to a point and then discontinue so they'll test negative. In other sports like football there are no tests for steroids that carry any penalties.

With the increasing emphasis on winning at all costs, there has been a surprising change in attitude among sports professionals. The American College of Sports Medicine is a top-level group of researchers and coaches in sports. They are officially opposed to steroids and no member would publicly endorse their use. Yet at their 1984 meeting in

San Diego, there was a surprising change of mood. At a symposium on drug use it was evident that steroid use had become so widespread that a resigned acceptance of the fact had been forced on the coaches. Coaches were talking about steroids as they had talked about vitamin supplements in earlier years. This was in striking contrast to previous symposiums when any usage was strictly and officially condemned. We are left in a curious situation where the officials prohibit them, the coaches tolerate them, and the athletes use them.

Increasing Awareness of the Dangers

William Taylor's *Anabolic Steroids and the Athlete* (McFarland & Co., 1982) and Bob Goldman's *Death in the Locker Room* (Icarus Press, 1984) were the first major books on the extent and hazards of steroid usage by athletes. *Sports Illustrated* has run a number of provocative articles on drug use that have alerted millions of readers to the dangers. More and more articles have been appearing in newspapers; here are some headlines from 1985:

- *Warning on Cancer Among Steroid Users*
- *A Death From Steroids*
- *Women Using Steroids Suffer Side Effects*
- *Steroids: A Problem of Huge Dimensions*

The public and the experts are more aware every day of the potentially dangerous results of chemical use. Despite all the warnings, drugs continue to be promoted and even glorified. Here's an example from the *Underground Steroid Handbook* in talking about HGH:

> *Wow, this is great stuff. It is the best drug for permanent muscle gains. It . . . makes your whole body grow . . . . This is the only drug that can remedy bad genetics, as it will make anybody grow. A few side effects can occur, however. It may elongate your chin, feet and hands, but this is arrested with cessation of the drug. Diabetes in teenagers is possible with it . . . . Massive increases in weight over such a short time can, of course, give you heart problems . . . . HGH use is the biggest gamble that an athlete can take, as the side effects are irreversible. Even with all that, we* LOVE *the stuff.*

Strength Coaches' Dilemma

Strength coaches—both in college and with professional teams—are caught in a bind. Even if they recognize the hazards and strongly disapprove, they know that many athletes are going to use them anyway.

I recently talked about this to a top-notch strength coach at a major university. He put it this way: "Everyone wants to play—to be as good as he can be. All the players have witnessed someone making definite gains through using steroids. And they think, 'I can't compete unless I use them,' or 'I can't make strength gains like those other guys unless I use the drugs.'"

He went on: "If we tell them the drugs are dangerous, they shouldn't use them, and we want nothing to do with it, it's like we're ostriches sticking our heads in the sand. Because they're going to go out and get who-knows-what drugs, use dosages that may be too high, or cycles or combinations that may be dangerous. So what we do, and I think this is true of many strength coaches, is to say, 'Look, here are the dangers of the drugs . . . If you *are* going to use them, however, here are some basic safety rules . . . .'"

I have seen three books that take the position that there is such a lack of information and so much *mis*information about anabolic steroids that it is better to publish the best available information in a responsible manner. These books are *Anabolic Steroids and the Athlete* by William N. Taylor, M.D. (McFarland & Co., Inc., Jefferson, N.C., 1982),

Anabolic Steroids and Sports by James E. Wright (Sports Science Consultants, Matick, Mass., 1978) and *The Practical Use of Anabolic Steroids With Athletes* by Robert Kerr, M.D. (Robert Kerr, M.D., San Gabriel, Calif., 1982).

Varying Opinions on Safety of Steroids

> *In recent years of working with anabolic steroids and thousands of patients, I've never seen any of these side effects happening to any of my patients. Now I don't mean that these medicines are absolutely safe; like any medication there is always a chance for side effects. But in my practice they have been extremely remote.*
>
> Dr. Robert Kerr, author
> *The Practical Use of Anabolic Steroids with Athletes*

Dr. Kerr recently stopped prescribing steroids for athletes, saying that he couldn't trust the athletes to only take what he recommended.

> *Athletes who take steroids are playing with dynamite. Any jock who uses these drugs is taking chances not just with his health but with his life.*
>
> Bob Goldman, author
> *Death in the Locker Room*

Fact: The United States Olympic Committee, the International Olympic Committee, the National Collegiate Athletic Association and professional sports leagues all ban the use of drugs by their athletes on both medical and ethical grounds. Medically, the premise is that any substance powerful enough to alter the body's system can have harmful side effects.

The reason for the opposing views on steroids is that in scientific research done to determine their safety and effectiveness, the results have been inconsistent and contradictory. No two individuals seem to respond to a drug (or an exercise) in the exact same manner. The increase in weight, muscle size, strength and "side effects" seen with steroids differ with each individual. There is a wide person-to-person variation in response to different types of steroids, dosages and schedules. The research to date seems to reflect only partially what is taking place with many steroid users. There have not yet been studies of long-range effects of steroid use.

Warning: Anabolic Steroids May Be Hazardous to Your Health

> *Side Effect: Any effect we do not want, the existence of which we will deny as long as we can.*
>
> Garrett Hardin, Sociologist

Evidence is starting to mount that to use anabolic steroids, one must pay a price. The side effects below are listed according to the principal organ or system affected. But keep in mind, the body functions as a whole: the *entire* body suffers when the function of any of its parts is impaired.

Side effects for males:

- Liver damage (The most commonly documented side effects are changes in liver function. Oral steroids cause more liver damage than injectibles.)
- Impaired thyroid and pituitary functions
- Impaired cardiovascular functions

- Increase in blood pressure or nervous tension
- Disorders of prostate gland
- Reduced reproductive processes (including atrophied testes)
- Increased body and facial hair, thinning hair on scalp
- Acne, skin rash
- Increased aggressiveness
- Changes in sexual desire (up, then down)
- Gastro-intestinal disorders
- Muscle cramps and spasms
- Headaches, dizziness, nose bleeds, drowsiness
- Gynecomastia (development of breast-like tissue in males), sore nipples

Many of these side effects seem to cease after the athlete stops using the drug. But no one really knows what the effects will be over 20 to 30 years.

Women and Steroids

If a woman uses anabolic steroids to raise her testosterone level, she will respond to training just as a man would and make similar gains in muscle mass. In addition to liver dysfunction, high blood pressure and other possible side effects experienced by men, women face these additional side effects from steroid use (the first two are unfortunately irreversible):

- Deepening of the voice
- Increase in facial and body hair
- Acne
- Clitoral enlargement
- Menstrual irregularities
- Increased collagen (the fibrous constituent of bone, cartilage or connective tissue)

Many physicians believe that anabolic steroids upset the body's natural hormone balance, particularly that involving testosterone. Normally, the hypothalamus (the part of the brain that controls many bodily functions, including water balance, sugar and fat metabolism, temperature, hormone secretion) monitors testosterone levels. If it finds them too low, it sends a signal to the pituitary gland to increase production. If it finds them too high, as in the case of steroid overload, it signals the pituitary to cease production. In some cases, when the athlete stops taking the drugs, the hypothalamus fails to get the system started again. This is where many of the side effects listed above occur.

You Can't Judge a Book by its Cover

In virtually all of today's major bodybuilding contests, the competitors, in spite of their superb physical appearance, are probably in poorer health than many people in the audience. This is because of the way they have abused themselves—primarily with drugs and unbalanced diets—getting into the condition necessary to be competitive world-class bodybuilders. A 19-inch biceps and a 52-inch chest do not represent good health if the athlete had to take heavy dosages of drugs over a long period of time to obtain such measurements.

   The same thing applies to strength athletes. Watching professional football games, have you noticed the size of the linemen's arms? Sometimes when I see the strength and power of those players, I wonder if the steroids they take to stay that strong will have any permanent after-effects. Will it turn out to be worth it?

In addition to anabolic steroids, those well-built bodies may contain such chemicals as:

- HGH (Somatotrophin): a hormone consisting of amino acids, extracted from the pituitary glands of human cadavers (and more recently synthetically derived) and capable of producing impressive gains in strength and size, as well as undesired and uncontrolled bone growth, diabetes and heart problems.
- HCG (Human Chorionic Gonadotropin): a complex hormone that is considered to increase not only muscle size, but also the size of blood vessels, or the "vascularity" desired by today's bodybuilders.
- Thyroid preparations, as well as diuretics or "water pills" to rid the body of excess fluid and help the user "cut up" (achieve better muscular definition) or make a weigh-in.

My Personal Feelings About Drugs

I personally feel that living as close as possible to nature, with wholesome food and sensible habits, will pay a thousand times more dividends in the long run than drug use. Of course, I'm talking as a 56-year-old who is no longer interested in competition. For young athletes, of course, the decision is a much more difficult one. How important are the gains and how hazardous are the risks? Only you can be the judge.

Is it possible to become a top-ranked bodybuilder or strength athlete without the use of steroids or other such aids? My answer is YES. True, you have to have a tremendous amount of natural talent and motivation, but it's possible.

Is it unethical to use such aids as anabolic steroids along with your training to achieve your goal? Some say it is simply a matter of choice. However, if you use steroids and compete against athletes who choose not to, either for ethical or health-related reasons, you *do* have an unfair advantage. Would you, for instance, think you had cheated if you took a 10 yard head start in a 100 yard sprint? But if you do not compete in sports, or if you only compete in a sports federation that supports drug use by banning all forms of testing (powerlifting has such a federation), and if you choose to abuse your body this way, it's your decision. If you're more concerned with what's immediately ahead than the long haul, that's also your decision.

In over three decades of continued bodybuilding on a daily basis and from working with literally thousands of people, I know from experience the importance of long-range health and fitness. As I've gotten older I've realized that I want to stay healthy and feel good for the rest of my life. If you abuse your body with *any* foreign substance that overloads the glands and organs, you're asking for trouble. In fact, you don't need a scientist to tell you that the more spectacular the "gains" from a drug, the higher price you'll end up paying in the long run. But isn't all life like that?

Physical health is seldom cherished until it is lost, and in the effort to regain it we begin to realize what we wasted and threw away. Please think twice before you risk your health and well-being. □

If You Quit

It's no disaster. Don't think, "Well, I missed a week so I've blown it—no sense starting over."

You can always start over. Remember the well-worn phrase, "Tomorrow is the first day of the rest of your life"? It's true. If you do quit, or if you *have* quit, tomorrow is a great time to get started again.

Look at it this way: you've had a little rest and now you can start fresh. Too many people get so psyched up about being regular with their workouts that if they stop—even for a short time—they think all is lost, that they've failed and so they quit.

Life is a series of ups and downs, starts and stops, mountains and valleys. No matter how many times you quit, you can always start again.

A BRIEF HISTORY OF RESISTANCE EXERCISE

By Terry Todd, Ph.D.
Professor of Physical Education, University of Texas at Austin

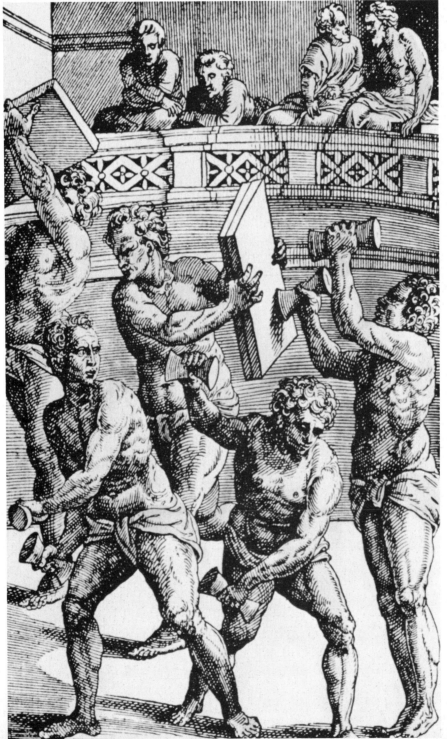

This Renaissance engraving illustrates some of the resistance exercises done before the time of Christ

erhaps the earliest record in existence of any form of resistance exercise is a drawing on the walls of a funerary chapel in Beni-Hassan in Egypt. This drawing, done approximately 4500 years ago, depicts three figures in various postures of raising overhead what appear to be heavy bags. The bags are lifted in what would now be termed a one-handed swing. Both the exercise and the shape of the bags are reminiscent of Indian club exercises.

As early as 1896 B.C., records can be found of feats of strength being practiced in what are now known as the British Isles. The early Irish or Tailtin Games included a form of weight throwing known as *rotheleas* or the *wheel feat*.

The Homeric poems also present early instances of weight throwing. According to the historian Norman Gardiner,

> *Throwing the diskos is one of the most popular diversions in Homer.... Odysseus proved his might by hurling a diskos heavier than any that the Phaeacians were wont to hurl.... Greece was a land of stones, and stones provided a natural weapon in war, and a natural test of strength....*

In the sixth century, B.C., training for strength was predominant in Greece. As Gardiner wrote,

> *The characteristic of the sixth century is strength. The typical athlete of the period is the strong man, the boxer or the wrestler. The object of the old gymnasts, says Philostratus, was to produce strength only, and in consequence of their healthy life the old athletes maintained their strength for eight or even nine Olympiads.*

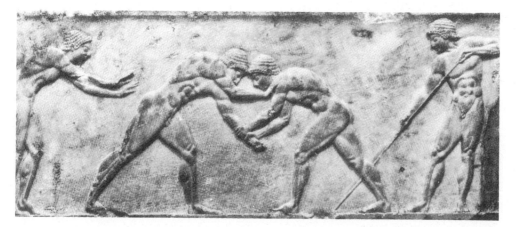

Relief from Greek statue base, late sixth century, B.C. showing athletes training. Left to right: Runner ready to start race; wrestlers; athlete testing point of his javelin.

Perhaps the most famous of these strength athletes was Milo, born in Crotone, in the district of Calabria in southern Italy, about 558 B.C. Milo is often credited with inventing progressive resistance because of his shouldering and carrying a growing heifer the full length of the stadium at Olympia, and doing so until it was four years old.

Strength was also depicted in the art of Greece in the sixth century B.C. Again, quoting from Gardiner,

When we turn to the records of art we still find strength the predominant characteristic of the period. We see this in those early nude statues, widely distributed throughout Greece and the islands. . . . In all of them we see the same attempt to render the muscles of the body, whether in the tall, spare type of the 'Apollo' of Tenea, or the shorter, heavier type of the Argive statues. It is in the muscles of the trunk rather than of the limbs that real strength lies, and it is the careful rendering of these muscles that distinguishes early Greek sculpture from all other early art. . . . The typical figure of the sixth century is that of the bearded Heracles (Hercules).

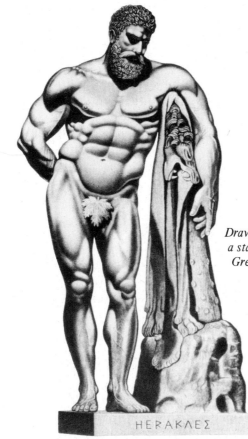

Drawing of the Farnese Hercules,
a statue from the sixth century, B.C.
Greece. By David P. Willoughby

Archaeological evidence exists to confirm the stories that strength was revered and weightlifting practiced during this era. Gardiner explains,

These stories of weightlifting have been strangely confirmed by discoveries in Greece. At Olympia a block of red sandstone was found, bearing a sixth-century inscription to the effect that one Bybon with one hand threw it over his head. . . . At Santorin, another such block has been found, a mass of black volcanic rock, weighing 480 kilos. The inscription on it, which belongs to the close of the sixth century, runs as follows: 'Eumastas the son of Critobulus lifted me from the ground.'

Evidence also points to the fact that implements such as the discus, the javelin and the *halteres*, or jumping weights, were used to increase health and strength. The *halteres* varied in size and shape and were evidently used in many exercise drills during the Greek period. It is safe to assume that the *halteres* are the progenitors of our modern dumbbell.

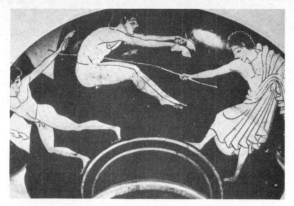

This drawing on a plate from the classical period in Greece shows two athletes using halteres—*the ancestors of our modern dumbbells. Halteres were used for various standard resistance exercises and also, as the drawing depicts, for broadjumping.*

Galen, the celebrated physician of the second century, A.D., was instrumental in developing systematic strength training exercises, using implements such as the *halteres.* His system included what we would now call heavy lifting, dumbbell training, and man-to-man isometric contraction exercises. Galen also recommended a number of exercises to enhance athletic power, or strength with speed.

These exercises were also used during the Roman period, although the grimly pragmatic attitude of the Romans dictated that any and all exercises be practical, with the aim of promoting prowess in battle. Besides the vigorous training of actual physical combat, gladiatorial training included such conditioning aids as chopping at a wooden post with weapons much heavier than those used in actual combat.

With the fall of the Roman Empire, the philosophy of Christian asceticism spread. The body was considered fit only for contempt and this attitude prevailed in one form or another for approximately a thousand years. During this dark period, all physical training had skill in warfare as its chief concern. However, while the actual practice of resistance exercise virtually ceased to exist, the writings of Galen and others explaining this form of exercise were preserved.

Renaissance and Rebirth

As early as 1531, Sir Thomas Elyot refers to Galen's system of lifting weights for exercise.

> *Touching such exercises as may be used within the house or in the shadow . . . as deambulations (walks), labouring with poises (weights) made of lead or other metal called in Latin* halteres, *lifting and throwing the heavy stone or bar.*

Another writer who touched on the subject of lifting weights was Joachim Camerarius, who, in 1544, published a brief dialogue on bodily exercise *(Dialogue de gymnasius).* Camerarius believed that boys should be encouraged to do exercises such as hanging from a bar, climbing a rope, lifting weights, and matching strength with an opponent in various ways.

And the French essayist Michel de Montaigne, writing in the 16th century of his father, leaves the following account indicating that resistance exercise was actively practiced at that time in Europe:

> *I have seen some hollow staves of his filled with lead which he was wont to use and exercise his armes withall, the better to enable himselfe to pitch the barre, to throw the sledge, to cast the pole, and to play at fences; with shoes with leaden soles, which he wore to ensure himselfe to leap, to vault, and to run.*

Gradually a rebirth of interest in things physical occurred and occasional notices were

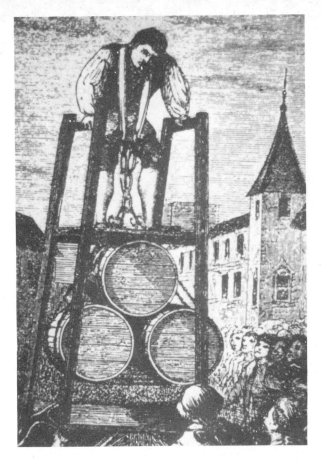

made of men of uncommon strength. Most of these accounts are sketchy in nature, however, for accurate reporting and scientific observation were the exception rather than the rule. The exception that proved the rule, however, was Dr. John Theophilus Desaguliers, who recorded the strength feats of Thomas Topham with the objectivity of a scientist conducting a laboratory experiment. Topham (shown at left) was born in 1710 in London and grew up to become a truly remarkable natural strongman.

Topham was approximately 25 years old at the time of his first public exhibition. He was 5'10" tall and weighed 195 pounds. At this exhibition he resisted the pull of a horse by bracing his feet against a low stone wall. The following announcement advertised one of Topham's exhibitions in the town of Derby:

> *By Desire of Several Gentlemen and Ladies at the Play-House in the Castle-Yard, on Tuesday next being the 10th of February, 1736.*

> *Mr. Topham the Strong Man from Islington performs all his Feats of Strength, as he did before the Royal Society in that Way: particularly to bend a large Iron Poker of three Inches Circumference over his naked Arm: he bends another Iron Poker of two inches and a Quarter around his neck: he fairly breaks a Rope that will bear two Thousand Weight.*

Topham's voice was suited to his freakish strength. He served for a time as soloist at St. Werburgh's Church in Derby, and his *basso profundo* was said to be "more terrible than sweet." It was said to be so deep and resonant as to be scarcely human.

Physical Education in the Schools

During the late 18th century there was great emphasis on physical education, the development of the body and "manly" exercises in the schools of Europe. Johann Gutsmuth, a German teacher, wrote his *Encyclopedia of Bodily Exercises* and is said to have laid the foundations for continental lifting with his invention of several new pieces of equipment.

Another German, Friederich Jahn (1778-1852) invented horizontal and parallel bars— the forerunners of the dipping and chinning bars used today. Jahn sponsored physical culture festivals where as many as 30,000 people would take part.

United States Backgound

An early reference to resistance exercise in the United States appears in a letter by Benjamin Franklin to his son in 1772.

London, August 19: 1772

(Dear Son)
  In yours of May 14th, you acquaint me with your indisposition, which gave me great concern. The resolution you have taken to use more exercise is extremely proper; and I hope you will steadily perform it. It is of the greatest importance to prevent diseases since the cure of them by physic is so very precarious. . . .
  . . . The dumbbell is another exercise of the latter compendious kind. By the use of it I have in forty swings quickened my pulse from sixty to one hundred beats in a minute, counted by a second watch; and I suppose the warmth generally increases with quickness of pulse.

Further evidence indicates that Franklin practiced dumbbell exercises even as an octogenarian. The evidence is presented in a letter quoted from biographer Carl Van Doren.

Franklin . . . wrote more and longer letters from 15 to 22 April (1786) than in any week since his return. '. . . I live temperately, drink no wine, and use daily the exercise of the dumbbell . . . .'

It was not until 1824, however, that Charles Beck arrived in New York from Germany and established the first gymnasium in the United States at the Round Hill School in Northampton, Massachusetts. Besides instructing pupils in gymnastic exercises, Beck advocated and taught exercises employing resistance training apparatus.
  Another true pioneer in the use of heavy resistance exercise in the United States was Dr. George Barker Windship. Born in Roxbury, Massachusetts, in 1834, he was educated at Harvard University, receiving his M.D. in 1857.
  He wrote the following in his introduction to weightlifting:

While at Rochester (Summer, 1854), as I was passing through the principal street, I met a crowd assembled about a lifting machine. On making trial of it, I found I could lift four hundred and twenty pounds. I had then been for four years a gymnast and I supposed my practice would have qualified me to make the crowd stare at my achievement. But the result was far from triumphant. I found what many other gymnasts will find, that main strength, *by which I mean the strength of the truckman and the porter, cannot be acquired in the ordinary exercises of the gymnasium.*

The "lifting machine" was his favorite form of exercise. It was an apparatus that approximated the "hand and thigh" lift, in which the bar is placed about six or eight inches above the knees, allowing the lifter to bend his knees and thus place most of the resistance on the hips and upper thighs, in the manner of a partial deadlift. Windship began to experiment with this form of exercise and as he got stronger, he traveled throughout the northern United States as well as part of Canada. He maintained that this form of heavy partial lifting was the best way to develop strength and therefore greater health. His motto was, "Strength is Health" and this lift became known as the "Health Lift."

Dr. Windship advocated the Health Lift as a means of promoting vigor, well-being, and freedom from disease. In the April, 1860, edition of *The Massachusetts Teacher*, he verbalized his remarkable and, for the most part, modern beliefs.

> *I was nearly seventeen years of age before I seriously undertook to improve my physical condition. I was then but five feet in height and a hundred pounds in weight. I was rather strong for my size, but not strong for my years, and my health was not vigorous. I am now twenty-six years, five feet seven inches in height, and one hundred and forty-eight pounds in weight. My strength is more than twice that of an ordinary man, and my health is as excellent as my strength . . . .*
>
> *During these nine years, while endeavoring to promote my physical welfare, I have made the following discoveries:*
> *. . . The stronger I became, the healthier I became . . . That I could gain faster in strength by forty minutes' gymnastic exercises once in two days, than by twenty minutes of the same daily . . . . That a person may become possessed of great physical strength without having inherited it . . . . That a delicate boy of seventeen need not despair of becoming in time a remarkably strong and healthy man.*

Growth in Britain and Europe

The expansion of weightlifting occurred in the British Isles and Europe as well as in the United States during this period, only earlier and at a much greater rate. There were gymnasiums, in fact, in use in the middle part of the 19th century which would rival anything seen today.

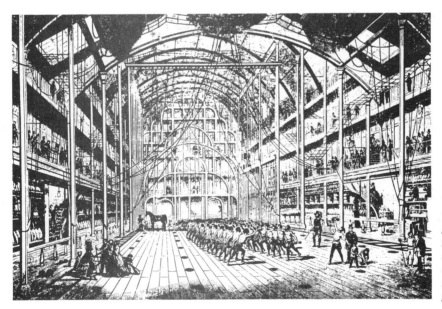

Triat's gym in Paris, 1854. Note rows of men doing dumbbell exercises and spectators in galleries.

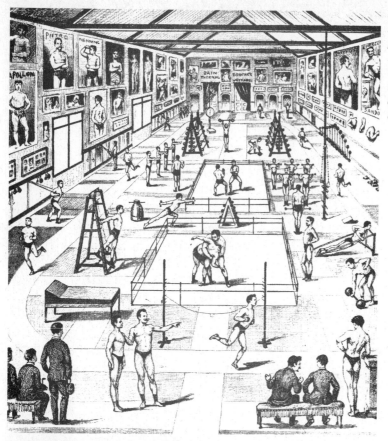

Professor Edmund Desbonnet's school of physical culture in Lille, France, 1885. Note the variety of exercising equipment. On the walls are posters of famous athletes.

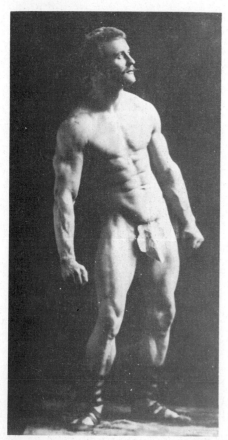

Hippolyte Triat's gym in Paris, for instance, was as enormous as it was popular, and Triat was famous for both his teaching and his physique. Most of the well-known strength athletes of the late 19th and early 20th century, of course, were professionals.

Foremost among these was a Prussian, Frederick Muller (1867-1925), who became famous as Eugen Sandow. Sandow first gained fame by a clever use of "test your strength" machines, then in vogue in Brussels. What Sandow did was use his great strength to overload and thus destroy the machines, an act which caused the police to put a "stakeout" on the repaired machines. As Sandow planned, the police saw him break a machine, but they had to release him when he explained that he had used the proper coin and was only following the instructions.

The resulting publicity boosted Sandow's career, but his big break came when he went to London in 1889 to challenge the successful strongman team of Samson and Cyclops. Sandow

Eugen Sandow, 1867-1925, whose phenomenal physique, strength, intelligence and promotional abilities made him the most famous bodybuilder in history.

jumped on the stage of the Westminster Theater, impeccably attired in evening wear. He challenged the two larger men, then whipped off his formal wear to reveal his magnificent physique. After defeating the strongmen, he was lionized and proceeded to make an excellent living touring the British theaters. His early acts were purely of the weightlifting variety, but artistically and dramatically presented. He toured the United States in 1893 and by then he had worked out acts in which he lifted and supported people, animals and heavy objects. He also posed in a lighted cabinet to accentuate his remarkable development.

One of the stops on Sandow's 1893 tour was the World's Fair in Chicago. There he joined forces with the promoter Florenz Ziegfeld. This partnership was of great benefit to both men, as Sandow was paid between $1500 and $3500 per week for his exhibitions during the fair. One of the interesting aspects of Sandow's Chicago appearances is that his physique and showmanship had a profound effect on a young physical culturist who saw him there—Bernarr MacFadden.

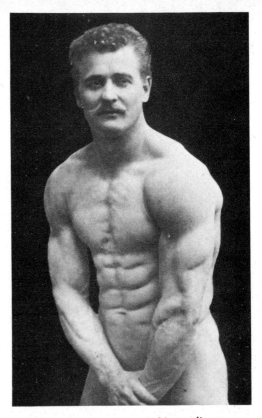

Sandow's musculature and skin quality gave him a look similar to Greek statues of white marble.

Feats of strength performed by Eugen Sandow. (1) The "human bridge." (2) The "bent press" with 2 small people inside the hollow spheres of the barbell. (3) The "Roman Column": Sandow would bring his body to an upright position holding either a barbell or a man. (4) A pony (about 350 lbs.) would be hoisted into place with a block and tackle and Sandow would walk across the stage. Drawings by David P. Willoughby.

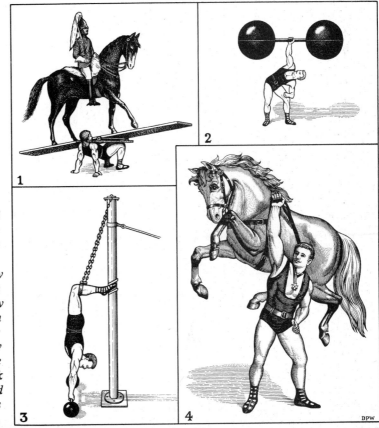

After seeing Sandow, MacFadden decided to try to make his living as an exponent of exercise and he soon began to build an empire that would far surpass anything seen up to that time. His magazine *Physical Culture*, for example, had a circulation of 400,000 in 1926, and it helped MacFadden amass a personal fortune of 30 million dollars by the late 1920s.

Strongwomen of the Past

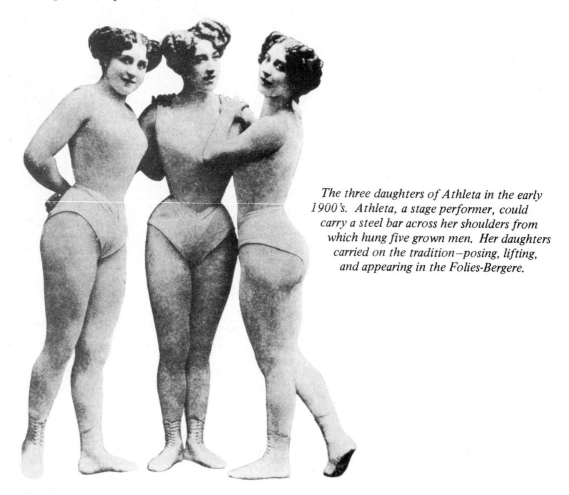

The three daughters of Athleta in the early 1900's. Athleta, a stage performer, could carry a steel bar across her shoulders from which hung five grown men. Her daughters carried on the tradition—posing, lifting, and appearing in the Folies-Bergere.

As far as women who performed "strong acts" are concerned, there were several who gained considerable stature—Athleta, Vulcana and Sandwina—but only one, Katie Sandwina, rose to the very top—appearing as a center ring attraction with the Ringling Brothers Circus. Born Katie Brumbach, this German amazon was billed as the "Strongest and Most Beautiful Woman in the World." At six feet and 200 pounds, Katie, who took the stage name Sandwina, was able to lift her 160-pound husband overhead with one arm and carry a 600-pound cannon around the ring on one shoulder. She also twisted horse-shoes, bent iron rods and is said to have once lifted 286 pounds over her head in a style called the "continental and jerk." Sandwina's strength was so awesome that many strongmen of the period would slink out of town under cover of darkness rather than risk the embarassment of being compared with this foremother of strength.

In the later years of the 19th century and early years of the 20th, several events conspired to damage and ultimately eliminate professional lifting. The chief factor was the industrial revolution, which affected all aspects of western culture. Industrialization removed vast numbers of people from the land and physical labor and made them less

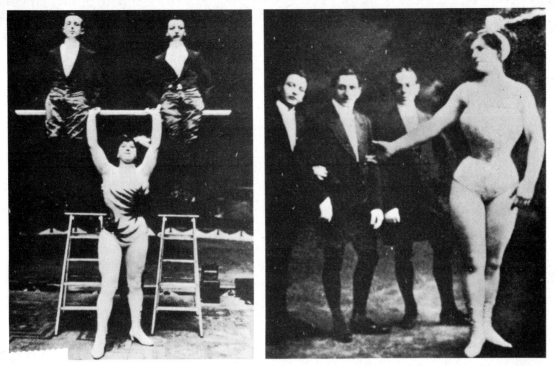

Katie Sandwina, the "Strongest and Most Beautiful Woman in the World." She was six feet tall, weighed 200 pounds and could lift her 160-pound husband overhead with one hand.

familiar with and dependent upon the physical side of their nature. As the professional strongman was obliged to draw paying crowds in order to exist, this declining knowledge of and interest in physical strength resulted in decreased attendance at strength displays. After 1910, the professional strongman became a rarity on the performing stage, and only such prominent and able athletes as Hermann Goerner, Ernest Cadine, Charles Rigulot, Sandwina, Warren Lincoln Travis, Ottley Coulter and Siegmund Brietbart were able to perform their acts with success. With the slow death of vaudeville around 1930, the era of the professional stage strongman came to an end.

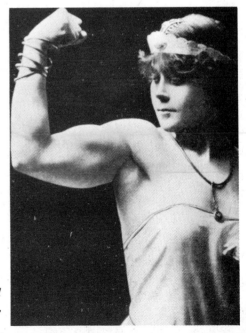

Kate Roberts, or Vulcana, an English Music Hall strongwoman who, although weighing 125 pounds, could lift 145 pounds overhead with one hand.

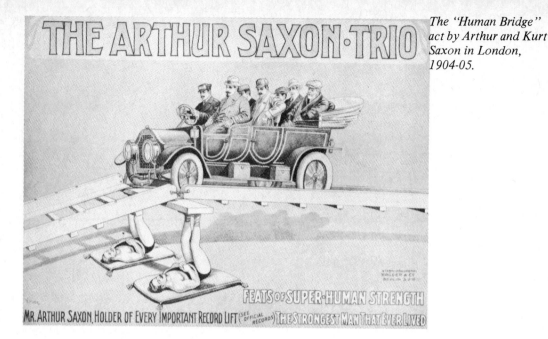

The "Human Bridge"
act by Arthur and Kurt
Saxon in London,
1904-05.

The Amateurs Take Center Stage

Another factor that influenced the demise of professional strongmen was the rising interest in amateur lifting. Many serious athletes were undoubtedly disgusted by the often preposterous claims of the professionals. This created within the non-professionals a desire to establish rules and regulations so that fair and honest competitions could be held and records could be verified. As the strength historian, David P. Willoughby, wrote:

> *(Amateur weightlifting) may be said to have 'come of age in 1891, when the 'Deutsche Athletik Sport Verband' (German Athletic Association) was founded in Duisburg.... The new association, in 1891, separated the lifters and wrestlers from the gymnasts or 'Turners,' and brought all the local 'Kraftsport' (strength-sport) clubs together under the direction of a*

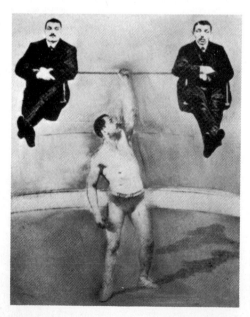

This rare photo shows Arthur Saxon lifting his brothers overhead with one hand. Using a twisting technique, called a bent press, to lift the bar from shoulder level up to arm's length, Saxon lifted 370 pounds—still a world record.

national governing body (with offices in Cologne). In 1900, the Association had a membership of over 300 clubs and over 12,000 athletes.
    . . . The first competition took place at Cologne in 1893. The weightlifting championship at that time was won by Johannes Schneider of Cologne. . . . Contemporary Austrian lifters, who trained in the same manner, formed a similar association, naming it the 'Osterreichisch Kraftsport Verband.'

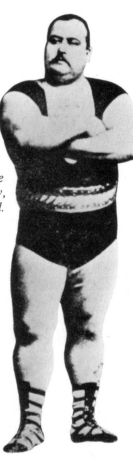

Louis Cyr, a colossal French-Canadian whose prime was in the late 1800's, was a specialist in feats of brute strength. In his day, he was widely considered to be the strongest man in the world.

Amateur lifting became increasingly popular and, in 1898, the first "world championship" was held. Willoughby wrote:

> *The year 1898 was an auspicious one in the annals of 'The Iron Game,' for it was then, for the first time, that a competition was organized to bring together the best amateur weightlifters of all nations in which competitive lifting was practiced. At that time, however, worthy competitors in this field were virtually restricted to continental Europe and the British Isles. The scene of the 1898 championship was to be the great sports-minded city of Vienna.*

Beginning in 1896, three of the first four modern Olympiads included weightlifting. Amateur lifting was also widely practiced at the turn of the century in France, where "clean" lifting (lifting in which the weight is taken to the shoulder in one motion rather than in two or more, as is the case with the "continental" style of lifting) was developed.
    Amateur lifting in Great Britain was also growing in the early years of the 20th century and, in 1911, the British Amateur Weightlifters' Association was formed, sponsored by the British publication, *Health and Strength.*

In the United States, open contests were seldom seen before the turn of the century. A rare exception was a gathering of strongmen in 1890, prompted by the *Police Gazette* magazine, which offered a large and valuable jewel-studded belt to the first man to raise a "dumbbell" of 1030 pounds.

Perhaps the most important figure in developing amateur lifting in the United States was Alan Calvert, who founded the Milo Barbell Company in 1902. As David P. Willoughby once wrote:

> *Perhaps the greatest single impetus ever given to weightlifting in this country was the establishing, in 1902, of the Milo Bar-Bell Company, in Philadelphia, and the subsequent popularizing of this form of training, both as a body-builder and as a sport, by the founder, Alan Calvert.*

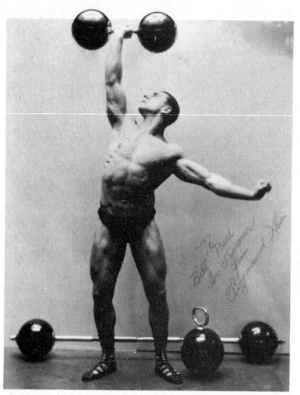

One-handed lifting was popular in the early 1900's and one of the best at it was Sigmund Klein. For many years Klein operated New York's most famous gym and it was filled with beautiful old barbells like those pictured here.

Calvert, who wrote such books as *Super Strength* and *The Truth About Weight-Lifting*, offered courses which were an honest attempt to teach the early 20th century seeker of strength the most modern and productive methods of training. He also offered the precedent-making plate-loading barbell, patterned after the Berg-Hantel barbell from Germany, as the main implement of his excellent course. Calvert spoke out strongly in favor of proper organization in weightlifting, and wrote:

> *Under the present system, where every professional and most amateurs feel at liberty to introduce special feats of their own devising, no man can train properly for a contest. In Europe, lifting contests are announced several weeks ahead of time. Every man who enters the contest is informed exactly which lifts will be on the program and he can train accordingly.*

By the middle 1920s, Calvert's words had created sufficient interest so that, under the direction of George F. Jowett, The American Continental Weightlifters' Association was formed. It was modeled after the British Amateur Weightlifters' Association and its rules were drafted by David P. Willoughby and Ottley Coulter. It recognized 60 lifts and six bodyweight divisions.

These organizations were gradually absorbed by the Amateur Athletic Union, which assumed control of United States lifting in 1927. This assumption of control by the Amateur Athletic Union resulted in the adoption of the French rules for lifting. This was done to enable the United States to qualify for admission into the *Federation Internationale Halterophile* or International Weightlifting Federation, which was formed in 1920 to promote and conduct international competition.

As the Olympic Games of 1912 and 1916 failed to include weightlifting, 1920 marked the rebirth of this sport in Olympic competition. But not all competitive lifting involves only the "Olympic" lifts. In fact, a type of lifting other than Olympic-style lifting is now

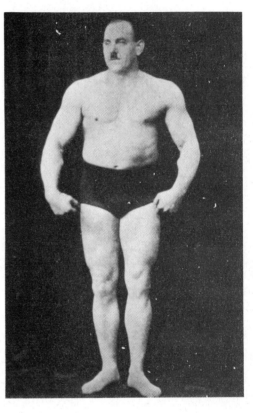

Herman Goerner, a German, set a world record in the one-hand deadlift with 727 pounds in 1920. Strength historian David P. Willoughby called it the single greatest feat of strength ever performed.

practiced on an increasing scale in quite a few countries, under the auspices of the International Powerlifting Federation.

The first official U.S. National Powerlifting Championship was not held until 1965, but this newer form of lifting now has at least ten times more participants than Olympic-style weightlifting. One of the chief reasons for the rapid rise in popularity of power-lifting is that, unlike weightlifting, little time need be spent on technique, as the power lifts—the squat, bench press and deadlift—are familiar to anyone who has ever trained with weights. Also, they are easy to perform and require mainly strength for success. The Olympic lifts, on the other hand, require a high degree of flexibility, balance and coordination—calling for proper training as a beginner as well as constant practice.

Bodybuilding

Another form of competition which indirectly involves the use of weights and resistance training is the often misunderstood activity in which men and women are judged on the basis of the excellence of their physiques. The modern physique competitors or body-builders all train with resistance exercise in order to attain the combination of huge musculature, proportion and muscular definition on which the contestants are judged. This form of "beauty" contest for men is perhaps even older than similar competition among women. The Greeks staged contests of this sort, and we know from the historical record that such competitions for men were part of the Panathenaean and Thesean festivals.

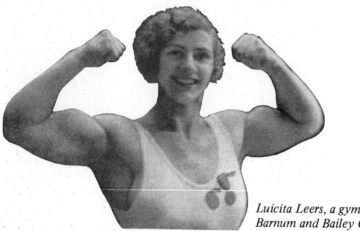

Luicita Leers, a gymnast with Ringling Brothers and Barnum and Bailey Circus, 1929-33.

The first known male physique contest in the U.S. was held in 1904, and was promoted by Bernarr MacFadden. It was held in New York City and it featured a division for women as well as men, with both divisions offering large cash prizes to the winners. Eugen Sandow sponsored physique contests in England, open to his pupils. The winners of these highly publicized contests received gold, silver and bronze statuettes for being what Sandow called "the best proportioned and developed men in the United Kingdom." Organized physique competitions gradually developed, and some of the yearly contests now being held began many decades ago. The contest for the title of Mr. Britain began even earlier than the Mr. America contest, which had its beginnings in this country in 1939. Other titles, such as *Le Plus Bel Athlete d'Europe,* began before the Second World War.

John Grimek, Mr. America in 1940 and 1941, Mr. Universe in 1948, Mr. USA in 1949.

The first truly international physique meet to be held was a "Mr. Universe" contest in Philadelphia, Pennsylvania, in conjunction with the World Weightlifting Championships in 1947. The winner of this title was Steve Stanko of the United States, an athlete who earlier gained fame by being the first man to achieve a total of 1000 pounds in the Olympic lifts.

Influence of Mail-Order Systems

Another significant factor in the history of resistance exercise has been the influence of mail-order systems of physical training. Pioneers in this field were Edmond Desbonnet of France and Theodore Siebert of Germany. They each developed systems very similar to present training courses. Both men began to work before the turn of the century and each was extremely active in the "iron game" for over fifty years. Sandow and MacFadden also sold early courses of resistance training through the mail.

Probably the most famous of all mail-order instructors, at least in today's world, is the late Angelo Siciliano or, as he is better known, Charles Atlas. He began selling his mail-order course in the early 1920s after having won a "perfect man" contest sponsored by Bernarr MacFadden. Although Atlas developed his physique by lifting barbells and dumbbells, he offered a course that used no apparatus, as he believed it would be easier to sell. His advertisements for "Dynamic Tension" have made the phrases "97 pound weakling" and "kicking sand in your face" familiar to millions of Americans. Untold numbers of young men who felt dissatisfied with their physical makeup saw in Atlas's advertisements a chance to build greater size and strength.

Another man who built a vast mail-order business in this country was Earle E. Liederman, whose volume of mail during the 1920s was so enormous that he employed approximately 150 secretaries in his office in New York.

A man who has had a far more profound effect on resistance training in the United States, through his publication from 1932 until 1986 of *Strength and Health* magazine, is the late Bob Hoffman, who was a tireless promoter of weight training for athletics and health. A more modest but still effective promoter of the iron game is Peary Rader, who published his honest and well-respected magazine, *Iron Man,* from 1936 to 1986.

In the last decade, Joe Weider—who publishes such magazines as *Muscle and Fitness Flex, Sports Fitness* and *Shape*—has dominated the field of weight training publications. And Joe's brother Ben is the founder and president of the International Federation of Bodybuilders, which now has affiliations in more than 100 countries. The Weider magazines and the IFBB have helped catapult people like Arnold Schwarzenegger, Lou Ferrigno and Rachel McLish to stardom.

Mail-order courses, interestingly enough, have grown in number but lessened in relative importance through the years. The main reasons for this are the increasing sales of barbells and other gymnasium equipment in virtually every sporting goods and department store, the enormous increase in physical education instruction in the schools of the United States, and the amazing growth, especially since World War II, of health studios.

Influence of Resistance Exercise in Rehabilitation

Before World War II, most of the information available on resistance exercise was found in mail-order courses and in the books and magazines in the field, many of which were commercially slanted. This type of empirical information, while often wholly honest and basically correct, was largely ignored by the medical profession and the physical education community. Following World War II, however, a series of medical experiments were carried out on resistance training and its applicability to rehabilitation. The results of these experiments, some of which were performed by Dr. Thomas L. DeLorme, an orthopedist, were an important step in revolutionizing the thinking of both doctors and

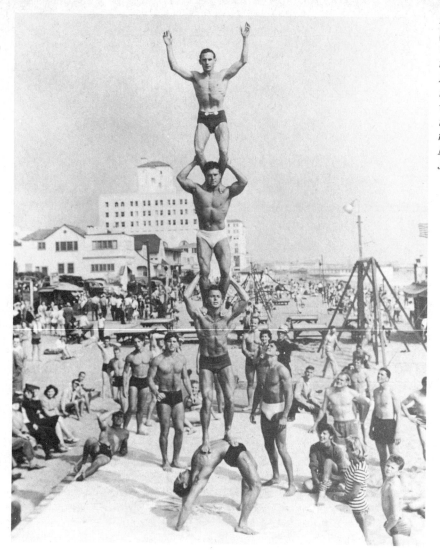

Harold Zinkin (bottom) disproving the musclebound myth at Muscle Beach, California, in the 1940's. Zinkin went on to invent the Universal Gym machine in 1957. Man next to top is Jack La Lanne.

physical education specialists concerning resistance exercise. As a result of his work and writing, Dr. DeLorme made the term "progressive resistance" famous.

As Dr. DeLorme's work became increasingly well-known, the use of progressive resistance exercise techniques for rehabilitative and adaptive measures expanded. Now, pre-operative, post-operative, chronic orthopedic, asthmatic, cardiac, postural, post-polio, neurological, general coordination and post-injury cases utilize this type of therapy.

Resistance Exercise and Athletics

For a variety of reasons, it was widely believed during the first half of this century that weightlifting would make a person "musclebound." Coaches and physical educators told athletes to avoid it at all costs. Even though articles appeared from time to time in lifting magazines arguing otherwise, the belief persisted. However, a few athletes who were either too stubborn to follow the teachings of their coaches, or sufficiently far-sighted to see the error in these teachings, continued to mix lifting and sports with beneficial results. As the results accumulated, a few physical educators and doctors began to see a pattern emerging from the eclectic hodge-podge of information on the subject by the late 1940s. This interest by professionals marked a turning point in the history of athletic conditioning as quality research began, and minds began to change. A study published by

Edward Chui in the *Research Quarterly* in 1950, for instance, concluded that a program of weight training seemed to increase athletic power to a greater extent than did a regular program of fitness training.

Another historically significant study, published by Zorbas and Karpovich in 1951 in the *Research Quarterly*, widened the wedge that would eventually split the knotty mass of myth and misinformation that existed in this area. The study, which was quite thorough, resulted in statistics which indicated that lifters were not slower than an average person, but faster. It should be added that a 1950s book, *Weight Training and Athletics* by Karpovich and Murray, had a profound effect on the willingness of coaches and physical educators to abandon the myth of the musclebound athlete.

The Future

It is not possible, of course, to predict the future with certainty by looking to the past for clues, but the past does offer us the best opportunity we have for seeing trends that may well continue in the years that lie ahead. The current popularity of resistance exercise, for instance, is so extraordinary that only those who were alert to such facts as the growing use of weights for sports, the changing attitudes about strength as an aspect of femininity and the increasing American interest in fitness, could have foreseen what has now come to pass.

Few bodybuilders in the 1940s or 1950s would have believed that by the 1980s pumping iron would become a passion shared by millions. And few weight-trained athletes of the same period would have been able to hide their amusement had anyone told them that by the '80s almost no top athlete in any sport would even *think* of neglecting his or her weight work. And fewer still weight trainers—of any sort—would have been willing, in the 1950s or 1960s, to admit the possibility of a future in which hundreds of thousands of women not only lifted weights but lifted them with passion and commitment.

Most people, in fact, who have watched the changing fortunes of exercise have been astonished by what they have seen, and the future may very well surprise us with equally dramatic changes, but it seems clear that an awareness of the contributions of the movers and shakers of the past can help us all to not only better guess the future but to profit from it as well by avoiding the mistakes of those who have gone before. □

APPENDIX

WEIGHT TRAINING PROGRAM (Photocopy for use in gym)

NAME: _____

DATE PROGRAM STARTED: _____

Exercises:	pg#	sets	reps	lbs.	sets	reps	lbs.	sets	reps	lbs.	sets	reps	lbs.	sets	reps	lbs.	sets	reps	lbs.	sets	reps	lbs.
1																						
2																						
3																						
4																						
5																						
6																						
7																						
8																						
9																						
10																						
11																						
12																						
13																						
14																						
15																						
16																						

Use this card along with any of the programs in the book.

LANGUAGE OF LIFTING

Abduction — Movement of a limb away from middle of body, such as bringing arm to shoulder height from hanging-down position.

Abs — Abbreviation for abdominal muscles.

Accommodating Resistance — Increasing resistance as lifter's force increases through range of motion. Nautilus machines are said to provide accommodating resistance.

Adduction — Movement of a limb toward middle of body, such as bringing arm to side from extended position at shoulder.

Adhesion — Fibrous patch holding muscles or other parts together that are normally separated.

Aerobic Exercise — (With oxygen) — Activity in which demands of muscle for oxygen are met by circulation of oxygen in blood. Distance running, cross-country skiing, distance cycling are aerobic activities.

AFWB — American Federation of Women Bodybuilders — group that administers women's amateur bodybuilding in America.

Agonist — Muscle directly engaged in contraction, that is primarily responsible for movement of a body part.

All-or-None — Muscle fiber contracts fully or it does not contract at all.

Anabolic Steroid — Synthetic chemical that mimics the muscle-building characteristics of the male hormone testosterone.

Anaerobic Exercise — (Without oxygen) — Activity in which oxygen demands of muscles are so high that they rely upon an internal metabolic process for oxygen. Short bursts of "all-out" activities such as sprinting or weightlifting are anaerobic.

Antagonist — Muscle that counteracts the agonist, lengthening when agonist muscle contracts.

APC — American Physique Committee, Inc. — group that administers men's amateur bodybuilding in America.

Arm Blaster — Aluminum or fiberglass strip about 5" x 24", supported at waist height by a strap around neck. Keeps elbows from moving while curling barbell or dumbbells or doing triceps pushdowns.

Atrophy — Withering away — decrease in size and functional ability of tissue or organs.

Baby's Butt — Indentation between the two heads of biceps muscles of very muscular athlete.

Back-Cycling — Cutting back on either number of sets, repetitions or amount of weight used during an exercise session.

Barbell — Weight used for exercise, consisting of a rigid handle 5-7' long, with detachable metal discs at each end.

Biomechanics — Science concerned with the internal and external forces acting on a human body and the effects produced by these forces.

Bodybuilding — Weight training to change physical appearance.

Buffed — As in a "finely buffed finish" — good muscle size and definition, looking *good.*

Bulking Up — Gaining body weight by adding muscle, body fat or both.

Burn — As in "going for the burn" — in endurance exercise, working muscles until lactic acid buildup causes burning sensation.

Cardiovascular Training — Physical conditioning that strengthens heart and blood vessels.

Chalk — Powder used on hands for secure grip.

Cheating — Too much weight used on an exercise, therefore relying on surrounding muscle groups for assistance in the movement; or changing joint angles for more leverage, as in arching back in bench press.

Circuit Training — Going quickly from one exercise apparatus to another and doing a prescribed number of exercises on each apparatus, to keep pulse rate high and promote overall fitness.

Clean — Lifting weight from floor to shoulder in one motion.

Clean and Jerk — Olympic lift where weight is raised from floor to overhead in 2 movements (see also SNATCH).

Clean and Snatch — One of 2 Olympic lifts where weight is raised from floor to overhead at arms' length in one motion.

Compound Training — Sometimes called "giant sets"; doing 3-4 exercises for same muscle, one after other, with minimal rest in between.

Concentric Contraction — When muscle contracts or shortens.

Crunches — Abdominal exercises — sit-ups done lying on floor with legs on bench, hands behind neck.

Curl-Bar — Cambered bar designed for more comfortable grip and less forearm strain.

Cutting Up — Reducing body fat and water retention to increase muscular definition.

Dead Lift — One of three powerlifting events (other two are squat and bench press). Weight is lifted off floor to approximately waist height. Lifter must stand erect, shoulders back.

Delts — Abbreviation for deltoids, the large triangular muscles of the shoulder which raise the arm away from the body and perform other functions.

Dip Belt — Large heavy belt worn around hips with chain at each end that can be attached to a barbell plate or dumbbell for additional resistance during certain exercises like dips.

Double (Split Training) Routine — Working out twice a day to allow for shorter, more intense workouts. Usually performed by advanced bodybuilders preparing for contests.

Drying Out — Encouraging loss of body fluids by limiting liquid intake, eliminating salt, sweating heavily and/or using diuretics.

Dumbbell — Weight used for exercising consisting of rigid handle about 14" long with sometimes detachable metal discs at each end.

Easy Set — Exercise not close to maximum effort, as in a warmup.

Eccentric Contraction — Muscle lengthens while maintaining tension (see p. 70).

Endurance — Ability of a muscle to produce force continually over a period of time.

Estrogen — Female sex hormone.

Extension — Body part (i.e. hand, neck, trunk, etc.) going from a bent to a straight position, as in leg extension.

Fascia — Fibrous connective tissue that covers, supports and separates all muscles and muscle groups. It also unites skin with underlying tissue.

Fast-Twitch — Refers to muscle cells that fire quickly and are utilized in anaerobic activities like sprinting and powerlifting.

Flex — Bend or decrease angle of a joint; contract a muscle.

Flexion — Bending in contrast to extending, as in leg flexions.

Flush — Cleanse a muscle by increasing the blood supply to it, removing toxins left in muscle by exertion.

Forced Repetitions — Assistance to perform additional repetitions of an exercise when muscles can no longer complete movement on their own.

Free Style Training — Training all body parts in one workout.

Gluteals — Abbreviation for *gluteus maximus, medius* and *minimus;* the buttocks muscles.

Hand Off — Assistance in getting a weight to starting position for an exercise.

Hard Set — Perform a prescribed number of repetitions of an exercise using maximum effort.

Hypertrophy — Increase in size of muscle fiber.

IFBB — International Federation of Bodybuilders, founded in 1946 — group that oversees worldwide men's and women's amateur and professional bodybuilding.

Isokinetic Exercise — Isotonic exercise in which there is ACCOMMODATING RESISTANCE. Also refers to constant speed. Nautilus and Cybex are two types of isokinetic machines, where machine varies amount of resistance being lifted to match force curve developed by the muscle (see pp. 63-64).

Isometric Exercise — Muscular contraction where muscle maintains a constant length and joints do not move. These exercises are usually performed against a wall or other immovable object (see pp. 63-64).

Isotonic Exercise — Muscular action in which there is a change in length of muscle and weight, keeping tension constant. Lifting free weights is a classic isotonic exercise (see pp. 63-64).

Kinesiology — Study of muscles and their movements.

Knee Wraps — Elastic strips about 3½" wide used to wrap knees for better support when performing squats, dead lifts, etc.

Lats — Abbreviation for *latissimus dorsi,* the large muscles of the back that move the arms downward, backward and in internal rotation.

Lean Body Mass — Everything in the body except fat, including bone, organs, skin, nails and all body tissue including muscle. Approximately 50-60% of lean body mass is water.

Lift Off — Assistance in getting weight to proper starting position.

Ligament — Strong, fibrous band of connecting tissue connecting 2 or more bones or cartilages or supporting a muscle, fascia or organ.

Lock Out — Partial repetition of an exercise by pushing the weight through only last few inches of movement.

Lower Abs — Abbreviation for abdominal muscles below the navel.

Max — Maximum effort for one repetition of an exercise.

Midsection — Muscles of abdominal area, including upper and lower abdominals, obliques and *rectus abdominis* muscles.

Military Press — Pressing a barbell from upper chest upward in standing or sitting position.

Muscle — Tissue consisting of fibers organized into bands or bundles that contract to cause bodily movement. Muscle fibers run in the same direction as the action they perform.

Muscle Head — Slang for someone whose life is dominated by training.

Muscle Spasm — Sudden, involuntary contraction of muscle or muscle group.

Muscle Tone — Condition in which a muscle is in a constant yet slight state of contraction and appears firm.

Muscularity — Another term for definition, denoting fully delineated muscles and absence of body fat.

Myositis — Muscular soreness due to inflammation that often occurs 1-2 days after unaccustomed exercise.

Nautilus — Isokinetic-type exercise machine which attempts to match resistance with user's force.

Negative Reps — One or two partners help you lift a weight up to 50% heavier than you would normally lift to finish point of movement. Then you slowly lower weight on your own.

Non-Locks — Performing an exercise without going through complete range of motion. For example, doing squat without coming to full lock-out position of knees or pressing a barbell without locking out elbows.

Obliques — Abbreviation for external obliques, the muscles to either side of abdominals that rotate and flex the trunk.

Odd Lifts — Exercises used in competition other than snatch and clean and jerk, such as squats, bench presses, barbell curls.

Olympic Lifts — Two movements used in national and international Olympic competitions: the SNATCH and the CLEAN AND JERK.

Olympic Set — High-quality, precision-made set of weights used for competition. The bar is approximately 7' long. All moving parts have either brass bushings or bearings. Plates are machined for accurate weight.

Onion Skin — Slang denoting skin with very low percentage of subcutaneous fat which helps accentuate muscularity.

Overload Principle — Applying a greater load than normal to a muscle to increase its capability (see p. 362-63).

Partial Reps — Performing an exercise without going through a complete range of motion either at the beginning or end of a rep.

Peak Contraction — Exercising a muscle until it cramps by using shortened movements.

Pecs — Abbreviation for *pectoral* muscles of the chest.

P.H.A. — Peripheral Heart Action — a system of training where you go from one exercise to another, with little or no rest, preferably alternating upper body and lower body exercises. Designed for cardiovascular training and to develop muscle mass.

Plyometric Exercise — Where muscles are loaded suddenly and stretched, then quickly contracted to produce a movement. Athletes who must jump do these, i.e. jumping off bench to ground, quickly rebounding to another bench.

Pose Down — Bodybuilders performing their poses at the same time in a competition, trying to outpose one another.

Power — Strength + speed.

Power Lifts — Three movements used in powerlifting competition: the squat, bench press and dead lift.

Power Training — System of weight training using low repetitions, heavy weights.

Progressive Resistance — Method of training where weight is increased as muscles gain strength and endurance. The backbone of all weight training.

Pumped — Slang meaning the muscles have been made large by increasing blood supply to them through exercise.

Pumping Iron — Phrase that has been in use since the 1950s, but recently greatly popularized. Lifting weights.

Quads — Abbreviation for *quadriceps femoris* muscles, muscles on top of legs, which consist of 4 parts (heads).

Quality Training — Training just before bodybuilding competition where intervals between sets are drastically reduced to enhance muscle mass and density, and low-calorie diet is followed to reduce body fat.

Repetition — One complete movement of an exercise.

Rep Out — Repeat the same exercise over and over until you are unable to do any more.

Reps — Abbreviation for REPETITIONS.

Rest Interval — Pause between sets of an exercise which allows muscles to recover partially before beginning next set.

Rest Pause Training — Training method where you press out one difficult repetition, then replace bar in stands, then after a 10-20 second rest, do another rep, etc.

Ripped — Slang meaning extreme muscularity.

'Roid — Slang for ANABOLIC STEROID.

Set — Fixed number of repetitions. For example, 10 repetitions may comprise one set.

Slow-Twitch — Muscle cells that contract slowly, are resistant to fatigue and are utilized in endurance activities such as long-distance running, cycling or swimming.

Snatch — Olympic lift where weight is lifted from floor to overhead, (with arms extended) in one continuous movement (see also CLEAN AND JERK).

Spot — Assist if called upon by someone performing an exercise.

Spotter — Person who watches a partner closely to see if any help is needed during a specific exercise.

Steroids — See ANABOLIC STEROIDS.

Sticking Point — Most difficult part of a movement.

Straight Sets — Groups of repetitions (SETS) interrupted by only brief pauses (30-90 seconds).

Strength — The ability of a muscle to produce maximum amount of force.

Strength Training — Using resistance weight training to build maximum muscle force.

Stretch Marks — Tears (slight scars) in skin caused if muscle or fat tissue has expanded in volume faster than skin can grow.

Striations — Grooves or ridge marks seen under the skin, the ultimate degree of muscle definition.

Super Set — Alternating back and forth between two exercises until the prescribed number of sets is complete.

Tendon — A band or cord of strong, fibrous tissue that connects muscles to bone.

Testosterone — Principle male hormone that accelerates tissue growth and stimulates blood flow.

Thick Skin — Smooth skin caused by too much fatty tissue between the layers of muscle and beneath skin.

Tone — See MUSCLE TONE.

Training Effect — Increase in functional capacity of muscles as result of increased (overload) placed upon them.

Training Straps — Cotton or leather straps wrapped around wrists, then under and over a bar held by clenched hands to aid in certain lifts (rowing, chin-ups, shrugs, dead lifts, cleans, etc.) where you might lose your grip before working muscle to desired capacity.

Training to Failure — Continuing a set until it is impossible to complete another rep without assistance.

Traps — Abbreviation for trapezius muscles, the largest muscles of the back and neck that draw head backward and rotate scapula.

Trimming Down — To gain hard muscular appearance by losing body fat.

Tri Sets — Alternating back and forth between 3 exercises until prescribed number of sets is completed.

Universal Machine — One of several types of machines where weights are on a track or rails and are lifted by levers or pulleys.

Upper Abs — Abbreviation for abdominal muscles above navel.

Variable Resistance — Strength training equipment where the machine varies amount of weight being lifted to match strength curve for a particular exercise — usually with a cam, lever arm or hydraulic cylinder. Also referred to as "ACCOMMODATING RESISTANCE."

Vascularity — Increase in size and number of observable veins. Highly desirable in bodybuilding.

Veining — See VASCULARITY.

Weight Training Belt — Thick leather belt used to support lower back. Used while doing squats, military presses, dead lifts, bent rowing, etc.□

BIBLIOGRAPHY

Aerobic Tennis by Bill Wright. Shelter Publications, Bolinas, CA, 1983.

Aerobic Weight Training—The Athlete's Guide to Improved Sports Performance by Frederick C. Hatfield, Ph.D. Contemporary Books, Chicago, IL, 1983.

Anabolic Steroids and Sports by James E. Wright, Ph.D. Sports Science Consultants, Natick, MA, 1978.

The Athlete's Guide to Sports Psychology: Mental Skills for Physical People by Dorothy V. Harris, Ph.D., and Bette L. Harris, Ed.D. Leisure Press, New York, NY, 1984.

Bodybuilding—An Illustrated History by David Webster. Arco Publishing, Inc., New York, NY, 1979.

Competitive Swimming Manual for Coaches and Swimmers by James E. Counsilman. Counsilman Co., Bloomington, IL, 1977.

The Complete Guide to Power Training by Frederick C. Hatfield, Ph.D. Fitness Systems, New Orleans, LA, 1983. Sports Conditioning Services, 5542 South Street, Lakewood, CA, 90713.

Death in the Locker Room—Steroids & Sports by Bob Goldman with Patricia Bush, Ph.D., and Dr. Ronald Katz. Icarus Press, South Bend, IN, 1984.

Essential Exercises for the Child-bearing Year by Elizabeth Noble. Houghton Mifflin Co., Boston, MA, 1982.

Exercise Physiology—Energy, Nutrition and Human Performance by William D. McCardle, Frank Katch and Victor L. Katch. Lea & Febiger, Philadelphia, PA, 1981.

Exercise Physiology—Human Bioenergetics and Its Applications by George A. Brooks and Thomas D. Fahey. John Wiley & Sons, Inc., New York, NY, 1984.

Fit or Fat by Covert Bailey. Houghton Mifflin Co., Boston, MA, 1978.

Fitness on the Road—Where to Stay to Stay Fit by John Winsor. Shelter Publications, Bolinas, CA, 1986.

Food For Sport by Nathan J. Smith, M.D. Bull Publishing Co., Palo Alto, CA, 1976.

Galloway's Book on Running by Jeff Galloway. Shelter Publications, Bolinas, CA, 1984.

Getting Built—A Women's Bodybuilding Program for Strength, Beauty and Fitness by Dr. Lynne Pirie with Bill Reynolds. Warner Books, New York, NY, 1984.

Getting Strong—A Woman's Guide to Realizing Her Physical Potential by Kathryn Lance. The Bobbs-Merrill Co., Inc., New York, NY, 1978.

How to Lower Your Fat Thermostat—The No-Diet Reprogramming Plan for Lifelong Weight Control by Dennis Remington, M.D., Garth Fisher, Ph.D., and Edward Parent, Ph.D. Vitality House International, Inc., Provo, UT, 1983.

Jane Brody's Nutrition Book—A Lifetime Guide to Good Eating for Better Health and Weight Control by Jane Brody. W. W. Norton & Co., New York, NY, 1981.

Keys to the Inner Universe—Encyclopedia of Weight Training by Bill Pearl. Bill Pearl Enterprises, Phoenix, OR, 1982.

The Lean Advantage by Clarence Bass. Ripped Enterprises, Albuquerque, NM, 1984.

Lift Your Way to Youthful Fitness—The Comprehensive Guide to Weight Training by Jan and Terry Todd. Little Brown & Co., Boston, MA, 1985.

Lisa Lyon's Body Magic by Lisa Lyon and Douglas Kent Hall. Bantam Books, New York, NY, 1981.

Listen to Your Pain by Ben E. Benjamin, Ph.D., with Gale Borden, M.D. Penguin Books, New York, NY, 1984.

Maggie's Back Book—Healing the Hurt in Your Lower Back by Maggie Lettvin. Houghton Mifflin Co., Boston, MA, 1976.

Over the Hill, But Not Out to Lunch! by Lloyd Kahn, Jr. Shelter Publications, Bolinas, CA, 1986.

Peak Performance—Mental Training Techniques of the World's Greatest Athletes by Charles A. Garfield, Ph.D., and Hal Z. Bennett. J.P. Tarcher, Inc., Los Angeles, CA, 1984.

Physiology of Exercise by Herbert A. deVries. Wm. Brown Co., Dubuque, IA, 1980.

Physiology of Fitness by Brian Sharkey. Human Kinetics Publishers, Inc., Champaign, IL, 1984.

The Practical Use of Anabolic Steroids with Athletes by Robert Kerr, M.D. San Gabriel, CA, 1982.

Pumping Iron II: The Unprecedented Woman by Charles Gaines and George Butler. Simon & Schuster, New York, NY, 1984.

The Rand McNally Atlas of the Body Ed. by Claire Rayner. Rand McNally & Co., New York, NY, 1980.

Reps!—Building Massive Muscle! by Robert Kennedy. Sterling Publishing Co., Inc., New York, NY, 1985.

Ripped—The Sensible Way to Achieve Ultimate Muscularity by Charles Bass. Ripped Enterprises, Albuquerque, NM, 1980.

Sports Psyching—Playing Your Best Game All of the Time by Thomas A. Tatko and Umberto Tosi. J.P. Tarcher, Inc., Los Angeles, CA, 1976.

Staying With It by John Jerome. The Viking Press, New York, NY, 1984.

Strength Training Principles—How to Get the Most Out of Your Workouts by Ellington Darden, Ph.D. Anna Publishing, Inc., Winter Park, FL, 1977.

Stretching by Bob Anderson. Shelter Publications, Bolinas, CA, 1980.

The Strongest Shall Survive—Strength Training for Football by Bill Starr. Port City Press, Inc., Baltimore, MD, 1978.

The Sweet Spot in Time by John Jerome. Avon Books, New York, NY, 1980.

Textbook of Medical Physiology by Arthur C. Guyton, M.D. W.B. Saunders Co., Philadelphia, PA, 1986. □

EXERCISE INDEX—DRAWINGS

You can use this index to look up any of the exercises in the book. Exercises appear *in this order* on the pages indicated. You can also take this index into the gym for ideas on the variety of exercises for specific body parts.

Abdominals ● *pp. 190-201*

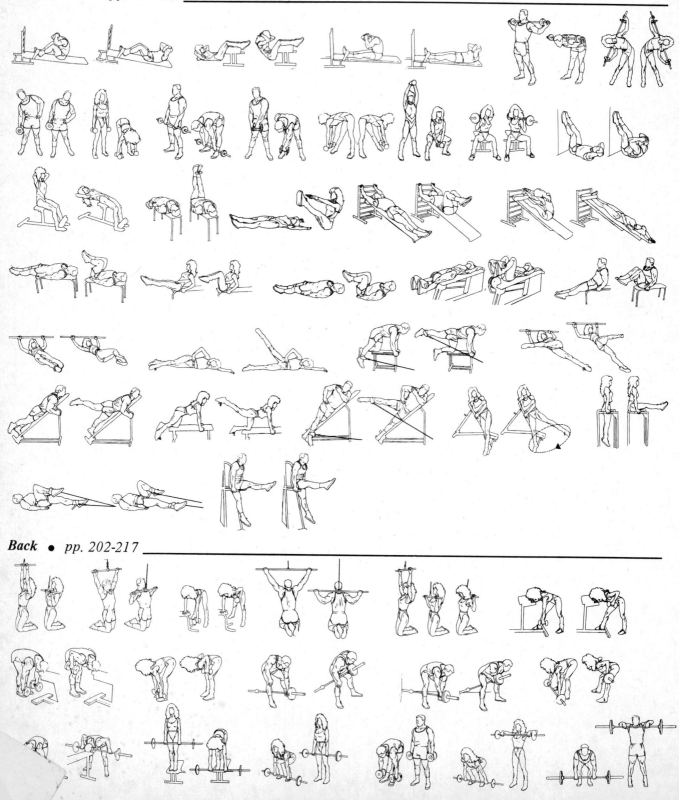

Back ● *pp. 202-217*

Back *(continued)* ● *pp.208-217*

Biceps ● *pp. 218-235*

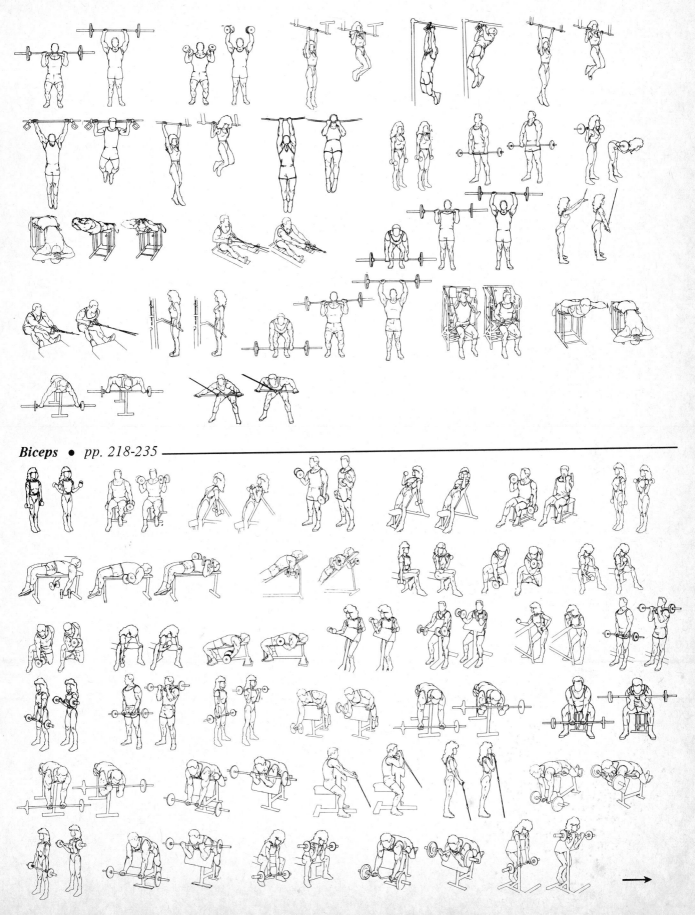

Biceps (continued) ● *pp.230-235*

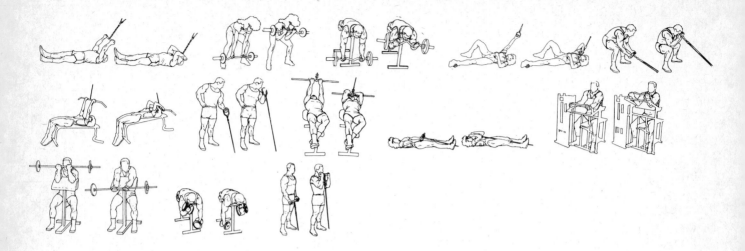

Calves ● *pp. 236-243*

Chest ● *pp. 244-257*

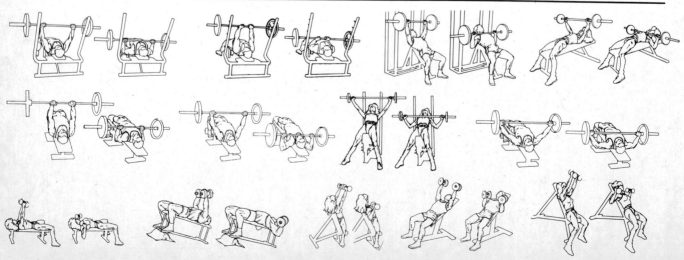

Chest *(continued)* ● pp. 249-257

Forearms ● pp. 258-265

Neck ● pp. 266-271

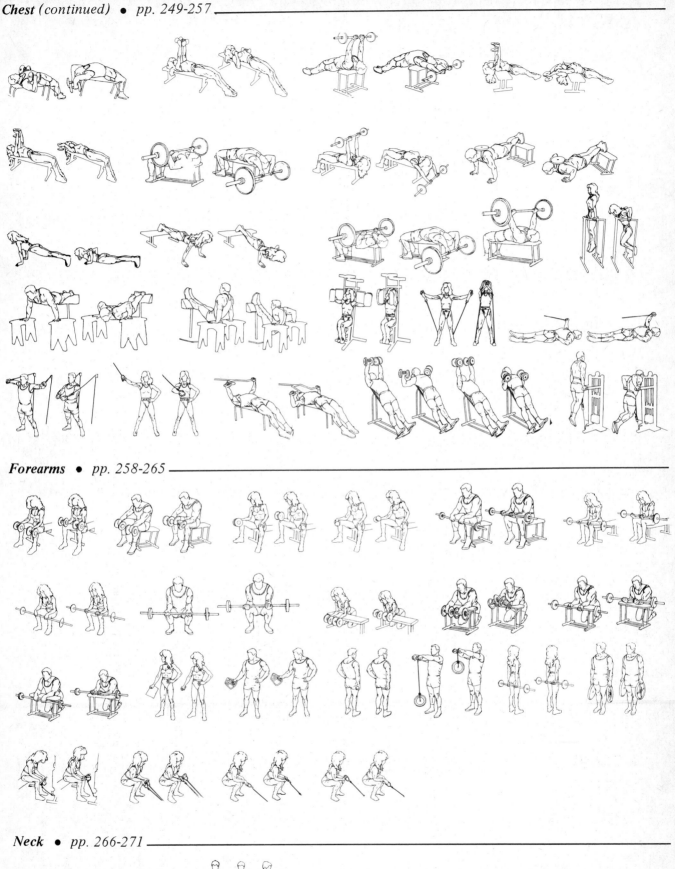

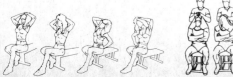

Neck (continued) ● pp.267-271

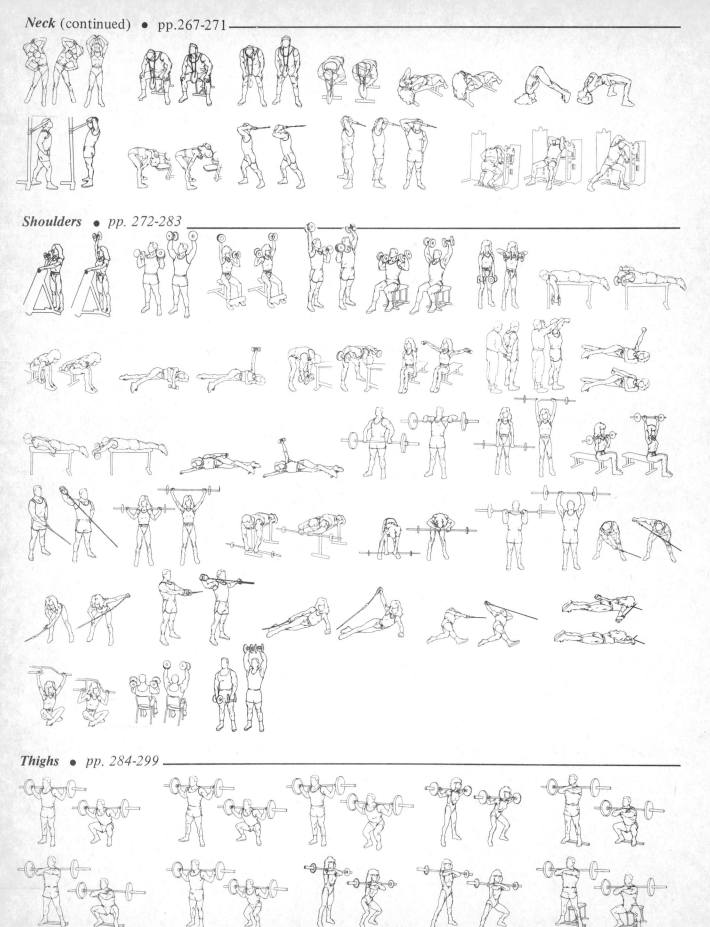

Shoulders ● pp. 272-283

Thighs ● pp. 284-299

Exercise Index — Drawings

Thighs (continued) • pp. 287-299

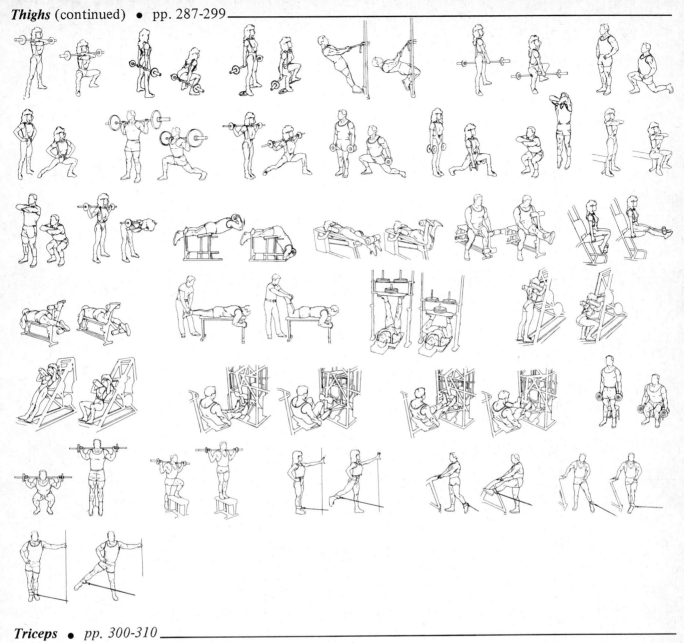

Triceps • *pp. 300-310*

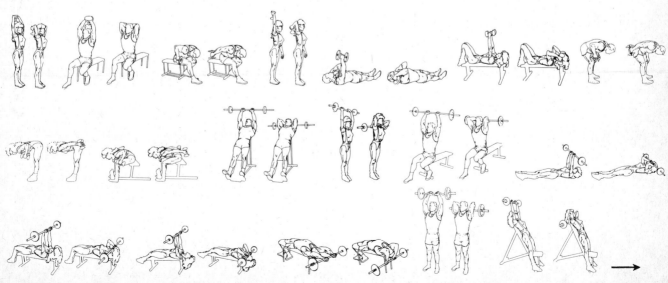

Triceps (continued) ● pp. 306 - 310

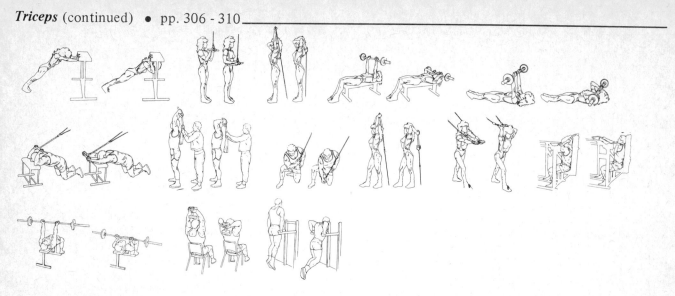

Nautilus Machine Exercises ● pp. 313 - 319

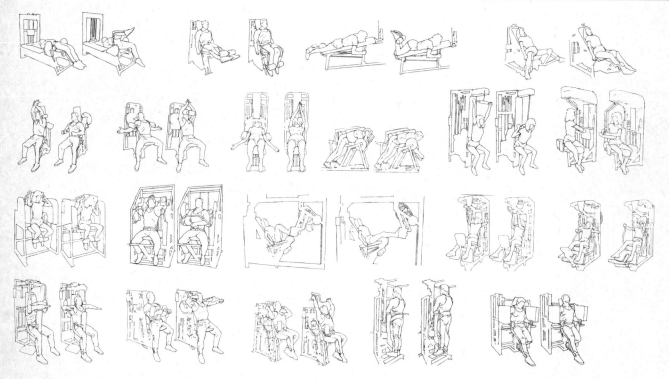

Universal Machine Exercises ● pp. 322 - 323

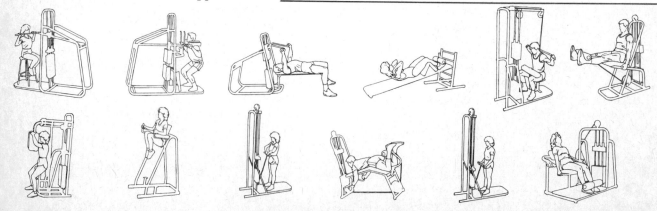

EXERCISE INDEX — TITLES

Back-Kick
-Incline Back-Kick, 199
-Kneeling Back-Kick, 199
-Kneeling Low-Pulley Back-Kick, 198

Bench Press
-Bench Press on Universal Machine, 256
-Close-Grip Barbell Bench Press, 244
-Decline Barbell Bench Press to Neck, 246
-Medium-Grip Barbell Bench Press, 244
-Medium-Grip Decline Barbell Bench Press, 246
-Medium-Grip Incline Barbell Bench Press, 245
-Wide-Grip Barbell Bench Press, 245
-Wide-Grip Decline Barbell Bench Press, 247
-Wide-Grip Incline Barbell Bench Press, 247

Bench Press, Triceps
-Reverse Medium-Grip Triceps Bench Press, 309

Bend to Opposite Foot
-Alternated Twisting Dumbbell Bend to Opposite Foot, 193
-Bend to Opposite Foot, 192

Calf Stretch
-Standing Calf Stretch Against Wall, 237
-Standing One-Legged Calf Stretch Against Wall, 237

Chin, Front
-Close-Grip Front Chin, 209
-Medium-Grip Front Chin, 210
-Reverse Close-Grip Front Chin, 211

Chin, Rear
-Medium-Grip Rear Chin, 211
-Wide-Grip Rear Chin, 210

Chin, V-Bar
-Close-Grip V-Bar Chin, 209

Compound
-Incline Compound, 257

Cross-Over
-Pec Cross-Over on High Pulley, 256

Curl, Barbell
-Flat Preacher Bench Close-Grip Barbell Curl, 227
-Flat Preacher Bench Medium-Grip Barbell Curl, 229
-Lying High Bench Close-Grip Barbell Curl, 227
-Lying High Bench Medium-Grip Barbell Curl, 226
-Scott Bench Close-Grip Barbell Curl, 234
-Seated Close-Grip Concentrated Barbell Curl, 226
-Standing Close-Grip Barbell Curl, 225
-Standing Close-Grip Barbell Curl Against Wall, 224
-Standing Medium-Grip Barbell Curl, 225

Curl, Dumbbell
-Flat Preacher Bench One-Arm Dumbbell Curl, 225
-Incline Alternated Dumbbell Curl, 219
-Incline Dumbbell Curl, 218
-Kneeling Concentrated Dumbbell Curl, 222
-Kneeling Isolated Dumbbell Curl, 221

-Lying High Bench Alternated Dumbbell Curl, 234
-Lying-Supine Dumbbell Curl, 223
-Lying-Supine 4x4x4 Dumbbell Curl, 220
-Seated Alternated Dumbbell Curl, 219
-Seated Concentrated Dumbbell Curl, 222
-Seated Dumbbell Curl, 218
-Seated Isolated Dumbbell Curl, 222
-Seated Scott Bench Two-Arm Dumbbell Curl, 223
-Standing Alternated Dumbbell Curl, 219
-Standing Dumbbell Curl, 220
-Standing One-Arm Dumbbell Curl Over Incline Bench, 224
-Standing Scott Bench One-Arm Dumbbell Curl, 223

Curl, Easy-Curl-Bar
-Flat Preacher Bench Close-Grip Easy-Curl-Bar Curl, 228
-Flat Preacher Bench Medium-Grip Easy-Curl-Bar Curl, 231
-Lying High Bench Medium-Grip Easy-Curl-Bar Curl, 230
-Scott Bench Close-Grip Easy-Curl-Bar Curl, 230
-Seated Close-Grip Easy-Curl-Bar Concentrated Curl, 231
-Standing Close-Grip, Easy-Curl-Bar Curl Against Wall, 224
-Standing Medium-Grip Easy-Curl-Bar Curl, 229

Curl, Inner Biceps
-Incline Inner-Biceps Curl, 221
-Seated Inner-Biceps Curl, 221
-Standing Inner-Biceps Curl, 218

Curl, Low Pulley
-Seated Scott Bench Bar Curl on Low Pulley, 228
-Squatting Concentrated Bar Curl on Low Pulley, 232
-Standing One-Arm Curl on Low Pulley, 232

Curl, Machines
-Lying Flat Bench Close-Grip Bar Curl on Lat Machine, 232
-Seated Medium-Grip Curl on Biceps Machine, 233
-Standing Bar Curl on Universal Machine, 228
-Lying Bar Curl on Universal Machine, 233

Curl, Thigh Biceps
-Assisted Thigh Biceps Curl, 294
-One-at-a-Time Biceps Curl on Leg Extension Machine, 293
-Thigh Biceps Curl on Leg Extension Machine, 292

Dead Lift
-Barbell Dead Lift, 206
-Stiff-Legged Barbell Dead Lift, 192
-Stiff-Legged Barbell Dead Lift off Bench, 206
-Stiff-Legged Dumbbell Dead Lift, 206

Deltoid Circle, Rear
-Lying Floor Low-Pulley Rear Deltoid Circle, 281
-Lying Rear Deltoid Circle, 276

Deltoid Lateral Pull
-Standing High-Pulley Rear Deltoid Lateral Pull, 280

Deltoid Pump
-Standing Deltoid Pump, 276

Deltoid Raise, Front
-Standing Dumbbell Straight-Arm Front Deltoid Raise, 283

Dips
-Dips, 253
-Dips with Weight, 257
-Feet Elevated Dip Between Stools, 310
-Reverse Grip Dip, 254

Fly
-Decline Dumbbell Fly, 248
-Incline Dumbbell Fly, 249

Forearm
-Hand-Gripper Forearm Exercise, 262
-Newspaper Hand and Forearm Exercise, 262

Good Morning
-Barbell Good Morning, 191
-Stiff-Legged Barbell Good Morning, 212

Hand Squeeze
-Rubber Ball Hand Squeeze, 262
-Standing Olympic Plate Hand Squeeze, 263

High Pull
-Medium Grip High Pull, 207
-Wide-Grip High Pull, 207

Hip Abduction, 299

Hip Adduction, 298

Hip Extension, 298

Hip Flexion, 298

Hip Roll, 197

Hyperextension
-Dumbbell Hyperextension, 292
-Hyperextension, 216
-Twisting Hyperextension, 213

Jefferson Lift, 288

Lat Pull-Down, Front
-Close-Grip Front Lat Pull-Down, 202
-Straight-Arm Close-Grip Lat Pull-Down, 214
-Wide-Grip Front Lat Pull-Down, 202

Lat Pull-Down, Front-to-Rear
-Medium-Grip Front-to-Rear Lat Pull-Down, 203

Lat Pull-Down, Rear
-Wide-Grip Rear Lat Pull-Down, 203

Lat Pull-In
-Seated Two-Arm High Lat Pull-In, 214
-Seated Two-Arm Low Lat Pull-In, 214
-Standing Bent-Over Wide-Grip Barbell Lat Pull-In on High Pulley, 216

Lat Pull-Up
-Lying High Bench Wide-Grip Barbell Pull-Up, 217

Lateral, 248
ley Chest Lateral, 256

-Incline Lateral, 248
-Low-Pulley Chest Lateral, 255
-Lying Low-Pulley One-Arm Chest Lateral, 255

Lateral, Side
-Bent-Over Low-Pulley Side Lateral, 280

Lateral Raise, Dumbbell-Held-to-the-Side
-Lying Floor Dumbbell-Held-to-the-Side Lateral Raise, 277

Lateral Raise, Side
-Lying Floor Side Lateral Raise, 276
-Seated Side Lateral Raise, 275

Leg Circle
-Incline Side Leg Circle, 200

Leg Crossover
-Lying Leg Crossover, 198

Leg Press, Machines
-Medium-Stance Lower-Pad Leg Press on Universal Machine, 296
-Medium-Stance Top-Pad Leg Press on Universal Machine, 296
-Wide-Stance Leg Press on Wall-Type Leg Press Machine, 294

Leg Pull-In
-Alternated Low-Pulley Leg Pull-In, 201
-Extension Machine Leg Pull-In, 197
-Flat Bench Leg Pull-In, 196
-Incline Leg Pull-In, 195
-Seated Flat Bench Leg Pull-In, 196

Leg Raise, Front
-Alternated Dip Stand Leg Raise, 201,
-Dip Stand Leg Raise, 201,
-Flat Bench Weighted Leg Raise, 200

Leg Raise, Side
-Incline Low Pulley Side Leg Raise, 200
-Lying Side Leg Raise, 198

Leg Tuck
-Seated Flat Bench Leg Tuck, 197

Lunge, Front
-Alternated Barbell Front Lunge, 289
-Barbell Front Lunge, 290
-Dumbbell Front Lunge, 290
-Freehand Front Lunge, 289

Lunge, Side
-Dumbbell Side Lunge, 290
-Freehand Side Lunge, 289

Neck Resistance
-Lying-Face-Down Barbell-Plate Neck Resistance, 269
-Lying-Supine Barbell-Plate Neck Resistance, 269
-Seated Freehand Neck Resistance, 266
-Standing Rubber-Inner-Tube Neck Resistance, 270
-Standing Towel Neck Resistance, 267

Neck Resistance, Buddy-System
-Lying Flat Bench Buddy-System Neck Resistance, 267
-Seated Buddy-System Neck Resistance, 266

Neck Resistance, Head Harness
-Lying Head-Harness Barbell-Plate Neck Resistance, 268

-Seated Head-Harness Barbell-Plate Neck
Resistance, 268
-Standing Head-Harness Barbell-Plate Neck
Resistance, 268
-Standing Head-Harness High-Pulley Neck
Resistance, 270

Neck Resistance, Machines
-Leg-Extension Machine Neck Resistance, 270
-Seated Neck Resistance on Paramount
Neck Machine, 271
-Standing Head-Harness Neck Resistance on Universal
Leg-Extension-Machine, 271

Power Clean
-Barbell Power Clean, 207
-Barbell Power Clean and Jerk, 215
-Barbell Power Clean and Press, 213

Press, Behind Neck
-Standing Barbell Press Behind Neck, 278

Press, Dumbbell
-Flat Dumbbell Press, 250
-Incline Dumbbell Press, 249
-Seated Back-Supported Palms-In Dumbbell Press, 282
-Seated Palms-In Alternated Dumbbell Press, 273
-Seated Palms-Out Dumbbell Press, 273
-Standing Palm-In One-Arm Dumbbell Press, 272
-Standing Palms-In Alternated Dumbbell Press, 273
-Standing Palms-In Dumbbell Press, 272

Press, Inner-Pec
-Inner-Pec Press on Inner-Pec Machine, 255

Press, Military
-Seated Barbell Military Press, 278
-Standing Military Press, 279

Press, Universal Machine
-Seated-Facing-Out Press on Universal Machine, 282

Pullover, Barbell
-Bent-Arm Barbell Pullover, 251
-Bent-Arm Barbell Pullover and Press, 253
-Close-Grip Straight-Arm Barbell Pullover
Across Bench, 250
-Medium-Grip Straight-Arm Barbell Pullover, 251

Pullover, Dumbbell
-Bent-Arm Dumbbell Pullover, 249
-Straight-Arm Dumbbell Pullover, 251
-Straight-Arm Dumbbell Pullover Across Bench, 250

Pullover, Machine
-Pullover on Nautilus Machine, 216

Push Press
-Barbell Push Press, 208
-Dumbbell Push Press, 208

Push-Ups
-Medium-Grip Push-Ups Between Stools, 254
-Medium-Grip Push-Ups, Feet on Bench, 252
-Medium-Grip Push-Ups on Floor, 252
-Weighted Medium-Grip Push-Ups, Feet on Bench, 252

Raise, Deltoid
-Lying Floor Low-Pulley Deltoid Raise, 281
-Standing Low-Pulley Deltoid Raise, 278

Raise, Front Barbell
-Bent-Over Close-Grip Straight-Arm Barbell
Front Raise, 279
-Standing Medium-Grip Front Barbell Raise, 277

Raise, Rear Deltoid
-Bent-Over Head-Supported Dumbbell Rear
Deltoid Raise, 275
-Bent-Over Low-Pulley Rear Deltoid Raise, 280
-Bent-Over One-Arm Rear Deltoid Raise, 282
-Lying Close-Grip Straight-Arm Barbell Rear
Deltoid Raise, 279
-Lying Floor Low-Pulley Across-Body Rear
Deltoid Raise, 281
-Lying on Floor Across-Body Rear Deltoid Raise, 275
-Lying Rear Deltoid Raise, 274
-Seated Bent-Over Rear Deltoid Raise, 274

Rowing, Barbell
-Bent-Over Head-Supported Wide-Grip
Barbell Rowing, 205
-Bent-Over Wide-Grip Barbell Rowing, 205
-Medium-Grip Barbell Upright Rowing, 277

Rowing, Dumbbell
-Bent-Over Dumbbell Rowing, 203
-Bent-Over Head-Supported Two-Dumbbell
Rowing, 204
-Bent-Over Two-Arm Dumbbell Rowing, 204
-Hand-on-Bench One-Arm Dumbbell Rowing, 202
-Standing Dumbbell Upright Rowing, 274

Rowing, Long Bar
-Standard Bent-Over One-Arm Long Bar Rowing, 204
-Standard Bent-Over Two-Arm Long Bar Rowing, 205

Shoulder Shrug
-Barbell Shoulder Shrug, 212
-Dumbbell Shoulder Shrug, 212
-Universal Machine Shoulder Shrug, 215

Side Bend
-Barbell Side Bend, 191
-Dumbbell Side Bend, 191

Sit-Up
-Bent Knee Sit-Up, 190
-Feet-Against-Wall Sit-Up, 194
-Heel-High Sit-Up, 190
-Incline Arms Extended Sit-Up, 195
-Jackknife Sit-Up, 195
-Over-a-Bench Sit-Up, 194
-Sit-Up, 190

Squat
-Flat-Footed Medium-Stance Barbell Squat, 284
-Flat-Footed Wide-Stance Barbell Squat, 284

Squat, Back
-Flat-Footed Wide-Stance Barbell Back Squat, 287

Squat, Breathing
-Barbell Breathing Squat, 286

Squat, Freehand
-Flat-Footed Medium-Stance Freehand Squat, 291

Squat, Front
-Flat-Footed Wide-Stance Barbell Front Squat, 287
-Heels-Elevated Medium-Stance Barbell Front
Squat, 285
-Heels-Elevated Wide-Stance Barbell Front Squat, 285

Squat, Hack
-Heels-Elevated Wide-Stance Barbell Hack Squat, 288
-Medium-Stance Hack Squat on Ram Thrust Machine, 295

Squat, Half
-Flat-Footed Medium-Stance Barbell Half-Squat, 284
-Flat-Footed Wide-Stance Barbell Half-Squat, 285
-Wide-Stance Half-Squat on Thrust Machine, 295

Squat, Jump
-Barbell Jump Squat, 297
-Freehand Jump Squat, 291

Squat, Sissy
-Close-Stance Sissy Squat, 288

Squat, to Bench
-Flat-Footed Medium-Stance Dumbbell Squat to Bench, 297
-Flat-Footed Medium-Stance Freehand Squat to Bench, 291
-Heels-Elevated Wide-Stance Barbell Front Squat to Bench, 287

Step-Ups with Barbell, 297

Thigh Extension on Leg Extension Machine
-One-at-a-Time Thigh Extension on Leg Extension Machine, 293
-Thigh Extension on Leg Extension Machine, 293

Toe Raise
-Lying Supine Toe Raise on Wall Leg Press Machine, 242
-Seated Barbell Toe Raise, 237
-Seated Lower Pad Toe Raise on Universal Leg Press Machine, 243
-Seated Negative-Resistance Toe Raise on Universal Leg Press Machine, 239
-Seated Toe Raise on Nautilus-Type Machine, 238
-Standing Barbell Toe Raise, 242
-Standing Toe Raise on Power Rack, 239
-Standing Toe Raise on Ram Thrust Machine, 241
-Standing Toe Raise on Wall Calf Machine, 238
-Toe Raise on Seated Calf Machine, 242

Toe Raise, Donkey
-Donkey One-Legged Toe Raise, 240
-Donkey Toe Raise, 240

Toe Raise, One-Legged
-Lying Face Down One-Legged Toe Raise on Wall Leg Press Machine, 239
-Seated Dumbbell One-Legged Toe Raise, 236
-Standing Dumbbell One-Legged Toe Raise, 236
-Standing Freehand One-Legged Toe Raise
-Standing One-Legged Toe Raise on Power Rack, 241
-Standing One-Legged Toe Raise on Ram Thrust Machine, 243

Triceps Curl, Barbell
-Incline Close-Grip Barbell Triceps Curl, 303
-Lying Floor Close-Grip Barbell Triceps Curl to Forehead, 304
-Lying-Supine Close-Grip Barbell Triceps Curl to Forehead, 304

-Lying-Supine, Close-Grip Barbell Triceps Curl to Chin, 304
-Seated Close-Grip Barbell Triceps Curl, 303
-Standing Close-Grip Barbell Triceps Curl, 303

Triceps Curl, Dumbbell
-Lying Floor One-Arm Dumbbell Triceps Curl, 301
-Lying-Supine Two-Arm Dumbbell Triceps Curl, 301
-Seated Back-Supported Dumbbell Triceps Curl, 310
-Seated Dumbbell Triceps Curl, 300
-Standing Dumbbell Triceps Curl, 300
-Standing One-Arm Dumbbell Triceps Curl, 301

Triceps Curl, Easy-Curl-Bar
-Incline Close-Grip Easy-Curl-Bar Triceps Curl, 305
-Lying Floor Close-Grip Easy-Curl-Bar Triceps Curl to Forehead, 307
-Lying-Supine Close-Grip Easy-Curl-Bar Triceps Curl to Forehead, 307
-Standing Close-Grip Easy-Curl-Bar Triceps Curl, 305

Triceps Curl, High Pulley
-Kneeling Concentrated Triceps Curl on High Pulley, 308

Triceps Curl, Low Pulley
-Standing Face-Away Low-Pulley One-Arm Triceps Curl, 306

Triceps Curl, Nautilus
-Triceps Curl on Nautilus Machine, 309

Triceps Curl, Towel
-Standing Towel Triceps Curl, 308
-Standing Towel Triceps Curl on Low Wall Pulley, 308

Triceps Extension
-Freehand Triceps Extension, 306
-Kneeling Head-Supported Close-Grip Triceps Extension on High Pulley, 307
-Seated Bent-Over One-Arm Dumbbell Triceps Extension, 300
-Seated Bent-Over Two-Arm Dumbbell Triceps Extension, 302
-Standing Bent-Over One-Arm Dumbbell Triceps Extension, 302
-Standing Bent-Over Two-Arm Dumbbell Triceps Extension, 302
-Standing Face-Away Two-Arm Bar Triceps Extension on High Pulley, 309

Triceps Kick Back
-Lying-Supine Close-Grip Barbell Triceps Kick Back, 305

Triceps Press-Down
-Standing Close-Grip Triceps Press-Down on Lat Machine, 306

Twist
-Seated Barbell Twist, 193

Warm-Up
-Warm-Up (Dumbbell Swing-Through), 193

Wrestler's Bridge , 269

Wrist Curl, Arms Extended
  -Standing Arms-Extended Wrist-Roller
  Wrist Curl, 263

Wrist Curl, Palms-Down
  -Palms-Down Barbell-Over-a-Bench Wrist Curl, 261
  -Palms-Down Two-Dumbbells Over-a-Bench
  Wrist Curl, 261
  -Seated One-Arm Dumbbell Palm-Down
  Wrist Curl, 259
  -Seated Palms-Down Barbell Wrist Curl, 259
  -Seated Two-Dumbbell Palms-Down Wrist Curl, 258
  -Squatting One-Arm Palms-Down Low-Pulley
  Wrist Curl, 265
  -Squatting Palms-Down Barbell Wrist Curl, 260

Wrist Curl, Palms-Up
  -Palms-Up Barbell Over-a-Bench Wrist Curl, 261
  -Palms-Up Two-Dumbbells Over-a-Bench
  Wrist Curl, 260
  -Seated One-Arm Dumbbell Palms-Up, Wrist Curl, 258
  -Seated Palms-Up Barbell Wrist Curl, 259
  -Seated Two-Arm Palms-Up Low Pulley
  Wrist Curl, 264
  -Seated Two-Dumbbell Palms-Up Wrist Curl, 258
  -Squatting One-Arm Palms-Up Low-Pulley
  Wrist Curl, 264
  -Squatting Palms-Up Barbell Wrist Curl, 260
  -Squatting Two-Arm Palms-Up Low Pulley
  Wrist Curl, 264
  -Standing Palms-Up Barbell-Behind-Back
  Wrist Curl, 263 □

INDEX

Abbenda, Joe, 352
accommodating resistance, *see* machines, isokinetic
acetaminophen, 369
actin, 360
Adams, Sam, 156
adaption, 362
aerobic exercises, *see* exercises, aerobic
aerobic vs. anaerobic fitness, 73
aging, 342
agonist/antagonist muscles, 70, 372
alarm, *see* stress, psychological
Alexeev, Vasily, 372
alignment (skeletal), *see* biomechanical position
all or none concept, 70
Alpine skiing, *see* skiing (downhill) programs
Amateur Athletic Union, 411
amenorrhea, 27
American Continental Weightlifters' Association, 410
American Orthopaedic Society for Sports Medicine (AOSSM), 338
amino acids, 375
amphetamines, 391
anabolic steroids, 388
    black market, 388
    dangers, 392-395
    Dianabol, 390
    effectiveness, 388, 392
    injectible, 390
    medical supervision, 388
    opinions, 393
    oral, 390
    placebo effect, 388
    protein synthesis, 390
    safety, 392
    side effects, 391-394
    spread, 391-392
    testing, 391
    women, 394
anaerobic exercises, *see* exercises, anaerobic
Anderson, Bob, 18, 326, 342
antagonist muscles, *see* agonist/antagonist muscles
anti-doping laws, 391
anti-inflammatory drugs, 369
anticipation, *see* quickness
anxiety, *see* stress (psychological)
arms, 177, 257, *see also* biceps; triceps
Ashley, Peter, 138
aspirin, 369
Athleta, 406
Athletes' Guide to Sports Psychology, The, 78
Atkins, John, 142
Atlas, Charles, 64, 413
atrophy, 70

B 12 (vitamin), 384
back, 178, 191, 198-199, 206-208, 212-213, 216
back injuries, 332
balance, *see* muscle, balance
ballistic movements, *see* movements (sports)
barbells, 64, 410
Barrilleaux, Doris, 28
bars, exercise, 401
baseball programs,
    in-season, 91
    off-season, 89
    pre-season, 90
basketball programs,
    in-season, 95
    off-season, 93
    pre-season, 94
Bass, Clarence, 54
Beal, Doug, 169
Beardsley, Eric, 9
Beck, Charles, 402
beginners, 33-34
beginning bodybuilding program, 82
bench press, 105-6, 125, 180
benches, exercises, 347
Berg-Hantel barbells, 410
biceps, 218-234, *see also* arms; exercises, biceps
bicycling, *see* cycling programs
biomechanical position, 62, 333, 372
blood pressure, 64, 344
blue-collar workers' program, 335
body fat, 27
bodybuilding, 411-413, *see also* posing; resistance training; weight training
bodybuilding,
    cautions, 52-53
    competitive, 44
    contests,
        1st international, 413
        early, 412
        Mr. America, 412
        Mr. Britain, 412
bodybuilding programs,
    advanced, 41-43
    beginning, 33, 37
        No. 1, 35
        No. 2, 36
    competitive, 44-47
    vs. general conditioning programs, 32
    intermediate, 38-40
Bortz, Dr. Walter, 342
bottom, 179
Bourne, Bob, 120
Bowen, Lori, 28
boxing program, 97-99
breathing, 19
Brignoli, Dougie, 340
British Amateur Weightlifters' Association, 410
Brody, Jane, 376
Brumbach, Katie, *see* Sandwina, Katie
burn-out, 339

bursitis, 367
butazone, 369
buttocks, *see* bottom

Calcium, 384-385
calories, 380
Calvert, Alan, 410
calves, 235-243
Camerarius, Joachim, 400
carbohydrates, 376
cardiovascular endurance, 57-58
cardiovascular training, 17, 33, 71-76, *see also* exercises, aerobic
catchers, 88
cheating, 66, *see also* techniques
chest, 180, 244-257, 314, 317
children, *see* injuries, children; weight training, children
Chui, Edward, 415
circuit training, 75, 106, 321-324
Colgan, Dr. Michael, 380
combat training, 400
Combes, Laura, 28
complementary proteins, 375, 384
complete proteins, 375, 384
compression treatment, 369
concentration, 77, 79, 177-180
concentric contraction, 70
conditioning, total, 71
confidence, 341
connective tissue, *see* ligaments; tendons
contraction, *see* muscles, contraction
cookbooks, vegetarian, 385
cortisone, 369
Coulter, Ottney, 411
Counsilman, Doc, 149
creatine phosphate (CP), 390
crew, *see* rowing programs
cross-country skiing, *see* skiing (cross-country) programs
Cybex machines, 64
cycling programs,
    endurance training, 100
    on-season, 102
    off-season, 101
    speed training, 100
    sprint training, 100
Cyclops, *see* Samson and Cyclops
Cyr, Louis, 409

Dance, aerobic, 86-87
deadlift, 125
DeLorme, Dr. Thomas L., 413-414
deltoids, *see* exercises, deltoids
Desaguliers, Dr. John Theophilus, 401
Desbonnet, Edmund, 404, 414
Deutscher Athletik Sport Verband, *see* German Athletic Association
developmental stretch, 326
diet, 27, 38, 41, 44, 183, 385
disaccharides, 376
discus, 399
distilled water, 379
diuretics, 395
downhill skiing, *see* skiing (downhill) programs
drugs, 391, 395

drugs, anti-inflammatory, 369
dumbbells, 64, 400, 402, 410
   see also free weights; halteres
Dunlap, Carla, 28
Dynamic Tension, 64, 413
   see also weight training, isometric

E asy stretch, 326
eccentric contraction, 70
education, physical, *see* physical
   education
electrolytes, 379
elevation treatment, 369
Elyot, Sir Thomas, 400
endurance, 64
   development, 17
   muscular, 57, 60
equipment, 413, *see also* free
   weights; machines
*Essential Exercises for the Child-
   Bearing Year*, 27
estrogen, 27
examination, medical, *see* medical
   examination
exercises,
   abdominals, 106-111, 190-201,
      316
      lower, 191, 194-197, 201
      upper, 190, 194-195
   aerobic, 62, 72-76, 84, 86-87,
      97, 105, 169, 183, 321
   anaerobic, 62, 73-74
   back, 191, 198-199, 206-208,
      212-213, 215-216, 313
   biceps, 218-234, 315
      inner, 218, 221
      lower, 223, 226-227, 229-231
      outer, 224-234
      upper, 232
   buttocks, 313, 317
   calves, 236-243, 291, 297, 319
   chest, 244-257
   deltoids, 272-283, 315, 317-318
      front, 272-275, 277-279,
         282-283
      outer, 272-273, 275-279,
         281-282
      rear, 274-276, 278-282
   forearms, 258-265
      inside, 258-261, 263-264
      outside, 258-261, 263, 265
   hands, 262
   hips, 198-200, 298-9
   isometric, 400
   lats, 202-205, 209-211, 214,
      216, 314-316
      lower, 202, 204-205, 209,
         211, 214
      upper, 202-203, 205,
         210-211, 214
   leg biceps, 206
   legs, 206-208, 213, 215
   lower back, 191, 198-199, 206,
      212-213, 216
   neck, 266-271, 319
   obliques, 191-193, 197-198,
      200, 298-299, 316
      rear, 298
   pectorals, 244-257, 314, 317
      inner, 255-256
      lower, 246-248, 254-255, 310

   outer, 244-248, 254
   upper, 244-245, 247-251,
      254-257
   plyometric, 68, 149, 169
   rhomboid, 318
   rib cage, 249-251, 253
   rotator cuff, 149
   shoulders, 272-283
   stretching, 327-330
      rules, 326
      summary, 330
   thigh biceps, 289-290, 292, 294,
      298, 313
   thighs, 206, 284-299, 317
      inner, 284-290, 294-295, 314
      outer, 284, 288, 298
      upper, 284-286, 291, 295-297,
         313
   trapezius, 212, 215, 274, 277,
      315, 318
   triceps, 257, 300-310, 315,
      317, 318
   Universal, 320-323
      see also weight training
exhaustion, 362

F ailure, 78
fast-twitch fibers, 62-63
fat,
   body, 27
   dietary, 376-377
fatigue fractures, 367
feats,
   Human Bridge, 405, 408
   Roman Column, 405
   wheel, 398
Federation Internationale
   Halterophile, *see* International
   Weightlifting Federation
Ferrigno, Lou, 413
fiber splitting (muscle), 360
fine tuning programs,
   arms, 177
   back, 178
   bottom, 179
   chest, 180
   legs, 181
   shoulders, 182
   stomach, 183
   tips, 177-83
fitness, 415
   basic qualities, 57
   work, 332-335
fitness kit, 142
Flex (periodical), 413
flexibility, 19, 58, 92, 97, 112
flexing, 49
focusing, 44
football program,
   in-season, 109-11
   off-season, 106-8
forced reps, 66, *see also* techniques
fractures, 339
Francis, Bev, 28
Franklin, Benjamin, 402
free weights, 64, 346-347, 350
   see also barbells, dumbbells
   auxiliary equipment, 346
   barbells, 346
   dumbbells, 347

   exercises for, 184-310
   Olympic barbells, 346

G alen, 400
Garfield, Dr. Charles, 77, 79
Gaskill, Steven, 138
general conditioning programs,
   82-83
   No. 1, 20-21
   No. 2, 22-23
   No. 3, 24-25
German Athletic Association,
   408-409
glucose, 376
gluteal muscles, *see* bottom
glycogen, 376
goalkeepers (soccer), 146
goals, 14-15, 33-34, 52
Goerner, Herman, 407, 411
Gold's Gym, 28
golf programs,
   in-season, 115
   off-season, 113
   pre-season, 114
Grimek, John, 8, 412
gymnastic programs,
   in-season, 119
   injury prevention, 116
   off-season, 117
   pre-season, 118
gymnasiums, 351-353
   19th century, 403
   commercial bodybuilding, 351
   first (U.S.), 402
   health studios, 351, 413
   home gyms, 82, 352-353, 355
   Nautilus, 351
   school weight rooms, 351-352
   spas, 351
   Triat's, 403-404
   YMCA, 351-352

H agerman, Topper, 142
Health and Strength (periodical),
   409
Health Lift, 403
health studios, *see* gyms
heart disease, 71
heat, 369
Hercules, 399
Hoffman, Bob, 413
home gym programs,
   barbell, 355
   dumbbell, 354
Homer, 398
hormone balance, 394
hormones, 390
Howard, John, 79, 100
Hugo, Victor, 342
human body,
   fuels, 374
   machine, 361
   systems, 358
Human Bridge, 405, 408
Human Chorionic Gonadotropin,
   (HCG), 395
Human Growth Hormone (HGH),
   392, 395
hyperplasia, 360
hypertrophy, 27, 70, 125
hyperventilation, 371
hypothalmus, 394

I ce hockey programs,
   in-season, 123
   off-season, 121
   pre-season, 122
ice treatment, 369
imagery, 79, *see also* focusing;
   visualization
incomplete proteins, 375
individuality, 70
industrial revolution, 406
infielders, 88
inflammation, *see* bursitis; injuries;
   tendinitis
injuries, *see also* rehabilitation
   children, 338
   chronic, 368
   dislocations, 367
   fractures, 339, 367
   lifting, 366
   lower back, 332
   prevention, 56, 106, 142,
      371-372
   rehabilitation, 56, 105, 370, 413
   shoulder, 182
   sprains, 366-367
   strains, 366-367
   treatment, 368-369
   weight training, 371
   work-related, 332
International Federation of
   Bodybuilders, 413
International Olympic
   Committee, 391
International Powerlifting
   Federation, 411
International Weightlifting
   Federation, 411
interval running, 169
Irish Games, 398
iron game, *see* weightlifting
Iron Man (periodical), 413

J ahn, Friedrich, 401
javelin, 399
Jones, Arthur, 349, 389
Jowett, George F., 410
jumping, *see* exercises, plyometric
jumping weights, *see* halteres

K arlsen, Torbjorn, 138
*Keys to the Inner Universe, An En-
   cyclopedia on Weight Training,* 8
kidney problems, 375
Klein, Sigmund, 410
Kono, Tommy, 9

L aLanne, Jack, 352, 414
lactic acid, 73, 367
lacto-ovo-vegetarianism, 383
LaSpina, Gina, 28
lats, *see* back; exercises, lats
laws, anti-doping, 391
Leers, Linda, 412
leg curls, 106-11
leg extensions, 106-11
legs, 181, *see also* calves; thighs
Liederman, Earle E., 413
lifting,
   everyday objects, 333-334
lifts,

continental, 409
partial, 402
ligaments, 361, 366, 370
Lisa Lyon's Body Magic, 28
lowering objects, 334
Lyon, Lisa, 28

M acFadden, Bernarr, 405-406, 412
machines,
   Biokinetic, 64
   biokinetic, 149
   Cybex, 64
   isokinetic, 349
   lifting, 402
   Nautilus, 64, 349-350
   strength testing, 404
   traditional, 348
   Universal, 320-323, 348, 414
macrominerals, 378
mail-order systems, 413-414
maturity (sexual), *see* puberty
McLish, Rachel, 28, 413
McMurtry, John, 142
meals, 377
measurements, 34
medical examinations, 14, 33, 71,
   344, 368
menstruation, 27
Mentzer, Mike, 349
middle age, *see* weight training,
   middle age
midfielders (soccer), 146
Milo Barbell Company, 410
Milo of Croton, 363, 398
mind/body integration, 77
minerals, *see* vitamins and minerals
mirror, 48
monosaccharides, 376
Montaigne, Michel de, 400
Moran, Gary T., 11, 15, 368
Morris, Bruce, 80
Morris, Jim, 11
motivation, 352
movement (sports), 350
Muller, Frederick, *see*
   Sandow, Eugen
multi-poundage system, 66 *see also*
   techniques
Muscle and Fitness (periodical), 413
musclebound myth, 414-415
muscles, 366
   balance, 60, 70, 372
   contraction, 70, 360
   fibers, 62-63, 359-360
   groups, 17
   growth, 360-364
   rehabilitation, 370
   tone, 33
   types, 358
   use and disuse, 70, 342-343
muscular endurance, 57, 60
myofibrils, 360
myofilaments, 360
myosin, 360

N arcissism, 41
National Strength Coaches
   Association (NSCA), 338
natural food, 381-382
Nautilus Machines, 349-350

Nautilus training,
   exercises, 313-319
   rules, 312
neck, 266-271
negative reps, 66, *see also*
   techniques
negative thinking, 78-79
nerves, 62, 360
Nilivar, 389
Noble, Elizabeth, 27
Nordic skiing, *see* skiing (cross-
   country) programs
nutrients, 374
nutrition, 374-385

O dysseus, 398
oil (skin), 50
Olympic barbells, *see* free weights
Olympic Games,
   ancient, 398, 412
   modern, 409, 411
   1972, 390
Olympic lifts, 411
organic food, 381-382
outfielders, 88
outside fullbacks (soccer), 146
over-50 program, 344
overhead (tennis), 153
overload principle, 53, 362-363
oxygen, 73

P almieri, Jerry, 172
Pan American Games (1983), 391
parents, 340-341
partial lifts, 66, 125, *see also*
   techniques
partners, *see* training partners
peaking, 125
Pearl, Bill
   anabolic steroids, 389
   astronaut trainer, 383
   early weight training, 8-9
   fitness store (Medford, OR), 11
   gym,
      Los Angeles, (CA), 10
      Pasadena, (CA), 349, 389
      Sacramento, (CA), 10, 348,
         377-378
   health food store, 377-378
   *Keys to the Inner Universe, An
      Encyclopedia on Weight
      Training,* 10-11
   Mr. Universe 1961, 389
      1967, 389
      1971, 79, 389
   Navy enlistment, 9-10
   physical training consultant, 383
   routine, 54
   vegetarianism, 382-383
Pearl, Judy, 10, 383
Pearl, Phil, 371
periodization, 68-69, 125
perspiration, 379
Peters, Don, 116
Peters, Mary, 26
Philostratus, 398
photographs, 34
Physical Culture (periodical), 406
physical education, 401, 413
physical examination, *see* medical
   examination

Physician and Sports Medicine (periodical), 338
physiology, 69-70
pitchers, 88
pituitary gland, 394
plate-loading barbells, *see* free weights, barbells
PNF, *see* proprioceptive neuro-muscular facilitation (PNF)
polysaccharides, 376
posing, 48-50
positive thinking, 78-79
Pound, Robin, M.S., 86, 130
power, 57
power clean, 105-106
powerlifting, 411
powerlifting programs,
   Monday, 126
   Tuesday, 127
   Thursday, 128
   Friday, 129
pregnancy, *see* women
prepubescence, *see* puberty
prevention, *see* injuries
Pritikin, Nathan, 377
progressive resistance training, 177, 362, *see also* weight training
proprioceptive neuromuscular facilitation (PNF), 67, 156
proteins, 374-376, 384
   deficiency, 375
   overload, 375
   synthesis, 390
puberty, 340
pulse rate, 74-75
pumping iron, *see* weightlifting
Pumping Iron II: The Unprece-dented Woman, 28
pyramid training, 65, *see also* techniques

Quadriceps, 100
quickness, 62, 415

R. I.C.E. treatment, 368, *see also* injuries
Rader, Peary, 413
Recommended Dietary Allowance (RDAs), 376, 380-381
record, workout, 14
rehabilitation, 105
   weight training programs for, 370
   weight training, 413
resistance, 62
resistance training,
   athletics, 414-415
   benefits, 415
   earliest record, 398
   early Greece, 398
   practical, 400
   progressive, 177, 382
   rocks and stones, 399
   Roman, 400
resistance, accommodating, *see* machine, isokinetic
rest, 15, 17, 33, 38, 41, 53, 125, 362, 368-369
Richardson, Horst, 146
risk factor (cardiovascular), 72
Rolf, Ida, 372
Roman Column, 405

Ross, Clancy, 8, 10
rotator cuff exercises, 88
rothelas, *see* wheel feat
routines (posing), 49
routines (workout), 335
rowing programs,
   in-season, 133
   off-season, 131
   pre-season, 132
running (distance) programs,
   in-season, 136
   off-season, 135
running, interval, 169

S. P.O.R.T. CORD, 142
Sanders, Roosevelt, 97
safety, 19
Samson and Cyclops, 404-405
Sandow, Eugen, 404-406
Sandwina, Katie, 406-407
Sansone, Tony, 352
Saxon, Arthur, 408
Saxon, Kurt, 408
scar tissue, 368
Schwarzenegger, Arnold, 28, 79, 413
Seay, Joe, 172
Selye, Dr. Hans, 362
serve (tennis), 153
Shape (periodical), 413
shoulders, 182, 272-283
Siciliano, Angelo, *see* Atlas, Charles
Siebert, Theodore, 413
Sime, Dave, 56
Simmons, Al, 6
sit-ups, 332-333
skiing (cross-country) programs,
   in-season, 141
   off-season, 139
   pre-season, 140
skiing (downhill) programs,
   in-season, 145
   off-season, 143
   pre-season, 144
sleep, *see* rest
slow-twitch fibers, 62-63
soccer programs,
   in-season, 148
   off-season, 147
Somatotrophin, *see* Human Growth Hormone (HGH)
soreness, 367
spas, *see* gymnasiums
specificity, 69, 116
speed, 64
split routines, 66-67
Sport Fitness (periodical), 413
sports training programs, *see* individual sports programs, e.g. boxing program
Stanko, Steve, 413
Starr, Bill, 104, 372
starvation, 375
static stretching, 156
Stern, Leo, 9-10
steroids, *see* anabolic steroids; testosterone
sticking point, 64, 349
stomach, 183, 190-201
stopper backs (soccer), 146

strength, 16, 57, 60, 62, 398-399
Strength and Health (periodical), 413
strength coaches, 392
stress (physical), 362, *see also* overload principle
stress (psychological), 53, 77, 362
stress fractures, 339
stretch reflex, 67
Stretching, 18
stretching, 105-106, 120
   developmental, 326
   easy, 326
   rules, 326
   static, 156
strikers (soccer), 146
stroke (tennis), 153
strongmen, 404-407
strongwomen, 406
success, 78
sugars, 376
super-stretching, 67
Superior Physique Association, 28
supersets, 65, *see also* techniques
supplements, vitamin and mineral, 377-378, 380-381
sweating, 379
swimming programs,
   in-season, 152
   maintenance, 152
   off-season, 150
   pre-season, 151
systems (human body), 358

Tailtin Games, *see* Irish Games
tanning, 50
target zone, 321
team sports, 338
techniques, 65, 125
tendinitis, 367, 370
tendons, 360, 366
tennis programs
   in-season, 153
   off-season, 154
   strokes, 153
tension movements, *see* movements (sports)
testosterone, 27, 390
thighs, 284-299
Tinerino, Dennis, 352
tips, 33
Todd, Jan, 69, 125
Todd, Terry, 69, 343, 398
tone, *see* muscles, tone
Topham, Thomas, 401
total conditioning, 71
trace minerals, 378
track & field programs,
   circuit weight training, 157
   decathletes
     in-season, 161
     off-season, 160
   heptathletes
     in-season, 161
     off-season, 160
   hurdlers,
     in-season, 159
     off-season, 158
   jumpers,
     in-season, 159
     off-season, 158

sprinters,
  in-season, 159
  off-season, 158
  throwers,
    in-season, 163
    off-season, 162
  vaulters,
    in-season, 161
    off-season, 160
training cycles, *see* periodization
Training Card, 417
training partners, 340-341, 352
training to failure, 39
Triat, Hippolyte, 404
triathlon programs, *see also*
  cycling, swimming, running
    (distance) programs
triathlon programs,
  in-season, 167
  off-season, 166
triceps, 300-319, *see also* arms
trisets, 65, *see also* techniques
Trusley, Pete, 8
Tylenol, *see* acetaminophen

Universal Aerobic Super Circuit, 321
Universal machines, *see* machines,
  Universal
urea, 375

Vascularity, 395
vaudeville, 407
vegans, 383-384
vegetarianism, 383-385
visualization, 77, 80
vitamins and minerals, 377-378,
  380-381, 384
volley (tennis), 153
volleyball programs,
  in-season, 171
  off-season, 170
Vulcana, 406-407

Walker, Herschel, 80
warmup, 106, 372, *see also*
  stretching
water, 378-379
Washington, Kermit, 92
water pills, 395
Weider, Ben, 413
Weider, Joe, 413
weight training, *see also* stretching
weight training, 169
  aerobic, 75
  aging, 342
  benefits, 338, 363-364
  children, 338-341
    benefits, 338
    equipment, 339
    program, 339
    reservations, 339

stress, 339
  concepts, 65-70
  dress, 33
  effectiveness, 324
  focusing, 33
  high intensity, 38, 65-66
  isometric, 63-64
  isotonic, 63-64
  methods,
    East German, 77
    Russian, 77, 389
  middle age, 342-344
  moderation, 92
  position, 18-19
  progressive, 177
  rehabilitation, 413
  sports,
    rep table, 61
    training chart, 60
  techniques, 18
  therapy, 414
  time, 41
  variety, 34, 38, 44
  warmup, 18
  weaknesses, 33
weightlifting, 409
  1st world championship, 409
  amateur, 408-411
  growth, 403
  organization, 410-411
  professional, 404-407
  progressive, 372
    see also resistance training;
      strongmen; strongwomen;
      weight training
Weinberg, Barry, 88
wheel feat, 398
white-collar workers' program, 334
Willoughby, David P., 411
Windship, Dr. George Barker,
  402-403
wings (soccer), 146
Wiren, Gary, Ph.D., 112
women,
  bodybuilding, 28
  bone structure, 27
  heavy resistance, 29
  pregnancy, 27
  toning body, 28
  weight training
  misconceptions, 26
    special considerations, 27
    see also diet; fat (body);
      strongwomen
work, *see* blue-collar workers'
  program; fitness, work; injury,
  work-related; white-collar
  workers' program
workouts,
  frequency, 15
  techniques, 65

wrestling programs,
  in-season, 175
  pre-season, 174
Wright, Bill, 153

Ziegfeld, Florenz, 405
Zinkin, Harold, 414 □

CREDITS

Publisher & Editor
Lloyd Kahn, Jr.

Contributing Editor
Daniel Rogoff

*Book Design
& Art Direction*
Drake Jordan

Production Editor
Marianne Orina

Research Editors
Robin Pound, M.S.
Dick Fugett

Typesetting
Trudy Renggli
Barrie Stebbings

Production Staff
Patricia Maloney
Helen Jordan
Barrie Stebbings
Susan Sanders

Pre-Production Design
David Wills

*Chief Proofreader
and Indexer*
Craig Ruffin Bailey

Assistant Proofreader
Chris Faville

Medical Drawings
Edna Indritz Steadman

Nutritional Consultants
Jim Coyne & Don Burns,
Nutritional Factors

PHOTOGRAPHY

Cover photo
Jack Fulton, San Rafael, CA

Cover Art & Airbrushing
Gary Fox, Mill Valley, CA

Sports Photos
Photo research by Budd Symes,
Budd Symes Photography, Los Angeles,
CA; Carrie Monaghan, Duomo Photo-
graphy, Inc., New York, NY; and Erin
O'Hearn, All-Sport Photography USA,
Inc., Chatsworth, CA

*Photos for "A Brief History of
Resistance Exercise"*
Todd-McLean Collection,
University of Texas, Austin, Texas

Photostats of Drawings
Marinstat Graphic Arts

Photo Developing & Printing
General Graphic Services, San Francisco, CA
North Bay Photo, San Rafael, CA
Professional Color Laboratory,
  San Francisco, CA

Color Separation, Cover
Focus 4, Belmont, CA

TYPESETTING & PRINTING
Type for body of book was set on an IBM
Electronic Composer run by a Pilara
2000 Word Processor
Type face for text is Press Roman
Headline type is Eras Demi Bold and
  Eras Bold

Typesetting headlines, programs, charts
Marinstat Graphic Arts, Mill Valley, Calif.

Special Thanks to
Bob & Jean Anderson/
Lynn Black & Universal Gym
Equipment, Inc., Cedar Rapids, Iowa/
Ruth Christian/Lesley Creed/
Jim Cron/Ellington Darden, Ph.D./
Jim Flanagan and Brenda Hutchins
of Nautilus Medical/
Sports Industries, DeLand, Florida/
Ted Di Sante/Pam Doyle/
John Gourgett, M.D., World Gym,
Kentfield, California/
Kathy Groover/Richard Harrington/
Frederick Hatfield, Ph.D./Chris Lund
Judy Pearl/Phillip Pearl/
Anne Reeves/John Sandler/Leo Stern
Terry Todd & Jan Todd/Bill Wright/
Chip Wright's Nautilus Training Center,
Medford, Oregon/

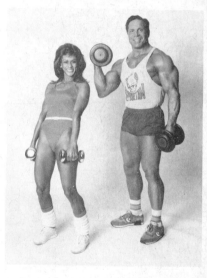

*Models for Exercise Drawings
and Cover Photo*
Breigh Kelley and Bill Pearl.
Breigh, born in Wahiawa, Hawaii was
Miss World Physique of 1985-86.
She is a singer and dancer, and a model.
She has been a bodybuilder for three
years, swims, cycles and attends non-
impact aerobic classes. Her husband
Rick is also an athlete and they live
in San Rafael, Calif. with their two
children, Kef and Ricky.

ABOUT THE AUTHORS

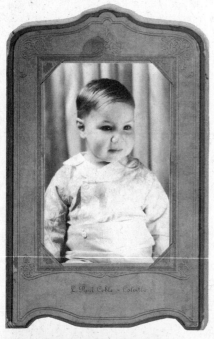

BILL PEARL was born in Prineville, Oregon on October 31, 1930. At age 14 he acquired his first set of weights and has lifted weights ever since. He was a star wrestler and football player in high school. He then joined the U.S. Navy and won the 13th Naval District Heavyweight Wrestling Championship and the Pacific Northwest All Comers Meet in 1951. He began training with gym owner Leo Stern in the early '50s in San Diego and he credits Stern with coaching him and helping him on the road to winning the following titles:

1953 Mr. Southern California
1953 Mr. California
1953 AAU Mr. America
1953 NABBA* Mr. Universe, Amateur
1956 Mr. USA, Professional
1956 NABBA Mr. Universe, Professional
1961 NABBA Mr. Universe, Professional
1967 NABBA Mr. Universe, Professional
1971 NABBA Mr. Universe, Professional
1974 WBBG** World's Best Built Man
1978 Entered into WBBG Hall of Fame

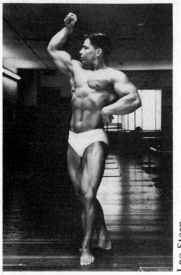
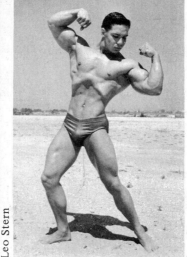
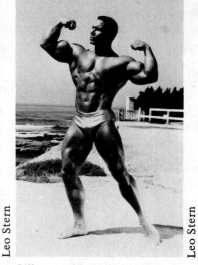

Photos of Bill in his early 20s in San Diego, California   *Bill at age 35, 1965*

Bill has run gyms in Sacramento, California and Los Angeles for over 30 years. He has personally coached more major contest winners than anyone else in history: his pupils have won 10 Mr. Universe titles and 8 Mr. America titles. Bill appears regularly at sports fitness conventions, bodybuilding contests and other invitational events. Notes on his career and photos appear in practically every book on bodybuilding today. He was the subject of a feature article by Terry Todd in *Sports Illustrated* in 1983.

Bill and his wife Judy recently moved to a small town near Medford, Oregon. They live on a four-acre ranch with fruit trees, two dogs, a cat, two tortoises and a parrot. In a barn behind the house Bill has set up his gym. He gets up at 3:00 a.m. to train six days a week. He first does some cardiovascular training and stretching and is then joined at 4:30 sharp by his training partners—including Judy, also a bodybuilder. Their workout lasts about 2½ hours.

*National Amateur Bodybuilding Association
**World Bodybuilding Guild

445

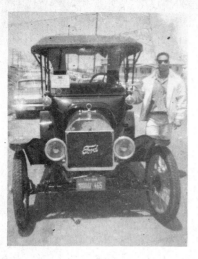

Bill has long been an admirer of the old strongman traditions. He used to blow up hot water bottles until they burst and can still tear two California license plates in half with his bare hands. This love of things old also shows in Bill's collection of antique cars—which he restores himself—including an 1899 Marlboro, a 1907 Model N Ford, a 1910 Stanley Steamer, a 1915 Model T Ford, a 1932 Ford Phaeton 4-door convertible and a 1949 Willy's Jeep.

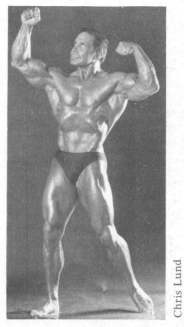

At age 56 Bill is still asked to pose in bodybuilding contests. In 1985 he appeared in Derby, England; Dusseldorf, Germany; and at several locations in the U.S. When he was introduced to present the trophies at the 1985 NABBA Mr. Universe contest in London, he received a standing ovation.

Bill at age 55, 1985

Chris Lund

GARY T. MORAN has a Ph.D. in Human Anatomy and Kinesiology (the science of human motion and movement) from the University of Oregon and a Master's Degree in Exercise Physiology from San Diego State University. He has been a consultant to university, professional and Olympic teams and athletes as well as to sports medicine centers, sports shoe companies and equipment manufacturers. He has published numerous research papers in sports medicine and has lectured in Europe, Canada and Australia. He lectures on Kinesiology at the University of San Francisco, is a Clinical Associate with the Motion and Performance Laboratory at the Ralph K. Davies Medical Center in San Francisco and is the Director of Sports Medicine at the Marin Foot Health Center in Mill Valley, California.

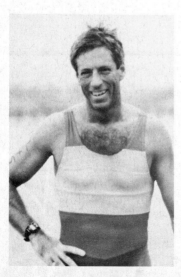

Gary was on the varsity tennis and track and field teams at the University of Bridgeport, Connecticut. He coached football, basketball, soccer and swimming and the cross-country and track teams at Concordia University in 1975-77 and was on the U.S. Navy Pentathlon team. He is an active runner, weightlifter, cyclist and triathlete. He has run a marathon in 2:48, competes in distance running events and triathlons and at a body weight of 154 bench presses 270 pounds. He is a Lieutenant Commander in the U.S. Naval Reserve and helped design the U.S. Navy Health and Physical Readiness program.□

446

MORE FITNESS BOOKS

from Shelter Publications

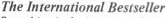

SHELTER

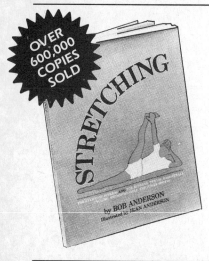

OVER 600,000 COPIES SOLD

The International Bestseller
Stretching is the important link between the sedentary life and the active life. It prepares you for movement, reduces soreness and prevents injuries. In the classic fitness book, Bob Anderson presents an easy-to-follow guide to stretching all parts of the body, with routines for 36 sports and activities.

"I use the book regularly and find it an extremely valuable resource."
    –Richard O. Keelor, M.D.
    The President's Council on Physical Fitness & Sports

"The best on the market. I use the exercises myself."
    –Art Ulene, M.D.
    The Today Show NBC TV

STRETCHING
By Bob Anderson; illustrated by Jean Anderson © 1980
192 pp. paperback $9.95
ISBN 0-394-73874-8
Distributed by Random House

A New Book For The Second Wave of Runners!
State-of-the-art running for the late-'80s. Olympic runner Jeff Galloway explains his secrets to running better, his revolutionary ideas on stress and rest, tells beginners how to get started sensibly and provides unique training charts for 10K races and marathons. Why you should run *farther* than the race *before* the race, why "carbo-loading" doesn't work, how to select the right shoes, how to use running to effectively burn off fat.

FASTEST SELLING RUNNING BOOK IN AMERICA

"An outstanding contribution to competitive running."
    –Kenneth Copper, M.D.
    Author, *Aerobics*

"Galloway not only knows his craft, but also has the rare ability to convey this knowledge through teaching."
    –Frank Shorter

Also recommended by Bill Rodgers, Dr. George Sheehan & Dr. Joan Ullyot

GALLOWAY'S BOOK ON RUNNING
By Jeff Galloway © 1984
288 pp. paperback $9.95
ISBN 0-394-72709-6
Distributed by Random House

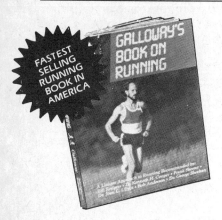

Once You're Over the Hill, You Pick Up Speed!
49 people over 40 talk about active lives: running, surfing, riding mountain bikes, swimming in the ocean, hang gliding, running in triathlons, tap dancing and lifting weights. These diverse and lively people share their training tips, eating habits and secrets to their fitness, longevity and lust for life. Ages 40 to 101. Amusing, provocative and inspirational.

"Delightful."
    –S.F. Chronicle

"I love the book."
    –Joanie Greggains
    Morning Stretch

"A treat."
    –Pacific Sun

OVER THE HILL, But Not Out To Lunch!
By Lloyd Kahn, Jr. © 1986
160 pp. paperback $9.95
ISBN 0-936070-05-6
Distributed by HPBooks

To order any of these books, send the listed price plus $2.00 postage and handling to Shelter Publications, Inc., P.O. Box 279, Bolinas, CA 94924. Write also for free catalog of Shelter books.

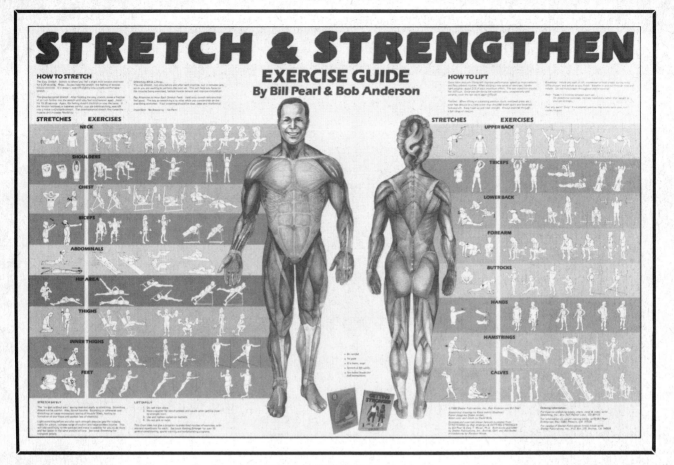

Brand new! Color coded ● 4-color wall poster ● 23" x 35" ● 2 stretches & 3 weight training exercises for each of 19 muscle groups - Scientifically accurate anatomical drawings - On plain paper or laminated with 3-mil vinyl and brass eyelets for durable reference use in gyms, recreation rooms or schools - $15.95 laminated - $10.95 100-lb paper (varnished) ● Plus $2.50 shipping and handling ● Order from Shelter Publications, Inc., Box 279, Bolinas, CA. 94924. Wholesale information upon request.

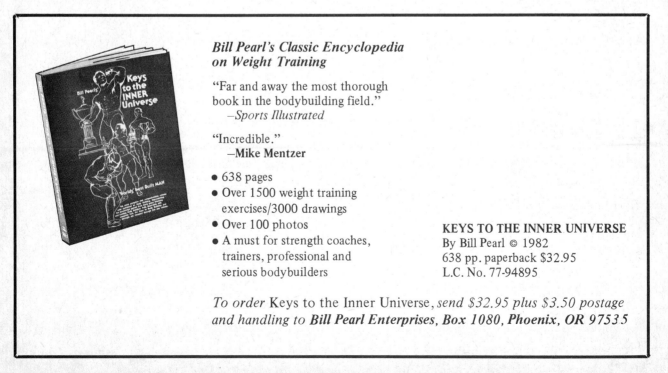

Bill Pearl's Classic Encyclopedia on Weight Training

"Far and away the most thorough book in the bodybuilding field."
—*Sports Illustrated*

"Incredible."
—**Mike Mentzer**

● 638 pages
● Over 1500 weight training exercises/3000 drawings
● Over 100 photos
● A must for strength coaches, trainers, professional and serious bodybuilders

KEYS TO THE INNER UNIVERSE
By Bill Pearl © 1982
638 pp. paperback $32.95
L.C. No. 77-94895

To order Keys to the Inner Universe, *send $32.95 plus $3.50 postage and handling to* **Bill Pearl Enterprises, Box 1080, Phoenix, OR 97535**

Note: Bill Pearl is available for talks, clinics and conventions. Call 503-535-3363.

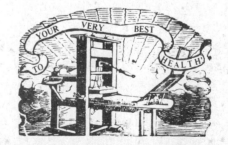

Shelter Publications, Inc.
P.O. Box 279
Bolinas, CA 94924